Childhood Feeding Problems and Adolescent Eating Disorders

Disturbances in eating arising in infancy, early childhood and adolescence are increasingly being recognised as a major source of distress and disturbance to young people and their families.

Childhood Feeding Problems and Adolescent Eating Disorders covers a wide spectrum of phenomena of variable clinical significance, ranging from variations of normal behaviour to serious clinical conditions such as failure to thrive and anorexia nervosa. In three sections, the following subjects are covered:

- Feeding and weight problems of early childhood
- Nature of anorexia nervosa and bulimia nervosa
- Treatment of anorexia nervosa and bulimia nervosa

The contributors discuss important issues such as the influence of maternal eating problems, the consequences of early feeding problems and the management of early onset anorexia nervosa.

This book will be an important resource for all the paediatricians, psychologists, psychiatrists, nurses, nutritionists and other health professionals concerned with the assessment and treatment of these major clinical problems.

Peter J. Cooper is Professor of Psychopathology at the University of Reading, honorary Consultant Clinical Psychologist with West Berkshire Health Authority and an honorary Senior Research Fellow in the Department of Psychiatry at Cambridge University. He is also a Co-Director of the Winnicott Research Unit.

Alan Stein is Professor of Child and Adolescent Psychiatry at the University of Oxford and an honorary Consultant in Child and Adolescent Psychiatry with Oxfordshire Mental Healthcare Trust.

Contributors: Ian W. Booth, Rachel Bryant-Waugh, Cynthia Bulik, Jacqueline Carter, Peter J. Cooper, Regina Cowan, Debra L. Franko, Jennifer A. Gray, Sophie Grigoriadis, Gillian Harris, David B. Herzog, Andrew J. Hill, Safia C. Jackson, Debbi Jonas, Allan Kaplan, Walter Kaye, Bryan Lask, Lisa R. Lilenfeld, Rochelle Martin, Traci McFarlane, Lynda Molleken, Marion Olmsted, Sheena Reilly, Gerald F. M. Russell, David Skuse, Sandy Sonnenberg, Alan Stein, Michael Strober, Kelly M. Vitousek, Heather Williams, Dieter Wolke, D. Blake Woodside, Helen Woolley, Kelli Young

Childhood Feeding Problems and Adolescent Eating Disorders

Edited by Peter J. Cooper and Alan Stein

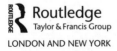
Routledge
Taylor & Francis Group

LONDON AND NEW YORK

First published 2006 by Routledge
27 Church Road, Hove, East Sussex BN3 2FA

Simultaneously published in the USA and Canada
by Routledge
270 Madison Avenue, New York, NY 10016

Routledge is an imprint of the Taylor & Francis Group, an informa business

Typeset in Times by
RefineCatch Limited, Bungay, Suffolk
Printed and bound in Great Britain by
TJ International Ltd, Padstow, Cornwall
Cover design by Richard Massing

This publication has been produced with paper manufactured to
strict environmental standards and with pulp derived from
sustainable forests.

British Library Cataloguing in Publication Data
A catalogue record for this book is available from the British Library

Library of Congress Cataloging in Publication Data
Childhood feeding problems and adolescent eating disorders /
   edited by Peter J. Cooper & Alan Stein.
       p. ; cm.
   Includes biographical references and index.
   ISBN-13: 978-0-415-37185-8 (hardcover)
   ISBN-10: 0-415-37185-6 (hardcover)
   1. Eating disorders in children. 2. Eating disorders in
adolescence. I. Cooper, Peter J. II. Stein, Alan.
       [DNLM: 1. Eating Disorders – therapy – Adolescent. 2. Eating
Disorders – therapy – Child. 3. Eating Disorders – therapy – Infant.
4. Feeding Behavior – Adolescent. 5. Feeding Behavior – Child. 6.
Feeding Behavior – Infant. WS 115 C5367 2006]
   RJ506.E18C45 2006
   618.92′8526 – dc22   2005043528

ISBN13: 978-0-415-37185-8 (hbk)

ISBN10: 0-415-37185-6 (hbk)

Contents

Contributors

Ian W. Booth Department of Paediatrics and Child Health, The Medical School, University of Birmingham, UK

Rachel Bryant-Waugh Mental Health Group, School of Medicine, University of Southampton, Royal South Hants Hospital, Southampton, UK

Cynthia Bulik Department of Psychiatry, University of North Carolina Medical School, Chapel Hill, North Carolina, USA

Jacqueline Carter University Health Network, Toronto General Hospital, and Department of Psychiatry, University of Toronto, Canada

Peter J. Cooper School of Psychology, University of Reading, Reading, UK

Regina Cowan University Health Network, Toronto General Hospital, and Department of Psychiatry, University of Toronto, Canada

Debra L. Franko Eating Disorders Unit, Massachusetts General Hospital, Harvard Medical School, Boston, Massachusetts, USA

Jennifer A. Gray Department of Psychology, University of Hawaii, Hawaii, USA

Sophie Grigoriadis University Health Network, Toronto General Hospital, and Department of Psychiatry, University of Toronto, Canada

Gillian Harris School of Psychology, University of Birmingham, Birmingham, UK

David B. Herzog Eating Disorders Unit, Massachusetts General Hospital, Harvard Medical School, Boston, Massachusetts, USA

Andrew J. Hill Academic Unit of Psychiatry and Behavioural Sciences, School of Medicine, University of Leeds, Leeds, UK

Safia C. Jackson Eating Disorders Unit, Massachusetts General Hospital, Harvard Medical School, Boston, Massachusetts, USA

Debbi Jonas University Health Network, Toronto General Hospital, and Department of Psychiatry, University of Toronto, Canada

Allan Kaplan University Health Network, Toronto General Hospital, and Department of Psychiatry, University of Toronto, Canada

Walter Kaye Department of Psychiatry, Western Psychiatric Institute, School of Medicine, University of Pittsburgh, Pittsburgh, Pennsylvania, USA

Bryan Lask Department of Psychiatry, St George's, University of London, UK; the Huntercombe Hospitals, Taplow, UK; and Regional Eating Disorders Service, Ulleval University Hospital, Oslo, Norway

Lisa R. Lilenfeld Department of Psychology, Georgia State University, Atlanta, Georgia, USA

Rochelle Martin University Health Network, Toronto General Hospital, and Department of Psychiatry, University of Toronto, Canada

Traci McFarlane University Health Network, Toronto General Hospital, and Department of Psychiatry, University of Toronto, Canada

Lynda Molleken University Health Network, Toronto General Hospital, and Department of Psychiatry, University of Toronto, Canada

Marion Olmsted University Health Network, Toronto General Hospital, and Department of Psychiatry, University of Toronto, Canada

Sheena Reilly La Trobe University, Faculty of Health Sciences, School of Human Communication Sciences, Bundoora, Melbourne, Australia

Gerald F. M. Russell The Priory Hospital, Hayes, UK

David Skuse King's College, University of London, and Institute of Child Health, Behavioural Sciences Unit, University College London, UK

Sandy Sonnenberg University Health Network, Toronto General Hospital, and Department of Psychiatry, University of Toronto, Canada

Alan Stein Section of Child and Adolescent Psychiatry, University of Oxford, Warneford Hospital, Oxford, UK

Michael Strober David Geffen School of Medicine, University of California at Los Angeles, Los Angeles, California, USA

Kelly M. Vitousek Department of Psychology, University of Hawaii, Hawaii, USA

Heather Williams Section of Child and Adolescent Psychiatry, University of Oxford, Warneford Hospital, Oxford, UK

Dieter Wolke The University of Zurich, Institute of Psychology, Zurich, Switzerland

D. Blake Woodside University Health Network, Toronto General Hospital, and Department of Psychiatry, University of Toronto, Canada

Helen Woolley Section of Child and Adolescent Psychiatry, University of Oxford, Warneford Hospital, Oxford, UK

Kelli Young University Health Network, Toronto General Hospital, and Department of Psychiatry, University of Toronto, Canada

Introduction

Peter J. Cooper and Alan Stein

Feeding and eating serve a range of biological, psychological and social functions in the life of the developing child. The biological function is clearly the most basic in that the child requires adequate nutrition not only to survive but to thrive physically and mentally. The psychological functions have received considerable attention. For example, it has been argued that even the timing of the first feed after the infant's delivery is significant: if this occurs soon after the birth while the child is in an alert state, breastfeeding is likely to go particularly well (MacKeith and Wood, 1977). Psychoanalytic theorists have stressed the importance of early oral experiences in the child's development of gratification and frustration; and authors from many intellectual traditions have argued for the emotional benefit of breastfeeding over bottlefeeding in the child's early development. Whatever the merits of these arguments there is no doubt that early feeding is important to the psychological development of infants since much of the early interaction between the baby and its mother and other caretakers centres on feeding. Indeed, feeding is essentially concerned with nurturance and, as such, is of fundamental significance to the child's experience of the world and his or her place in it. Feeding and eating also play an important role in the social life of the child. Meals are usually timed when the family is together and are the focus of much of family life. Furthermore, much social interaction outside the family occurs during mealtimes and this context therefore serves a wider socialising function.

Given the central role feeding and eating play in the life of a developing child, it is not surprising that deviations or disturbances in feeding and eating are not only a problem for the individual but can cause great anxiety within the family. Thus, when a child presents to the clinician with an eating or feeding problem, adequate management depends on viewing this problem in its wider familial and social context. This applies not only to consideration of aetiological factors, but to factors that may be the sequelae of the eating difficulties which themselves come to maintain them.

Feeding difficulties are a common problem in childhood (Dunn, 1980; Eppright *et al.*, 1969). They cover a wide spectrum of phenomena of variable clinical significance, ranging from variations of normal behaviour such as mild faddiness, to conditions of major developmental significance such as failure to thrive. Many of these disorders have their origins in a combination of both difficulties within the child (e.g. neuro-developmental, temperamental) and parental handling problems. In other cases, feeding difficulties may be the expression of general difficulties within the family. The feeding difficulties of early childhood are not as well studied as adolescent disorders of eating but their importance has been increasingly recognised in recent years.

The eating disorders anorexia nervosa and bulimia nervosa, which typically have their onset in adolescence, have been the subject of a substantial body of research. These disorders exact a considerable toll in human suffering. The physical complications arising from the disordered eating habits and the disturbance in body weight are manifold. Indeed, recent long-term follow-up evidence on patients with anorexia nervosa has revealed an alarmingly high mortality rate from the disorder – in the region of 10–15 per cent. Concomitant depressive symptoms are a prominent feature of these patients and suicide accounts for much of the mortality. Even when the physical complications are minimal and there is little mood disturbance, these disorders severely limit and restrict normal human development and functioning. Thus, it is common in outpatient clinics to see relatively mild cases of anorexia nervosa presenting in their mid-twenties with a ten-year history. These young people's lives have been dominated by their preoccupations with food, eating, body shape and weight, and they have consequently largely missed the normal experiences of ordinary adolescence and young adulthood, particularly in the area of interpersonal relationships. Bulimia nervosa has similar wide-ranging adverse repercussions. Again, even in relatively mild cases, the psychological toll is considerable. These young people are plagued by guilt and burdened by shame. Their self-esteem is consequently low and their interpersonal lives are correspondingly adversely affected. Given the major negative impact of these disorders, it is a cause for concern that they have such a high prevalence and may be increasing in incidence in developed countries (Szmukler et al., 1986; Lucas et al., 1999).

In recent years there has been considerable interest in refining the diagnostic criteria for the eating disorders, elucidating their clinical features and developing and evaluating treatments. Much progress has been made on all these fronts. There has been rather less systematic attention paid to the processes by which these disorders come about. Research on risk factors has largely been retrospective in nature (Fairburn et al., 1999). However, in order to advance knowledge of the causal chains implicated in the aetiology of these conditions, and of the risk and protective factors that operate, longitudinal research is necessary (Rutter, 1988).

One important issue which arises is whether there is any relationship between feeding difficulties in the first years of life and the eating disorders of late childhood and adolescence. There is a major gap in knowledge about the early experiences of patients with eating disorders. There have been suggestions that the quality of early care in this group is peculiarly poor and reports of gross neglect and even frank abuse are common (Palmer *et al.*, 1990; Welsh and Fairburn, 1994; Vize and Cooper, 1995). There have also been suggestions that the early experience of feeding is disturbed in these patients and that there exists a continuity in pathology between childhood disturbance in eating and adolescent onset of anorexia nervosa or bulimia nervosa (Marchi and Cohen, 1990). The evidence for this is meagre, and clearly this is an area which demands research attention.

The chapters contained in this book concern the nature, development and clinical management of feeding problems and eating disorders in children and adolescents. They are organised in three sections. The first section contains five chapters concerned with the feeding and weight problems of early childhood. In Chapter 1, Sheena Reilly, David Skuse and Dieter Wolke describe the nature and consequences of feeding problems in infancy. They describe the normal development of feeding and the development of oral motor skills. The types of feeding difficulties are discussed (including refusal to eat, colic and vomiting), and their relation to other infant behaviours, such as sleeping and crying, is considered. Finally there is a discussion of specific feeding difficulties (such as rumination and colic). In Chapter 2, the same authors deal with the prevention and management of feeding problems. They begin by providing guidelines for the management of the three basic stages and transition periods of early feeding (i.e. breast- and bottle-feeding, introduction of solids and the development of mealtime behaviours). A major part of this chapter concerns a description of the behavioural treatment approach developed by the team at Great Ormond Street Hospital in London for the management of feeding problems amongst children with cerebral palsy. There is also a section on artificially fed infants with recommendations on how best to reinstate oral feeding. In Chapter 3, Gillian Harris and Ian Booth provide an account of the feeding problems encountered in pre-school children. They note the high prevalence of such disorders, pointing out that some problem with food refusal is reported by the great majority of parents with pre-school children. After defining some key terms, the relation between chronic food refusal and non-organic causes of failure to thrive is discussed. A major section deals with the organic and non-organic causes of feeding problems and their interrelationship. The assessment of these problems is discussed and, in an appendix, a detailed Feeding Assessment Form is provided. Finally, guidelines for management are outlined which draw on a wide spectrum of therapeutic strategies. In Chapter 4, Andrew Hill reviews the research literature on the nature and prevalence of body dissatisfaction and dieting in children. He highlights the evidence for the very early appearance of body shape concerns in children in western societies, and the associated dieting behaviours, especially in girls. The role of the media, families and peers in the promotion of these concerns and behaviours is considered and the role of primary prevention and health promotion programmes is discussed. In Chapter 5, the final chapter of the first section, Alan Stein, Helen Woolley and Heather Williams deal with an issue which has only recently become the object of systematic research attention, namely the impact on infants of having a mother with an eating disorder. They review the mechanisms by which eating disorders affect parenting and child development, and discuss their clinical implications.

The second section of this book contains three chapters on the nature of anorexia nervosa and bulimia nervosa. In Chapter 6, Gerald Russell provides an account of anorexia nervosa of early onset and its impact on puberty. He provides a brief account of the epidemiology of anorexia nervosa and a review of what is known about its aetiology. He suggests a classification of the disorder into pre-pubertal, pre-menarchal and post-pubertal, thereby alerting clinicians to the risk of pre-pubertal anorexia nervosa delaying the onset of puberty. He gives an account of the clinical features of early onset anorexia, highlighting its impact on particular aspects of pubertal development. Finally, he provides a discussion of the course and outcome of these disorders together with an outline of prognostic factors. In Chapter 7, David Herzog, Safia Jackson and Debra Franko provide an account of the epidemiology, clinical features, course and outcome and medical complications of both classic anorexia nervosa of adolescent onset and bulimia nervosa. They also review the evidence on risk and prognostic factors for these disorders, highlighting the 'front-line' role of the paediatrician in detection and management.

In Chapter 8, the final chapter of this section, Michael Strober, Lisa Lilenfeld, Walter Kaye and Cynthia Bulik provide a comprehensive review of family and twin studies of anorexia nervosa and bulimia nervosa. This includes a review of molecular genetic studies; and family studies of comorbidity. They conclude by considering the implications of the genetic evidence for elucidating the inherited diathesis in these disorders.

The final section of this book contains five chapters concerned with the treatment of anorexia nervosa and bulimia nervosa. In Chapter 9, Bryan Lask and Rachel Bryant-Waugh discuss the management of anorexia nervosa of early onset. They stress the need for an integrated comprehensive treatment programme to be instituted early in the development of the disorder before it becomes entrenched. They provide clear practical guidelines for the management of these patients, as well as advice on how to cope with the families, and deal with a range of clinical issues including the decision about whether outpatient or inpatient treatment is most appropriate. In Chapter 10, Kelly Vitousek and Jennifer Gray provide a comprehensive review of outpatient treatments for anorexia nervosa and the evidence supporting their use. They highlight problems encountered in delivering outpatient services to this patient group and possible solutions. Particular attention is paid to the issue of patient motivation and how it can be maximised, and dealing with issues of specific therapeutic concern. Finally, a careful analysis of the advantages of outpatient care is provided. In Chapter 11, Peter Cooper considers the outpatient management of bulimia nervosa. He provides a brief review of treatment using antidepressant medication, but most emphasis is given to cognitive behaviour therapy for this disorder. He provides a description of the structure and content of this treatment and reviews the evidence for its efficacy. He also reviews promising recent work on the delivery of this treatment through self-help manuals. In Chapter 12, Marion Olmsted, Traci McFarlane, Lynda Molleken and Allan Kaplan describe the day hospital programme for eating disorders that was initiated by the Toronto General Hospital twenty years ago. As well as describing the structure and content of this programme, they consider indications and contraindications for this form of treatment. Finally, in Chapter 13, Blake Woodside, Sandy Sonnenberg, Kelli Young, Debbi Jonas, Jacqueline Carter, Allan Kaplan, Rochelle Martin, Regina Cowan and Sophie Grigoriadis describe the inpatient treatment programme developed by them and their colleagues over many years in Toronto. They review the changes that have taken place in the hospital management of anorexia nervosa over the last sixty years, emphasising the shift away from single approaches to the development of individual programmes for each patient which use a multitude of therapeutic strategies. They describe the development of the Toronto programme, providing a detailed description of the programme components, dealing with the features specific to the management of this patient group as well as more general therapeutic aspects. They finally provide guidance on specific clinical issues (such as self-harm).

The purpose of this collection is to provide an account of the phenomena encountered in infants with feeding problems and children and adolescents with eating disorders, as well as a description of the main methods of clinical management for these disorders. We hope that this volume will serve to help paediatricians, psychiatrists, psychologists, nutritionists and other health professionals who deal with these patients in their diagnosis and management of these major clinical problems.

References

Dunn, J. (1980) Feeding and sleeping. In: M. Rutter (ed.) *Scientific Foundations of Developmental Psychiatry*. London: Heinemann Medical Books.

Eppright, E.S., Fox, H.M., Fryer, B.S., Lamkin, G.H. and Vivian, V.M. (1969) Eating behaviour of preschool children. *Journal of Nutrition Education*, 1, 16–19.

Fairburn, C.G., Cooper, Z., Doll, H.A. and Welsh, S. (1999) Risk factors for anorexia nervosa: three integrated case-control comparisons. *Archives of General Psychiatry*, 56, 468–476.

Lucas, A.R., Crowson, C.S., O'Fallon, W.M. and Melton, L.J. (1999) The ups and downs of anorexia nervosa. *International Journal of Eating Disorders*, 26, 397–405.

MacKeith, R. and Wood, C. (1977) *Infant Feeding and Feeding Difficulties*. Edinburgh: Churchill Livingstone.

Marchi, M. and Cohen, P. (1990) Early childhood eating behaviours and adolescent eating disorders. *Journal of the American Academy of Child and Adolescent Psychiatry*, 29, 112–117.

Palmer, R.L., Oppenheimer, R., Dignon, A., Chaloner, D.A. and Howells, K. (1990) Childhood sexual experience with adults reported by women with eating disorders. *British Journal of Psychiatry*, 156, 699–703.

Rutter, M. (1988) Longitudinal data in the study of causal processes: some uses and some pitfalls. In: M. Rutter (ed.) *Studies of Psychosocial Risk: The Power of Longitudinal Data*. Cambridge: Cambridge University Press.

Szmukler, G.I., McCance, C. McCrane, L. and Carlson, I.H. (1986) Anorexia nervosa: a case register study from Aberdeen. *Psychological Medicine*, 16, 49–58.

Vize, C. and Cooper, P.J. (1995) Sexual abuse in patients with eating disorders, patients with depression and normal controls: a comparative study. *British Journal of Psychiatry*, 167, 80–85.

Welsh, S. and Fairburn, C.G. (1994) Sexual abuse and bulimia nervosa: three related case-control comparisons. *American Journal of Psychiatry*, 151, 402–407.

Chapter 1

The nature and consequences of feeding problems in infancy

Sheena Reilly, David Skuse and Dieter Wolke

Introduction

The human infant, like other infant mammals, depends completely upon a social relationship for its nutritional requirements and for the maintenance of life and its physical well-being (Lipsett *et al.*, 1985). The earliest relationship between the infant and caregiver may serve a number of different purposes quite apart from the importance of that interaction for the supply of adequate and appropriate nutrition. The relationship may serve as a basis of social dialogue, and the quality of action during feeding may reflect the nature and quality of parent–infant interaction in other settings as well (Wolke, 1994, 1996). The style of the interpersonal relationship during feeding will be influenced by the individual characteristics of both the infant and the caregiver, and if problems develop during the course of that feeding interaction there may be implications for the style and quality of their relationship in other (non-feeding) contexts, as well as for subsequent feeding behaviours, including preferences and aversions (Lindberg, 1994).

The relative neglect of feeding as an issue central to early child development is puzzling. In an editorial in the journal *Developmental Medicine and Child Neurology* Bax (1989) suggested that the reason why feeding has received little attention in the developmental psychology and paediatric literature is because it is treated so extensively in childcare books that the subject does not seem to be a 'respectable one' for the clinician or research worker to investigate. He goes on: 'A glance at the work of nutritionists, gastroenterologists and even dieticians . . . shows that none of them discusses the problem of actually getting food into the child.' Bax examined the bibliography of the journal and discovered that in previous years there had been very few publications in the journal regarding infant feeding: one paper in 1986, none in 1987 and two in 1988. Bax issued a challenge to all health professionals involved in paediatrics to pay increased attention to infant feeding.

Recently we have seen the publication of numerous specialist textbooks devoted to the management of feeding problems, the publication of a specialist journal devoted to dysphagia, as well as a plethora of journal articles. Some names stand out as being major contributors to our understanding of infant feeding, such as James Bosma, whose work spans over thirty years of study of the anatomy and physiology of feeding (e.g. Bosma et al., 1967; Bosma, 1977, 1986), Erika Gisel (e.g. Gisel and Patrick, 1988) and Suzanne Evans-Morris, who has made a particular study of the feeding difficulties of infants with cerebral palsy (e.g. Evans-Morris, 1977a, 1977b, 1985).

Early feeding and the success of feeding development in the infant depend upon the organisation of a number of interacting biological and psychological systems in which nutritional requirements, developmental attainments, internal sensations such as hunger and satiety, and cultural pressures impinge upon the child. It is not possible to discuss sensibly the nature and range of feeding problems encountered in infancy without first discussing the normal developmental phases to be observed. The success of the infant's feeding relationship for normal growth and health is dependent upon a number of self-regulatory processes, and also upon a caretaker who is sufficiently responsive to that infant to provide requisite environmental modifications. The infant is born with the capacity to emit a repertoire of signals which indicate needs and which are intended to evoke the appropriate response from the caregiver (Adoph, 1968). A lack of capacity for self-regulation would render the infant's very survival at risk; normal development is contingent upon the infant's ability to signal his or her needs clearly and unambiguously.

Endogenous or constitutional factors comprise a complex repertoire of reflexes and behaviour patterns which are well suited to the task of acquiring food and ingesting it. There are complex schemas of rooting, sucking and swallowing responses which take advantage of the presence of a caregiver who can feed the child responsively, and whose own psychological and physiological resources are normally well coordinated with the infant's physiognomic and behavioural characteristics. In the earliest days the infant is motivated primarily by reflexive and biologically programmed behaviours in order to seek food. In the first few months of life caregivers respond adaptively to their infant's needs and must recognise and respond appropriately to their infant's repertoire of behaviours. Feeding problems are particularly likely to develop when either the infant's endogenous programming is faulty in some way, compromising the clarity of these signals or the coherence of the pre-programmed behaviours, or when the caregiver is for some reason unable accurately to identify or respond to the infant's particular needs (Wolke, 1994). There is a subtle interrelationship between these two major variables which puts a proportion of infants at relatively 'high risk'. The feeding relationship could thus be seen within the framework of a transactional model (Emde, 1987): constitutional factors (such as the coherence of foetal development, the duration of gestation, and perinatal and postnatal factors that might affect subsequent psychomotor performance) interact with environmental conditions and emerging social, emotional and cognitive abilities that may or may not act in concert with the reflexive developments which are age-appropriate.

The development of ingestive behaviour

Any discussion of feeding problems in infancy should begin with mention of the development of swallowing *in utero*. Foetal swallowing is thought to contribute to several critical developmental processes including the regulation of amniotic fluid volume and composition, the acquisition and re-circulation of solutes from the foetal environment, and the maturation of the foetal gastro-intestinal tract. Controversy surrounds the role of foetal swallowing and voiding in the regulation of amniotic fluid volume. Nevertheless some interesting facts remain. First, the volume of fluid swallowed is strongly correlated with the volume of the fluid within the amniotic cavity. Second, there is marked increase in foetal swallowing in association with increasing gestational age: an 18-week-old foetus swallows 4–11 ml of fluid per day, whereas near-term foetuses (38–40 weeks) have a mean swallowing rate of 198 ml per day (Abramovich *et al.*, 1979). Finally, ultrasound studies have demonstrated that the human foetus can chew, swallow and regurgitate during intrauterine life (Bowie and Clair, 1982), and that the presence of foetal vomiting *in utero* may be associated with gastrointestinal obstruction.

These studies demonstrate that oral-motor and pharyngeal activity increases throughout gestation (Humphrey, 1964; Hack *et al.*, 1985), indicating that the motor program for sucking and swallowing appears to function well before term thereby providing the foetus with a range of early experiences *in utero*.

There is growing support from both animal and human studies to suggest that prenatal nutritional deprivation may be associated with increased risk of disease in adulthood (e.g. Barker and Martyn, 1992). The materno-foetal pregnancy environment may be influenced by regulatory mechanisms which control ingestive behaviour; furthermore, foetal swallowing might be modulated by a variety of factors including neuro-behavioural state changes and might be further influenced by hypoxia, hypotension and plasma osmolality changes. Although speculative, there are also suggestions that foetal swallowing might be regulated by the development of appetite sensation, salt appetite and the development of taste. Animal studies have demonstrated that altered osmotic environments modulate not only swallowing activity but also the development of adult sensitivities for thirst and arginine vasopressin secretion and responsiveness.

Therefore, future work with human foetuses will have important implications for foetal and adult dipsogenic regulation. The suggestion that regulatory mechanisms such as the development of appetite, salt and taste sensation are susceptible to influences in the pregnancy environment will alter our concept of the development of ingestive behaviour during the postnatal period. Prenatal constitutional factors may play a far greater role than previously expected.

Learning processes in infancy

Although infants have traditionally been viewed as capable of only reflexive behaviours at birth there is increasing evidence that very young infants, including newborns, can learn the contingencies between their own responses and the consequences they produce. These behavioural changes are not elicited, nor are they a reflection of the general behavioural arousal. In full-term newborns the rapidity of acquisition is specific to the nature of the response and reinforcer and the task parameters. Responses associated with feeding, for example, are learned very rapidly even by newborns (Rovee-Collier, 1987), in particular those associated with aversive experiences. Conditioning procedures have yielded evidence of robust retention of memories after hours, days and even weeks in extremely young infants. The young infant is prepared quite early to take in and learn from a wide range of stimulation, and to associate some experiences with others. Infants of 8 to 12 weeks of age, given the appropriate training conditions, can remember for periods of up to fourteen days without the benefit of a reminder. There is considerable evidence that, by 3 months of age, not only are infants capable of learning the contextual cues, but for periods of days or even weeks after that learning experience those contextual cues can selectively influence retrieval (for review see Rovee-Collier, 1987).

The cry of the human infant is highly effective in eliciting nurturance and bodily contact (Bernal, 1972) and it induces anticipatory milk let-down and increased breast temperature of the lactating mother (Vuorenskoski *et al.*, 1969). In general, newborns are hedonic creatures responding to the incentive-motivational properties of reinforcers with motor changes in behaviour, such as sucking and swallowing, and autonomic changes (Lipsitt *et al.*, 1985). Both the foetus and newborn have functioning chemosensory systems and within a few hours of birth infants are sensitive to subtle changes in gustatory stimulation and have pronounced preferences for sweeter fluids (e.g. Crook, 1979). While taste preferences for sweet foods, salty foods and milk appear to be influenced by a substantial genetic component, exposure of the foetus *in utero* to flavours in the amniotic fluid and human milk may also contribute to later preferences (Mennella and Beauchamp, 1998). In addition, postnatal maturation of the infant's sensory system is vulnerable to many other experiential influences.

There is normally a close and communicative interaction between a mother and her infant. During feeding the two individuals are responsive to one another and communication between them is warm and relaxed. All the child's sensory receptors become activated, and begin to integrate information from eyes, ears, nose, touch and movement. The development of normal feeding behaviour in infancy is also influenced by the transactional relationship between the infant's and the caregiver's behaviour. The crucial variables include, first, how the nutrition that is offered to the child is presented; second, how the nutrition is accepted by the child; and, third, the caregiver's reaction to how that offering is accepted. The infant's behavioural response during feeding may be an expression of underlying maturation, reflecting the integrity of the autonomic, motor and state subsystems and their transaction with the environment. If problems develop in the feeding relationship they can mirror difficulties elsewhere in the relationship at that time, but can also serve as a pointer to potential problems developing in the future.

Feeding and growth in early infancy

The first six months or so of life is a period of tremendous growth in terms of weight gain: in the first half of the first year after birth the rate at which the child is gaining weight is greater than it will ever be again until puberty, and of course must be sustained by an adequate intake of a diet rich in protein and calories. Relative deficiencies in protein or energy intake at this time are likely to have profound effects upon attained weight for age. The velocity of growth in terms of length is also at a peak shortly after birth, but in this case there is a more gradual diminution over the first two years or so. The rate of growth remains relatively constant until puberty from 6 months, in terms of weight gain, and from 2 years in terms of linear (skeletal) growth. In order to sustain this remarkable rate of growth in infancy the infant needs an adequate supply of calories, energy intake seemingly being the most common limiting factor upon growth, at least within the developed world. The proportion of energy (caloric) intake that is used for growth is higher during the first four to five months after birth than it ever is again: for a period of about five months after birth, in full-term infants, growth accounts for more than 8 per cent of normal energy intake but at no subsequent stage is it more than 5 per cent (Widdowson, 1973). Stunted growth due to chronic early malnourishment may be reversed in later years by a plentiful supply of food; but the longer the early period of under-nutrition the briefer the subsequent period of so-called 'catch-up growth' and the smaller the ultimate size of the child (Widdowson, 1973).

There is considerable individual variability in energy needs. Healthy babies who are being breastfed may consume a daily volume of milk at any given age that varies across a two- to threefold range (e.g. Whitehead and Paul, 1981). This variance cannot simply be accounted for by the differences in size of babies or by differences in their velocity of growth. Whitehead (1985) demonstrated that, at least from 2 to 8 months after birth, standard rates of growth can be achieved on energy intakes that are substantially smaller than the current recommended dietary allowances (Department of Health and Social Security, 1979). Towards the end of the first year there is closer correspondence with the WHO/FAO recommendations, possibly because of increased activity levels (FAO/WHO/UNU, 1985).

Historical trends in infant feeding

During the last decade there have been major changes in infant feeding practices. The first seventy years or so of the twentieth century saw a progressive fall in the use of human lactation as the normal way of feeding a young baby (Whitehead *et al.*, 1986). During 1911–1915, 70 per cent of American infants were reported to be breastfed at the time they left hospital (Hirschman and Butler, 1981). Even at 9 months of age the proportion was still as high as 30 per cent. However, by 1946–1950, the corresponding levels had fallen to only 24 per cent and 1 per cent respectively. Quite clearly there had to be a correspondingly high proportion of infants who were consuming cow's milk based formulae, and there is evidence to suggest that solid foods were being given at increasingly early ages. By the 1970s, 80 to 95 per cent of British babies were receiving non-milk solids by 3 months of age (Whitehead *et al.*, 1986). This however fell steadily to 68 per cent in 1990 and 55 per cent in 1995 (Foster *et al.*, 1997), the changes reflecting the recommendations prevailing at the time the two surveys were undertaken.

Babies are said to adjust their volume of intake to the caloric density of the feed, so the daily fluid intake of babies fed over-concentrated feeds is reduced (Whitehead *et al.*, 1986). Despite reduced water intake, caloric intake is, in such circumstances, higher than that of infants fed formulae of lower caloric density. Reduced water intake may have the effect of making infants especially vulnerable to changes in external water balance, and also renders them unable to tolerate long periods without feeding, giving rise to the common complaint that infants fed in this way never seem to be satisfied (Taitz, 1974). Studies on serum osmolality suggested that such babies were in a state of mild hypertonicity. The fault lay not with artificial feeding itself, but with the way in which mothers were preparing the infant feeds. Inappropriate methods of preparation led to solute loading and excessive caloric density. However, a further problem may have been the introduction of sucrose to increase the sweetness and hence to raise intake.

The trends in infant feeding practices between 1910 and the early 1970s are now being reversed. A comparison of the Office of Population Censuses and Surveys (OPCS) studies carried out since 1975 shows the proportion of babies put to the breast has steadily increased, with a statistically significant increase between 1990 and 1995 (with 66 per cent of babies breastfed in the UK). This welcome trend is also found in at risk infants such as very low birthweight children (Wolke and Meyer, 1998; Gutbrod *et al.*, 1999). The associations between initiation of breastfeeding and maternal characteristics remain similar to previous surveys where mother's educational level, age and previous feeding experiences are all strong predictors of breastfeeding. In contrast, infant behavioural features such as sleeping through the night and excessive crying are associated with earlier termination of breastfeeding (Wolke, 1994; Wolke and Meyer, 1998; Gutbrod et al., 1999).

Breastfeeding and growth

Exclusive breastfeeding is encouraged in early infancy because of known nutritional benefits and immunologic protection. In addition, it is said to promote improved emotional bonding and fulfil both maternal and infant psychological needs. The length of time that an infant can fulfil its nutritional needs from breast milk or infant formula alone varies considerably from baby to baby (Ahn and Maclean, 1980; Hitchcock et al., 1981). It is known that in breastfeeding, infants' milk (and energy) intake per kilogram body weight falls in the first half of infancy. There is also less rapid weight gain from the third month, and this is especially marked if the infant is not fed solids until after 4 months of age (Wolke, 1994). There is likely to be a wide range in the duration of time for which exclusive breastfeeding is adequate, because infants vary in their requirements and mothers vary in the amount and composition of milk they produce (FAO/WHO/UNU, 1985).

The immunologic protection provided by human milk is well known. Epidemiological studies demonstrate a relationship between exclusive breast-feeding (4 months or longer) and a decrease in childhood onset diabetes mellitus, Crohn disease and childhood cancers (especially acute leukaemia). Infants breastfed exclusively for six months have also been shown to have a lower than average predicted onset of allergic symptoms (e.g. eczema, infant onset asthma and rhinitis) (Bender, 1985). In a prospective study of infants living in south-east Queensland, the incidence of reported diarrhoea and/or vomiting in breast-, bottle- and mixed (breast and bottle) fed infants was compared from birth up to 1 year of age (Eaton-Evans and Dugdale, 1987). Up to 6 months, infants who were given breast feeds, with or without other milks, had less diarrhoea and vomiting than those given bottle feeds alone. Breastfeeding seemed to protect the infant against possible introduced infection even when other milk was given along with the breast milk. After 6 months, breastfeeding did not reduce the incidence of gastrointestinal infections. In an epidemiological study of the Canadian Eskimo, exclusively breastfed infants were found to be at reduced risk for the development of 'positional otitis media' (Lawrence, 1995). Exclusive breastfeeding fell in this population and infants bottlefed from the first month of life experienced a ten times greater incidence of severe otitis media than those infants breast-fed exclusively for 8 months or more. Whilst the protective qualities of human milk have always been thought to play a role, more recent research suggests that infant position (being placed in a more supine position or propped up for a bottle) and the high negative intra-oral pressure necessary to extract milk from a bottle may contribute to the presence of milk in the Eustachian tube (Lawrence, 1995).

Although breastfeeding is a natural biological process, it is neither instinctive nor simple (Wolf and Glass, 1992) and breastfeeding alone is not always adequate for infant growth, particularly when it is prolonged. In some cases breastfeeding may be associated with failure to thrive (Davies, 1979). Fawzi *et al.* (1998) suggested that undernourished children were more likely to have experienced prolonged breastfeeding and that the children of poor or illiterate mothers were more likely to be affected than children of affluent or literate mothers. The authors proposed that poorer complementary feeding among the breastfed children might in part explain this difference amongst children from poorer households.

Lawrence (1989) proposed a diagnostic flowchart for the evaluation of infants who fail to thrive at the breast. The chart highlights the complex nature of breastfeeding problems when weight gain is poor. Wolf and Glass (1992) discuss the importance of the interrelated nature of the breastfeeding dyad and the fact that attention is required to the physical and emotional/behavioural status of both mother and infant. Even though a problem may develop with just one component of breastfeeding, other aspects very quickly become affected and additional problems may arise. Fretful, irritable infants may be more difficult to breastfeed, and there is at least anecdotal evidence that a history of constant crying and irritability can be associated with excessively frequent and brief feeds. As a result the infant in question becomes increasingly relatively malnourished and a vicious cycle can be established. There may be associated colic and vomiting, and the infants are light in relation to their length, although skinfold thickness is in the low normal range. Davies (1979) has proposed that inadequate milk production is unlikely to be the explanation in every case. The process of feeding in such cases becomes tense and unpleasant for the mother and as a result infants may receive too few calories because feeding is terminated before the fat-rich 'hind milk' is ingested.

Maternal worry and tiredness can adversely influence the production of milk, by interfering with the neurohumeral 'let-down' reflex (Davies, 1979). The breast may not be emptied, because the infant has a weak suck or does not latch on correctly, leading to increased duct pressure, pain for the mother and interference with the let-down process.

Breastfeeding may also lead to failure to thrive, in the sense of poor weight gain, in a second group of apparently contented yet chronically underfed infants who give the impression of being satisfied after feeds. For these infants there may be excessively long intervals between feeds, with lengthy periods of sleep at night (Keane *et al.*, 1988). The problem here may be mothers who do not respond to their infant's needs, but to their demands. A relatively undemanding baby who, at just a few weeks of age, is prepared to sleep for twelve to fourteen hours at a stretch without a feed may be a delight to its mother, but will almost certainly fail to receive sufficient energy intake in a twenty-four-hour cycle to promote a normal rate of growth.

There are numerous 'infant causes' for breastfeeding problems and these are discussed in some detail by Wolf and Glass (1992). Briefly, some of these may include oral-motor dysfunction (e.g. poor tongue tip elevation, tongue retraction, poor central grooving of the tongue, excessive jaw excursion, inadequate mouth opening), structural abnormalities (small or recessed jaw), behaviour and state irregularities (e.g. infant temperament) and endurance irregularities (e.g. the baby who tires easily).

When the diagnosis is made of an infant who is failing to thrive at the breast it is important to take a careful feeding history, and also to confirm by test-weighing over a period of 24 to 48 hours that less than adequate amounts of breast milk are being taken in. An evaluation of the child's oral-motor function is essential.

When a breastfed baby appears hungry the first response is usually to increase the frequency of breast feeds. It is inappropriate to breastfeed a baby according to a strict timetable, and mothers who do so are more likely than those who feed on demand to stop breastfeeding in the early weeks. Frequent suckling stimulates the mother's secretion of prolactin which, in turn, contributes to an increased milk supply. If milk is regularly and frequently emptied from the breast by suckling, breast engorgement rarely occurs. The frequency of 'on demand' feeds may rise to two-hourly in the early days; but, towards the end of the first week of life, the milk supply becomes adjusted to the baby's demands and these become less frequent. If a mother breastfeeds, no other fluid should be given to the baby. If the mother responds to the infant's demands by giving formula feeds instead of extra breastfeeds it is likely her supply of breast milk will not increase to meet her baby's demands and she will find she does indeed have 'insufficient milk'. However, successful lactation can often be reestablished even after a week of no suckling (Llewellyn-Jones, 1983).

Although breastfeeding is desirable, it should not be supported to the exclusion of other options, given the consequences of poor growth in early infancy (Skuse *et al.*, 1994). Other options are available and the child's nutritional intake should be considered paramount.

Development of oral and pharyngeal skills in infancy

As highlighted earlier in this chapter, the development of oral and pharyngeal skills begins *in utero*. The normal infant is born with a well-established motor program for sucking and swallowing and with anatomic features that are well adapted to feeding success and safety. In fact the infant is perfectly designed to use a suck or suckle feeding pattern whilst held in a recumbent position. However, throughout infancy and early childhood, subtle structural changes in the shape, size and relationship of the oral cavity and the pharynx take place. These do not occur in isolation but alongside major developmental changes in the central nervous system and experiential learning. The resulting increase in motor control enables the infant to gradually adopt a more upright position, to adapt to increasing changes in their diet and the manner in which it is delivered.

Achievements in feeding (e.g. suckling, sucking, chewing, biting, swallowing) take place in a sequential process (Evans-Morris, 1985). There is little doubt that the evolution of the qualities of oral-motor skills needed for skilled and refined control during feeding is influenced both by individual rates of maturation and by feeding experiences (e.g. the textures of foods). During the first three months after birth, the full-term infant has a repertoire of reflexes that are able to ensure survival by means of the acquisition of nutrition. These include rooting, mouth opening, biting and lateral tongue movement. In addition, there is a series of protective reflexes (gag, cough and reflex closure of the airway) which ensure that the infant can feed safely while using the same conduit, the pharynx, to not only transport the liquid bolus but also to breathe. Successful feeding is highly dependent on this series of reflexive actions over which the neonate has little or no control. The reflexes may be elicited individually but most successfully integrate together. Neurological control is exerted at the subcortical level via the brainstem.

The rooting and perioral rooting reflex consist of orienting responses of the head and lips to assist the infant in locating the source of nourishment. At birth, and for the first two to three weeks of life, the baby demonstrates the side-to-side head-turning responses that consist of the head turning alternately towards and away from the stimulus (nipple) (Lewis, 1982). In addition, the lips orientate towards the stimulus while the mouth opens reflexively to receive the nipple or teat. In these earliest days the infant suckles on the nipple: suckling (also called a lick-suck movement) is a reflex feeding activity regulated at the subcortical level, probably in the medulla or pons. It consists of an extension and retraction pattern of the tongue because of limited room within the oral cavity. Sucking differs slightly in that the body or dorsum of the tongue moves up and down in time with the mandible to extract more liquid. At the same time the lips close tightly around the nipple/teat and increased negative pressure is created. The baby may use a mixture of sucking and suckle feeding up to the age of 6 months when sucking tends to predominate as the more efficient method for food intake. Each infant has a unique suckling pattern of bursts and pauses which occur in a stable pattern. Respiration patterns vary with infant age and stage of development but are always well coordinated with swallowing. During nutritive sucking most infants utilise a 1:1:1 suck–swallow–breathe pattern, with one such sequence once per second (Comrie and Helm, 1997), although some may sequence two or more sucks before pausing to breathe or swallow. By about 6 months, however, the infant has learnt to use much longer sequences of sucking, swallowing and breathing. Safe feeding requires precise coordination of the pharyngeal and laryngeal musculature in order to fulfil the two contradictory functions of airway maintenance for breathing and airway protection for swallowing.

Not surprisingly this feeding behaviour may not be fully developed in pre-term infants who are less efficient at safe feeding than full-term neonates. Bosma (1985) discusses several natural biological protection mechanisms that may be reduced in the premature infant. Some of these include a musculo-skeletal system that does not support the required postures for feeding, a lack of strength and endurance required to maintain feeding, impaired or immature neurological control and poor structural stability. In addition, many premature infants have additional medical problems which may compromise respiration (e.g. tracheomalacia and/or laryngomalacia), as well as gastrointestinal and cardiac problems and many other complications which may directly affect feeding.

Early sucking and swallowing difficulties may present as isolated symptoms or in association with other neurological signs in children who later develop cerebral palsy or a variety of other neurological conditions. They can be a subtle indicator of central nervous system dysfunction and of structural abnormalities. For example, a child with a tracheoesophageal fistula may have difficulty feeding safely and a child with a cleft lip and/or palate may not be able to suck efficiently.

Weaning

Weaning is the process by which the infant's food is changed from predominantly milk or formula to that of a solid diet (Lebenthal, 1985). Parents and physicians feel there are advantages to the early feeding of solid foods. For example, it has been claimed that the infant is more likely to sleep through the night (Lebenthal, 1985). Some parents also believe that the early introduction of weaning foods facilitates the development of speech by exercising oral structures and improved teething. A baby food company recently adopted this concept very successfully by claiming that feeding stage two baby foods (containing lumps for chewing) would help baby to speak. It has also been alleged that the early introduction of solid foods may encourage the development of taste and later acceptance of a varied diet.

An interesting and important body of research has emerged over the past five to ten years regarding children's experience and eating behaviours. The work of Leanne Birch has demonstrated clearly that children do not eat what they do not like. Similarly it has been shown that infants have an innate preference for sweet tastes and will reject sour or bitter foods (Cowart, 1981), and quite early in infancy develop a preference for salt, at 3–4 months. In consuming foods they like children select energy-dense foods which are high in fat or carbohydrate (Birch and Fisher, 1996).

In contrast, however, we have almost no information about children's acceptance of and ability to manage different food textures. There does appear to be a sensitive period between about 3 and 6 months of age, during which infants are relatively receptive to new gustatory experiences, and a sense of familiarity with a wide range of tastes and textures introduced at that time may facilitate the process of weaning and enhance the later introduction of a varied mixed diet. For some time now there has been a belief that the longer a child is breastfed the more difficult it is to get him or her to take ordinary food (Illingworth and Lister, 1964). While this may apply to some infants who are exclusively breastfed it now appears to be an outdated concept as more recent studies show that breastfed infants show greater acceptance of a novel food than formula-fed infants (Sullivan and Birch, 1994). This is thought to be due to the fact that breastfed infants have a variety of early experiences of flavour because different flavours are ingested by their breastfeeding mothers and present in the breast milk.

The seminal paper by Illingworth and Lister (1964) recommended that children should be given solids to chew when they are developmentally ready, usually around 6–7 months of age. They proposed that infants who were not given solids that needed chewing at that time would probably be excessively difficult about taking them later. Feeding problems would result, with refusal to accept lumpy foods, and even vomiting. This opinion is widely accepted despite the lack of supporting empirical evidence. The oral-motor skills necessary for munching and chewing emerge between 5 and 8 months of age although certain components of chewing can be demonstrated in infants as young as 7 days (Sheppard and Mysak, 1984). Chewing is dependent on sensory feedback combined with reflexes interacting to produce this complex motor pattern (Miller, 1999). It is a learned motor response that develops postnatally and is highly dependent on maturation of the central nervous system and eruption of primary dentition (although some controversy surrounds this concept).

The introduction of solid foods is, in our culture, coincident with the commencement of spoon feeding. On initial presentation of spooned food the infant reacts by trying to suckle as with the teat/nipple. They may repetitively protrude and retract their tongue and lose a great deal of the purée offered, at the same time producing some very expressive facial gestures. Many parents interpret this behaviour as the infant expressing their dislike of the food offered. However, the infant requires time to adjust to a more mature spoon feeding pattern which includes using the upper lip to remove food from the spoon. Of equal importance is the fact that the acceptance of new foods does not come immediately and eight to ten exposures may be necessary to induce acceptance in young infants (Birch and Fisher, 1996).

By the age of 9 months the infant has not only learned more sophisticated methods of using both lips and teeth or gums to remove food from the spoon but now has more refined tongue movements which extend beyond the simple extension and retraction present at 6 months. The infant at this age may still find it difficult to accurately grade mouth opening in order to match the configuration of spoon and food, and the mouth tends to be opened too wide in what seems to be virtually an orienting response. This improves rapidly and by 12 months most infants are able to grade the amount of mouth opening, and gauge it according to the quantity of food about to be received and the implement being used to convey it.

When more highly textured foods (either smooth foods containing lumps or thick purées) are introduced, there may be some initial gagging and coughing. The infant has become used to smooth textures and may be confused by a lump which works its way to the back of the tongue or a lump of food that is swallowed whole. Once again the infant must develop a new set of oral skills to manage these foods more efficiently. The introduction of solid foods which require munching (up and down movements of the jaw) or chewing (lateral and rotary movements of the jaw) is not dependent on dental eruption. Many infants are able to gum rusks, crackers or biscuits well before their teeth appear and in fact the role of the teeth is thought to be overrated in the chewing process. Of far greater importance is the smooth and coordinated range of movements performed by the tongue to move the food around the mouth and prepare it for swallowing in conjunction with a range of jaw movements.

At some stage during the first twelve months cup drinking is introduced to the majority of infants. As with the introduction of spooned foods the infant initially experiences considerable difficulty and may cough and choke as they are unable to control the faster flow of the liquid. Cup drinking requires extra demands in that the child cannot use the same suckle/suck pattern and must adapt the manner in which a swallow is triggered and coordinate respiration accordingly. It is not surprising that it can take a few attempts to get it right. A stable and steady mandible (jaw stability) is required and the child may bite on the rim of the cup to achieve this. Tongue movements change; the intrinsic muscles of the tongue alter tongue configuration to create a reservoir for the liquid and to collect up liquid that has spread under the tongue and around the mouth. The liquid is then propelled backwards in preparation for swallowing.

By 18–24 months infants have acquired the ability to manage a huge variety of tastes and, textures and providing they have been exposed to a range of foods, can manage an adult diet (they may have some minor difficulty with grinding fibrous meat). Gisel (1992), however, states that oral-motor skills do not fully mature until 6 years. It is not clear whether transitional feeding is a necessary step in learning to chew or prepare foods orally. The conventional method of progressing children though the transitional stages outlined above is based on belief in child rearing practices rather than empirical evidence (Stevenson and Allaire, 1991). For example, in other cultures children are not progressed through the same weaning process and may be weaned directly from breastfeeding to solid foods (Millard and Graham, 1985).

Infant feeding problems: a community perspective

Relatively little work has been done on the development of infant feeding problems and their consequences within a community context. An exception to this is the work of Margareta Dahl who conducted a series of studies in ten child health clinics in the urban district of Uppsala in Sweden (Dahl and Sundelin, 1986, 1987a, 1987b, 1987c). She studied a sample of fifty infants aged between 3 and 12 months, with a view to identifying the nature, correlates and consequences of feeding problems. In the course of a home visit an interview was conducted, the infant had a physical examination and the mealtime was observed. The feeding interaction was assessed by a schedule developed by the authors. Feeding problems were judged to be present when three criteria were fulfilled. First, both the child health clinic nurse and the parent considered that the child presented a consistent feeding problem of some kind. Second, the feeding problem had been present continuously without interruption for at least one month. Third, the primary help which had been given at the child health clinic, in the form of medical and psychological advice and treatment, had eliminated the problem. The number of infants found to have feeding problems, as a proportion of the population at risk, was 1.4 per 100 infants. Altogether fifty infants met case criteria and thus constituted the initial study material, comprising twenty-six girls and twenty-four boys with ages from 3 to 12 months (mean age 7 months). The mean duration of the feeding problems was found to be five months. The problems they presented with were refusal to eat (56 per cent), colic (18 per cent), vomiting (16 per cent), and other miscellaneous difficulties (10 per cent). At the time of examination most (82 per cent) case infants were underweight for their age, 46 per cent were more than one standard deviation below the mean (50th population centile of weight for age) and 14 per cent were at or more than two standard deviations below the mean.

The feeding behaviours of the infants actually observed during mealtimes varied according to the nature of the problem. Those who were said to be 'refusals to eat' ate slowly with many interruptions, and their mother attempted to control the feeding by tempting, distracting or even forcing the child to eat. Dahl attempted to sub-classify this group into those who refused all kinds of food (mean age 7 months), those who accepted breast milk only (mean age 9.5 months), and those who refused only solid food (mean age 8 months). Overt difficulties in the interaction between mother and child were striking only in the refusal to eat group. Most of the infants with colic ate eagerly in a tense and impatient manner and the infant controlled the feed. Overall, 14 per cent of the children who were seen had some form of physical disorder which was thought to be contributing to the feeding problem, and in 6 per cent there was a serious organic disease or disorder (e.g. congenital heart disease) which had not been detected until the time of this investigation. Dahl and Sundelin reported (1987a) that a substantially greater proportion of parents with infants with feeding problems reported feeding difficulties in their own childhoods than would be expected by chance. Infants who were first enrolled in the study at a median age of 7.3 months were seen again at a median age of 10 months and again at approximately 2 years. In total forty-two out of fifty children were followed up, comprising all those who did not have a significant organic disease, and excluding any who were premature. Twenty-five of the forty-two subjects who were followed up had formerly been refusing to eat; nine had had colic, seven had had vomiting, and one child displayed 'hyper-irritability at mealtimes'. Controls drawn from the same health district, matched for age, size and residential area, but who showed no feeding difficulties, were seen in the follow-up study. At the three-month follow-up sleeping problems were far more frequent among the refusal to eat group (40 per cent) than among the controls (4 per cent). By the two-year follow-up the rate of sleeping problems was rather similar in both groups (around 30 per cent). The sleeping problems of children with feeding difficulties had an earlier onset and persisted for a longer time than those of the controls.

At the age of 2 years 36 per cent of the refusal to eat group had a persistent feeding problem. In none of the children in the original colic group had the problem persisted, although two out of eight children in the vomiting subgroup continued to have difficulties.

After the onset of symptoms the standard deviation scores of attained weight and length decreased significantly in the children who had been refusing to eat, and in those with vomiting (Dahl and Sundelin, 1987a). The rate of weight gain was significantly lower in the refusal to eat group than in the comparison group. At 2 years of age the weights of the children with vomiting had recovered and had shown complete catch-up growth. The risk of growth impairment was greatest in those children who refused all food, or all food except breast milk.

In a more recent study, Dahl and colleagues (1994) followed-up the twenty-five children they had earlier identified with refusal to eat (RTE). Eighteen of these children (seven boys and eleven girls), now attending primary school and still resident in the district, were reinvestigated, and compared to a comparison group. The mean age of the children in the comparison group was 9.5 years and in the refusal to eat group 9.6 years. Information was collected from teacher and parent questionnaires, from child health records and parent completed questionnaires about the child's current eating behaviour and general behaviour. The number of problematic eating behaviours was reported to be far greater, both at school and at home, in the RTE children. No differences were found between the groups in respect to general behaviour, health problems or growth (weight and height). The study's findings are important as they provide new evidence of a link between early problematic eating behaviours, such as refusal to eat, and the persistence of such problems in later childhood. Dahl *et al.* (1994) raise the important question of whether these problems can precede eating disorders in adolescence and adulthood.

Relationships between feeding, sleeping and crying

At 3–4 months of age many infants still wake in the night, and it is often thought that they do so because they are hungry (Tuchman, 1988). Breastfed infants tend to wake more frequently than artificially fed infants (Wolke *et al.*, 1998). They also have fewer total hours sleep per twenty-four-hour cycle during the first two years of life (Keane *et al.*, 1988; Lucas and St James-Roberts, 1998). In 1990, Walloo *et al.* considered whether night waking might be due to excessive heat rather than related to feeding. They found that 3- to 4-month-old babies who were breastfed were more likely to wake their parents within four hours of sleep onset, although they did not wake more often than artificially fed babies over the course of the whole night. The authors did find evidence that heavily wrapped babies wake more often and many of these were observed by their parents to be sweating. This suggests that the sleep disturbance may have been due, in part, to their being uncomfortably warm.

Night feeds are the bane of many parents. The observation that the technique of feeding may have an important influence on sleep patterns has been made both in a longitudinal direct observation study (Wright, 1981) and via interview (Wright *et al.*, 1983); bottlefed infants established a more socially acceptable pattern of feeding at an earlier age than breastfed infants. Why should the night feeding pattern differ between the two groups? By 2 months of age the diurnal pattern for breastfed infants is one of large meals in the early morning and small meals at the end of the day. At 4 months the pattern switches to large meals at the end of the day, allowing the infant to cope with a prolonged period of night starvation. It is likely that the night waking of bottlefed infants will be regarded by mothers as more of a problem than the same pattern of behaviour in breastfed infants, and one way in which they try to get around it is to introduce solid foods. Macknin *et al.* (1989) conducted a survey to discover whether the introduction of cereals before bedtime did indeed affect infants' sleep patterns, but found no consistent tendency for one group to have a higher proportion of infants who slept through the night than the other. They concluded that the majority of infants in their study slept six consecutive hours at night by 12 weeks of age and eight consecutive hours at night by 20 weeks of age regardless of whether or not cereal was introduced.

Feeding and temperament are rarely considered together. Yet many determinants of crying and feeding problems may overlap, making their relative contributions to these behaviours hard to separate (Wolke, 1994; Barr *et al.*, 1989). For example, mothers who report excessive crying problems, colic or difficult temperament may also feed their children differently (Wolke *et al.*, 1995a, 1995b; Lucas and St James-Roberts, 1998). Indeed, in view of the fact that crying is frequently interpreted as indicative of hunger or 'insufficient milk', it may be used as a reason for changing the feeding regime (e.g. Forsyth *et al.*, 1985a). A recent prospective study (Barr *et al.*, 1989) found that choice of feeding at birth and perceived temperament at 2 weeks were only weakly associated with crying and fussing behaviour assessed at 6 weeks.

Parents of children who have problems in feeding, sleeping and crying may suffer feelings of anxiety, distress and a lack of self confidence, and these effects may be long-lasting. In a prospective study of all singletons born within a year at a Newhaven (CT) hospital over a four-month period, Forsyth *et al.* (1985a, 1985b) found that about one-third of mothers felt their infants had had either moderate or severe problems with feeding difficulties, excessive spitting, excessive crying or colic during the first four months of infancy. More mothers of formula fed than breastfed infants reported spitting as a problem; but the frequency of excessive crying, colic and feeding difficulties was similar in the two groups. Forsyth *et al.* comment that the fact that such a large proportion of these infants were felt to have problems suggests that some mothers regard as disorders behaviours that are normal. In this respect the findings from a questionnaire administered in the early postnatal period were revealing. Mothers' reports of concerns about potential feeding problems as soon as a few days after birth predicted which infants subsequently would be considered to have difficulties, but only in the breastfeeding group. These findings emphasise that it is important not to label the infant as the 'one with the feeding problem', since the presentation of problems to the clinician reflects a combination both of the actual disorder plus the perception by the parent of that disorder.

Rumination

Rumination is defined in DSM-IV as a disorder of infancy or childhood characterised by the bringing up (persistent regurgitation) of previously digested food which is then re-consumed. The disorder is present for a duration of at least one month following a period of normal functioning and in the absence of any known causal organic disorder (American Psychiatric Association, 1993). Rumination differs from vomiting in a number of distinctive ways. First, it is voluntary and not associated with acute illness or disease or associated with nausea. Second, it seems to be pleasurable (to the ruminator). Third, it is self-induced either by the placing of fingers or other objects in the mouth, or by less visible tongue movements or voluntary contraction of the tongue muscles. Prevalence estimates include 0.7 per cent in a sample of infants referred to an acute-care paediatric hospital (Kanner, 1972) and 6–9.6 per cent in long-stay institutions for the learning disabled (Singh, 1981; Ball *et al.*, 1974). The incidence is thought to be five times higher in males than in females (Mayes *et al.*, 1988).

Persistent rumination may produce medical complications such as malnutrition, dehydration and gastric disorders. In extreme cases, it may lead to death. A diagnosis of rumination should be clearly differentiated from gastro-oesophageal reflux (the involuntary return of the stomach contents into the oesophagus) which may produce in some children similar symptomatology, particularly in the learning disabled population. Historically, learning disabled children and adults were thought to be particularly prone to rumination, although in recent years a much higher incidence of gastro-oesophageal reflux has been identified in this population. Rogers *et al.* (1992) found a high prevalence of gastro-oesophageal abnormalities in institutionalised adults with severe learning difficulties. Presumably chronic regurgitation and vomiting in some of these individuals had been attributed to challenging behaviour and rumination rather than any underlying organic cause.

The aetiology of rumination seems uncertain, although hypotheses can broadly be divided into two types. First, there are psychodynamic explanations focusing on allegedly unsatisfactory mother–infant relationships in which the infant is said to be seeking internal gratification because of a lack of stimulation. In these cases there may be a physiological predisposition to regurgitation such as gastro-oesophageal reflux. Second, explanations based on learning theory emphasise the consequences of the behaviour, focusing especially on attention as a powerful positive reinforcer and maintaining factor. There is little empirical evidence for either theory.

Treatments of various sorts have been attempted and are reviewed by Winton and Singh (1983). The results have been generally consistent with other studies that have attempted to reduce undesirable behaviours in young children. Positive punishment procedures usually produce the most rapid effects even in subjects with whom other procedures have formerly been ineffective.

Pica

Pica is defined in DSM-IV (American Psychiatric Association, 1993) as a childhood eating disorder characterised by the developmentally inappropriate and persistent eating of non-food or non-nutritive substances for a period of at least one month. Culturally appropriate eating practices are excluded from this definition (see Kedesdy and Budd (1998) for a detailed discussion of inclusion/exclusion criteria). Pica has serious health consequences (intestinal obstruction, parasitic infection, poisoning – e.g. ingestion of materials with high lead concentration) and can be life threatening. Children may ingest a range of non-nutritive substances, including paper, dirt, toiletries, pens and pencils. The prevalence of pica is said to be around 37 per cent (Robinschon, 1971), and is age-dependent with a steady decline (from 35 per cent to 6 per cent) occurring between the ages of 1 and 4 years. One study reports a link between the persistence of pica in childhood and the later development of bulimia (Marchi and Cohen, 1990), suggesting that the presence of pica may be indicative of a general tendency towards indiscriminate or uncontrolled eating.

Pica in children is usually attributed to broad causes such as diet (e.g. as a result of nutritional deficiencies such as iron or zinc), infant constitution (e.g. developmental delay), caregiver characteristics (e.g. caregiver competency or maternal deprivation) or systemic factors (e.g. deprived home environment). Very little is known about intervention to reduce pica from empirical studies. Clearly there is a 'normal stage/range' during which pica occurs in childhood and this is associated with the intense mouthing and exploration of objects during infancy and early childhood. Persistence of this behaviour beyond the appropriate developmental stage is abnormal. There is some debate as to whether pica behaviour in the young infant justifies parental or professional concern. Robinschon (1971) suggests a three-stage process for developing an appropriate guide for intervention: first, development of improved interview techniques to enable health professionals to better identify pica behaviour; second, education of professionals to observe for pica behaviour; and third, monitoring children with increased risk for development of pica, such as those with identified developmental delay.

For a more detailed discussion on clinical guidelines for evaluation of and intervention for rumination and pica, readers are directed to a chapter written by Kedesdy and Budd (1998) who present case studies to illustrate their theories.

Colic

In early infancy, paroxysmal crying, which is not helped by the usual nursing procedures and which is sometimes associated with excessive gas in the abdomen, is a common complaint (Wolke et al., 1994; Wolke, 1993). This condition is often known as infantile colic and its reported frequency ranges between 16 and 30 per cent (Hide and Guyer, 1982; Illingworth, 1954, Forsyth et al., 1985a). The cause is unknown (Stahlberg, 1984). Although many attributes, such as flexing of legs occurring after feeds, have been used to characterise colic (Forsyth, 1989), there is little evidence for organic origin or indeed that flatulence or abdominal pain have to be present (Barr, 1990, 1995). The now widely accepted definition of colic is the 'rules of three' (Wessel et al., 1954): fussing and crying for three hours per day on at least three days per week for at least three weeks (Wolke, 1994). Although there is no universally accepted definition of colic the diagnosis is based on paroxysms of intense inconsolable crying usually starting after feeding, which occur most often during the evening hours and which are associated with other symptoms such as turning red, flexing of the legs, and abdominal distension. Symptoms tend to become worse throughout the day (Forsyth, 1989).

Inconsolable crying induces despair in parents and leads to decreased confidence in their own parenting abilities. Little is known about the best way to manage the problem. Colic usually begins in the first two to four weeks of life and persists through to the third or fourth month. It has been thought that the abdominal distension and excessive flatus are due to air swallowing. On the other hand, some believe that colic is a distinct and possibly pathological phenomenon, and that the excessive crying and associated symptoms are part of an adverse reaction to milk.

Over the past twenty to thirty years there has been burgeoning opinion that colic may be due to some specific allergic reaction to the protein content of milk; or, on the other hand, that milk intolerance is due to partial malabsorption of lactose (e.g. Jakobsson and Lindberg, 1983; Lothe et al., 1982). Intestinal brush border lactase activity is maximal in the prenatal period but, depending on the ethnic background of the infant, it may either remain high throughout life or diminish markedly from 3 to 5 years of age (see Lebenthal, 1985). About 10 to 20 per cent of North Europeans are lactose intolerant, and 80 to 90 per cent of the world's population are lactose intolerant. The notion that lactose intolerance is a significant problem for normal infants in the western hemisphere is exemplified by a recent prospective study of healthy newborn infants in Newhaven (CT) (Forsyth et al., 1985a). Twenty-six per cent of formula-fed infants followed by paediatricians in private practice had had their artificial feeds changed to non-cow's milk containing formulae by 4 months of age.

Several studies have attempted to eliminate cow's milk from the diet of colicky infants (e.g. Jakobsson and Lindberg, 1983; Lothe et al., 1982; Evans et al., 1981) but contradictory results have been found. It should be pointed out that the alleged intolerance to cow's milk that precipitates attacks of colic includes not only milk consumed by the infant but that consumed by the mothers of breastfed infants (Jakobsson and Lindberg, 1983; Lothe et al., 1982).

Forsyth (1989) attempted to conduct a study improving on the methodological deficiencies of previous research. He ran a randomised double blind trial with three changes of formula, for each of four four-day periods. Colicky infants alternately received a casein-hydrolysate milk (regarded as hypoallergenic, e.g. Knights, 1985) or a formula containing cow's milk. On the whole, there were more clinically significant responses to the casein-hydrolysate formula than to cow's milk. There had been three formula changes in total but only one in seventeen infants responded in the expected direction on all three occasions. Forsyth concluded that although colic may improve with the elimination of cow's milk formula the effect diminishes with time. There have been several studies in recent years (see Wolke and Meyer, 1995, for a review); however, they were mostly based on referred patients of parents who suffer themselves with atopic problems.

In conclusion, infantile colic is a short-lived disorder of heterogeneous origin, and it is probable that one of its causes is food allergy or intolerance (Sampson, 1989); but food allergy or intolerance is probably the cause of symptoms in less than 10 per cent of colicky infants. Wolke and Meyer (1995) suggested that if parent management counselling of persistent crying (Wolke et al., 1994) is not successful, then cow milk protein intolerance should be seriously considered and properly (multiple challenges) evaluated as a second course of action. So, a two- to three-month trial of hypoallergenic formula may be warranted in some instances. Parents should not be left with the idea that the infant will have lifelong food allergy problems; food allergy or intolerance in very young infants is often short-lived (Bock, 1987). More than one food antigen trial will be necessary to establish a causal relationship between food ingestion and the development of symptoms.

Gastro-oesophageal reflux

Gastro-oesophageal reflux (GOR) is recognised as an important clinical problem in young children. GOR is the involuntary return of gastric contents into the oesophagus. It is an occasional physiological event in normal adults and children but is pathological when its frequency and duration increase or when complications arise. Although recurrent vomiting and regurgitation are the clinical hallmarks of GOR their absence does not exclude the diagnosis (Sullivan and Brueton, 1991). Other symptoms typical of the clinical picture of a child with gastro-oesophageal reflux may include: irritability, food refusal, fussy, faddy eating behaviour (including taking a limited range of tastes and textures) and poor sleeping patterns. The older child may complain of symptoms suggestive of dyspepsia or heartburn or of food being stuck.

The causes of GOR fall into two groups: primary causes (anatomic or physiological), and causes secondary to other diseases such as metabolic disorders, food allergy, etc. (Davies and Sandhu, 1995). There are a number of important mechanisms that control GOR and they include: the lower oesophageal sphincter, the intra-abdominal segment of the oesophagus, the gastro-oesophageal angle of His, the mucosal rosette in the lower oesophagus and the pinchcock effect of the diaphragmatic crura (Sullivan and Brueton, 1991). These anatomical relationships, together with the coordinated peristaltic clearance of the distal oesophagus, prompt gastric emptying to prevent significant reflux of the gastric contents (Sullivan and Brueton, 1991). A defect of any of these components may result in GOR.

The frequent reflux of acidic gastric contents into the oesophagus causes a persistent burning sensation that quickly becomes associated with eating and drinking, even in very young babies. The oesophageal mucosa is not designed to be bathed in acid and persistent acid reflux may lead to painful oesophagitis, akin to battery acid splashed onto the skin. This understandably makes eating unpleasant, causing the infant or child to cry, refuse to open their mouth, and use other tactics to communicate a dislike of eating because of the consequences. The consequent psychological impact of this on both the child and carer may be profound. Some children remain food refusers or fussy, faddy eaters many years after their GOR has been treated, despite behavioural intervention.

The consequences of GOR can have a major impact on a child's health and development and include growth failure, dysphagia, stricture formation, haematemasis, iron deficiency anaemia, recurrent respiratory infections, apnoea, coughing and choking, stridor and, in the most severe cases, sudden infant death (Werlin *et al.*, 1980). Paton *et al.* (1988) found evidence for gastro-oesophageal reflux extending to the upper oesophageal or laryngeal level in a sample of eighty-two infants and children. Their subjects comprised: twenty-two infants who had had a 'near miss' for sudden infant death syndrome (SIDS); twelve siblings of previous SIDS victims; a miscellaneous group of forty-four children presenting with symptoms that were not life threatening (choking, wheeziness, recurrent vomiting); and four infants with mental retardation. The mean age of their sample was 0.36 years (range 0.03–1.79 years). Only sixty-one (9.6 per cent) of the episodes of gastro-oesophageal reflux in their sample, as measured by radionuclide scanning, were associated with vomiting, defined as the appearance of milk at the mouth. The absence of vomiting clearly does not preclude appreciable gastro-oesophageal reflux.

Bray and colleagues (1977) vividly describe a variety of clinical presentations of the condition. They report the history of a 3-month infant with extreme irritability and vomiting that began in the neonatal period, together with failure to thrive. This infant tended to hold his head to one side. Another child presented at the age of 2 months regurgitating her foods regularly. She stopped gaining weight and became very irritable. Symptoms of rapidly laboured respiration at 2.5 months led to hospitalisation and treatment for what turned out to be aspiration pneumonitis. The child also had a peculiar posture, holding her head cocked to the left. Several other similar cases with this often severe and intermittent head cocking trait are also presented by Bray *et al.* (1977). In several cases there was associated rumination with eructation and re-swallowing of the stomach contents, and repetitive thrusting movements of the tongue. Respiratory symptoms may be associated with spitting up, gagging, choking, and the inadvertent inhalation of stomach contents. The vomiting seen after feeds in infants with gastro-oesophageal reflux seems on occasion to be associated with episodes resembling seizures and can be accompanied by apnoea, cyanosis, and stiffening. These are probably aspirations (Bray *et al.*, 1977).

In the child with neurological disease or significant developmental delay GOR is not always readily identifiable, yet has been found to be extremely common (GOR was identified in up to 75 per cent of patients with cerebral palsy in a study by Abrahams and Burkitt (1970)). Such children may adopt bizarre posturing and dystonic movement patterns (Sandifer's syndrome is a rare but well described manifestation of GOR) which are mistakenly believed to be part of their neurological condition but are in fact occurring because of

GOR. Similarly, some sudden, jerky movements with stiffening of the limbs may need to be differentiated from seizure activity which can appear very similar.

The gold standard for documenting GOR is twenty-four-hour pH monitoring. This involves placement of a small thin pH probe through the nose to an area just above the lower oesophageal sphincter (the probe position is verified by X-ray). The probe is connected to a small box which records all lower oesophageal activity during the twenty-four-hour period. In addition the infant's activities are recorded and can be correlated during later analysis with the acidity of the lower oesophagus. The working group on GOR (the European Society of Paediatric Gastroenterology and Nutrition – ESPGAN) have published a protocol for lower oesophageal pH monitoring which contains detailed information about the procedures and interpretation of the results. A reflux episode is defined as when the lower oesophageal pH falls below pH 4.0. The total number of reflux episodes, and the length and frequency of episodes, are measured as well as the ability of the oesophagus to clear the reflux. Although the barium swallow with delayed imaging may also be used to detect GOR it has major limitations, notably the necessary restriction of exposure time to minimise the radiation dose, thereby increasing the likelihood of missing intermittent episodes. The barium study has been shown to be an unreliable method of assessing for GOR as the examination occurs over a very short period of time and the results may be misleading (Martin *et al.*, 1992). A range of treatment options are currently recommended and include:

- Thickened feeds
- Postural adjustment
- Dietary modifications
- Antacids
- H2, blockers
- Proton pump inhibitors

Uncomplicated cases of GOR may respond to thickened feeds, dietary modifications and/or postural adjustment such as positioning the infant in a prone position with the head elevated. Dietary modification usually consists of advice regarding a 'little and often' feeding regime to decrease the amount lost through vomiting. It may also include avoidance of particular types of food (e.g. fizzy drinks or spicy foods). Antacids are often used in conjunction with the above treatments. However, when these methods fail to alleviate the symptoms then medication may be introduced. In the child with neurological disease, medical management consisting of triple therapy (a combination of a prokinetic agent, an H2 receptor agent and an antacid) is nearly always required. Dietary and postural interventions are usually ineffective in this group. Surgical treatment (such as a Nissen fundoplication) is sometimes warranted when full medical treatment has failed (Spitz *et al.*, 1993). For a full discussion of the diagnosis and treatment of GOR readers are referred to a review paper by Davies and Sandhu (1995).

Dysfunctional feeding in the neonatal period

As highlighted earlier in this chapter, the newborn infant is well equipped to feed safely and successfully and indeed has been practising these skills for some weeks *in utero*. The gestational age needed for the establishment of coordination of sucking, respiration and swallowing ranges from 34 to 37 weeks (Braun and Palmer, 1985). In infants over 34 weeks gestation abnormalities of suckling and swallowing are not likely to be the result of immaturity, and usually have a pathological basis (Hill and Volpe, 1981). Persistently dysfunctional feeding behaviour in the full-term infant can be seen as an early marker for later neuro-developmental morbidity. There would be a high index of suspicion surrounding any infant with impaired sucking and/or swallowing in the neonatal period. Such infants would be monitored closely as their impaired feeding skills are most likely to be indicative of neurological damage.

The structural integrity of the oropharynx, hypopharynx, pharynx, larynx and oesophagus is an important prerequisite to safe and efficient feeding. Structural defects such as a cleft of the larynx or a tracheo-oesophageal fistula will seriously affect feeding. However, in the absence of any neurological or neuromuscular problem the baby will usually feed well once a repair is undertaken, although there may be other long-term problems associated with the structural defect.

In 1985 Braun and Palmer developed a system for neonatal oral-motor assessment (NOMAS – Neonatal Oral-Motor Assessment Scale). They studied a sample of infants between 35–46 weeks corrected age and a postnatal age at the time of testing of 7.6 weeks. The technique employed by Braun and Palmer was to get the infants to suck on a machine they christened the suckometer, which could measure both nutritive sucking (NS) and non-nutritive sucking (NNS). Sucking pressures were measured, the aim being to assess oral-motor components during sucking, including rate, rhythmicity, consistency and degree of jaw excursion, direction/range/motion and timing of tongue movements, and tongue configuration. Although the sample was rather small (n = 11) and no reliability information is presented, the authors maintained that the system enabled a distinction to be made between infants with disorganised, dysfunctional, and normal feeding behaviours. Disorganisation of sucking was defined as a lack of rhythm of the total sucking activity, rather than the incoordination of fine movements comprising a single response. Dysfunction was defined as interruption of the feeding process by abnormal movements of the tongue and jaw.

Six of their sample had known intraventricular haemorrhages which had been diagnosed by cranial ultrasound. Three of these were found to have abnormal oral-motor behaviours of one sort or another. Oral-motor dis-organisation and dysfunction were also found in two of three infants with known birth asphyxia. In this study oral-motor dysfunction was associated with generalised hypotonia, although hypotonia from various causes was no more commonly associated with oral-motor examinations that were normal than with those that were abnormal. The authors nevertheless suggest that both oral-motor disorganisation and dysfunction appear to be acquired (e.g. from brain damage at birth) and perhaps reflect a more widespread involvement of the CNS in some, but not all, of those infants with hypotonia from various causes.

Premature infants are less efficient at safe feeding than full-term infants; infants born at less than 34 weeks gestation have the greatest difficulty as they are unable to coordinate their respiration with sucking and swallowing. The more premature the infant the longer it will be dependent on tube feeding. Many premature infants have a range of associated medical and neurological problems involving the respiratory and digestive system. Furthermore, cardiac problems, neurological sequelae and hypoxic ischemic events make the premature infant vulnerable, the result being that the ability to feed safely and efficiently is considerably reduced. The very nature of the many problems likely to arise in the premature infant alter the baby's sensory experiences, particularly in the sensitive orofacial region. Repeated insertion of feeding tubes and suctioning equipment provides the infant with aversive oral experi-ences which are very different form those of the full-term infant. In addition, prolonged intubation and the presence of tracheomalacia or laryngeomalacia may compromise respiration and have a direct effect on feeding experience and efficiency. Such infants are at risk of developing tactile defensiveness and oral hypersensitivity.

Oral-motor dysfunction and failure to thrive

It has often been reported that the condition of failure to thrive is due pri-marily to maternal rejection and neglect (e.g. Patton and Gardner, 1963). However, a critical appraisal of the evidence suggests that a more balanced view should be taken of the role of the caregiver–child relationship (Skuse et al., 1985). The infant makes an important contribution to the relationship, and feeding problems may exacerbate tensions and lead to a negative cycle of interaction, which resolves when the problems are recognised and treated (Palmer et al., 1975). Lewis (1982) suggested that oral-motor abnormalities can contribute to failure to thrive in infancy, and described difficulties with sucking, chewing and swallowing, tongue thrusting, involuntary tonic biting of the spoon or nipple, excessive drooling and an intolerance of the textures of developmentally appropriate food. She commented that such problems may lead to prolonged feeding and also considered contextual features that might be important: for example, inappropriate positioning during feeding. Selley and Boxall (1986) have described 'incoordination of the feeding mechanism' as a possible cause of failure to thrive, which is susceptible to treatment with an intra-oral appliance.

Mathisen and colleagues (1989) administered a structured oral-motor assessment to nine, 1-year-old 'non-organic failure to thrive' infants and compared them to a group of healthy children. The case children and controls were presented with a variety of foods of different textures, graded from liquid (e.g. apple juice) through purées (e.g. fromage frais) and semi-solids (e.g. fresh fruit salad) to firm solids (e.g. oatcake biscuits). There were two options of food at each level of consistency; if the infant rejected the first, the second was substituted. The feeding assessment procedure was video-recorded and subsequently the video-recordings were analysed. Case infants were found to have oral-motor dysfunction (OMD) associated with developmental delay and the OMD was considered to be similar to that seen in neurologically impaired infants. Several features shown by the case infants were consonant with the view of Accardo (1982) that many infants with non-organic failure to thrive are 'minimally neurologically abnormal'. However, only tentative conclusions could be drawn because of the small sample and the fact that the children had been identified by health visitors for the study.

In a further study, a much larger sample (n = 94) of infants was studied (Reilly et al., 1999). Forty-seven infants with non-organic failure to thrive (NOFT) were matched to a comparison group of the same age (mean age 14.6 months; range 12 to 17 months). A previously validated assessment of oral-motor function, the Schedule of Oral Motor Assessment – SOMA (Reilly et al., 1995), was administered to each child. In addition, information about early feeding history and current methods of feeding was obtained from parent interview. A significant proportion (n = 30) of the NOFT children were found to have some degree of oral-motor dysfunction, with seventeen scoring in the moderate to severely impaired range on the SOMA. Neuro-developmental assessments revealed that the children with significantly impaired oral-motor skills tended to have higher abnormality scores for both fine and gross motor function and higher scores on a scale measuring congenital anomalies. We argued that the children with significantly impaired oral-motor skills had a subtle but unidentified neuro-developmental disorder and that higher prenatal and perinatal adversity scores suggest that this subgroup may indeed be biologically more vulnerable from birth.

Further evidence of neuro-developmental abnormalities in children who fail to thrive was provided by Ramsey et al. (1993) in their study of thirty-eight infants with NOFT and twenty-two with organic failure to thrive. The histories of the children with so-called NOFT were suggestive of an oral sensorimotor impairment reported to be present from birth or even early infancy. An objective assessment of oral-motor functioning was not included

in the study; however, Ramsey and colleagues (1993) described many characteristics suggestive of OMD during their observations of the children's
mealtimes. Significant proportions of the children studied were reported to
have a history of sucking difficulties, abnormal duration of feeding times,
poor appetite, delayed texture tolerance and difficult feeding behaviour. The
study concluded that despite the fact that no diagnostic label had been
applied to the NOFT children many had histories and developmental profiles
suggestive of minimal neurological impairment.

These studies have contributed significantly to our knowledge of failure to
thrive in infancy. First, they provide evidence to suggest that continued use of
the label 'non-organic' to describe this subgroup of children who fail to thrive
is no longer appropriate. Second, they strongly suggest that a balanced view
should be taken of the role of the caregiver–child relationship in failure to
thrive (Skuse et al., 1985). Recognition of the contribution the infant makes
is vital. Finally, they suggest that further study of oral-motor function in the
context of the child's overall development is necessary, although this would
necessitate a prospective study.

Conclusion

We have mentioned evidence that a thorough analysis of feeding problems
in infancy must not only take account of the overt behaviour, and the
psychological causes and correlates of that behaviour, but also certain developmental and biological characteristics of the child in question. However,
infant feeding disorders must also be viewed from a developmental perspective, and the individual characteristics of the child as well as of the caregiver
should be taken into account when assessing possible precipitating and
maintaining factors. Emerging evidence suggests that the foetal environment
may also play an important role in the development of taste and later
eating patterns. Some relevant individual difference biological factors, as
they pertain to the infant, have already received a great deal of attention
(e.g. infantile colic) whereas others have been virtually ignored in the general
run of paediatric and psychological literature (e.g. oral-motor dysfunction).

References

Abrahams, P. and Burkitt, B.F. (1970) Hiatus hernia and gastro-oesophageal reflux in
    children and adolescents with cerebral palsy. Australian Paediatric Journal, 6,
    41–46.
Abramovich, D.R., Garden, A., Jandial, L. and Page, K.R. (1979) Fetal swallowing
    and voiding in relation to hydramnios. Obstetrics and Gynecology, 54, 15–20.
Accardo, P. (1982) Growth and development: an interactional context for failure to
    thrive. In P. Accardo (ed.) Failure to Thrive in Infancy and Early Childhood:
    A Multidisciplinary Team Approach. Baltimore: University Park Press, 3–18.

Adolph, E.E. (1968) Origins of physiologic regulations. New York: Academic Press.

Ahn, C.E. and Maclean, W.C. (1980) Growth of the exclusively breast fed infant. *American Journal of Clinical Nutrition*, 33, 183–192.

American Psychiatric Association (1993) *Diagnostic and Statistical Manual of Mental Disorders – 4th edition*. Washington, DC: APA.

Ball, T.S., Hendricksen, H. and Clayton, J. (1974) A special feeding technique for chronic regurgitation. *American Journal of Mental Deficiency*, 78, 486–493.

Barker, D.J. and Martyn, C.N. (1992) The maternal and fetal origins of cardiovascular disease. *Journal of Epidemiology and Community Health*, 46, 8–11.

Barr, R.G. (1990) The early crying paradox: a modest proposal. *Human Nature*, 1, 355–389.

Barr, R. (1995) The enigma of infant crying: the emergence of defining dimensions. *Early Development and Parenting*, 4, 225–232.

Barr, R.G., Kramer, M.S., Press, I.B., Boisjoly, C. and Leduc, D. (1989) Feeding and temperament as determinants of early infant crying/fussing behavior. *Pediatrics*, 84, 514–521.

Bax, M. (1989) Editorial: eating is important. *Developmental Medicine and Child Neurology*, 31, 285–286.

Bender, A.E. (1985) The quantity and quality of breast milk – WHO. *Journal of the Royal Society of Health*, 105(6), 226.

Bernal, J. (1972) Crying during the first 10 days of life, and maternal responses. *Developmental Medicine and Child Neurology*, 14, 362–372.

Birch, L.L. and Fisher, J.A. (1996) The role of experience in the development of children's eating behaviour. In E.D. Capaldi (ed.) *Why We Eat What We Eat: The Psychology of Eating*. Washington, DC: APA, 113–141.

Bock, S.A. (1987) Prospective appraisal of complaints of adverse reactions to foods in children during the first 3 years of life. *Pediatrics*, 89, 683–688.

Bosma, J.F. (1977) Structure and function of infant oral and pharyngeal mechanisms. In J. Wilson (ed.) *Oral Motor Function and Dysfunction in Children*. Chapel Hill: University of North Carolina, 33–38.

Bosma, J.F. (1985) Postnatal ontogeny of performances of the pharynx, larynx, and mouth. *American Review of Respiratory Disease*, 131, S10–15.

Bosma, J.F. (1986) Anatomy of the infant head. Baltimore: Johns Hopkins University Press.

Bosma, J.F. (1992) Pharyngeal swallow: basic mechanisms, development and impairments. *Advances in Otolaryngology Head and Neck Surgery*, 6, 225–275.

Bosma, J.F., Grossman, R.C. and Kavanagh, J.F. (1967) A syndrome of impairment of oral perception. In J. Bosma (ed.) *Symposium on Oral Sensation and Perception*. Springfield, Ill.: Charles C. Thomas, 1967, pp. 318–335.

Bowie, J.D. and Clair, M.R. (1982) Fetal swallowing and regurgitation: observation of normal and abnormal activity. *Radiology*, 144, 877–878.

Braun, M. and Palmer, M.M. (1985) A pilot study of oral-motor dysfunction in 'at risk' infants. *Pediatrics*, 5, 13–25.

Bray, P.F., Herbst, J.J., Johnson, D.G., Book, L.S., Ziter, F.A. and Condon, V.R. (1977) Childhood gastrooesophageal reflux: neurologic and psychiatric syndromes mimicked. *Journal of the American Medical Association*, 237, 1342–1345.

Comrie, J.D. and Helm, J.M. (1997) Common feeding problems in the intensive care nursery: maturation, organisation, evaluation and management strategies. *Seminars in Speech and Language*, 18, 3.

Cowart, B.J. (1981) Development of taste perception in humans: sensitivity and preference throughout the life span. *Psychological Bulletin*, 90, 43–73.

Crook, C.K. (1979) Taste perception in the newborn infant. *Infant Behaviour and Development*, 1, 49–66.

Dahl, M. and Sundelin, C. (1986) Early feeding problems in an affluent society: i) Categories and clinical signs. *Acta Paediatrica Scandinavica*, 75, 370–379.

Dahl, M. and Sundelin, C. (1987a) Early feeding problems in an affluent society: ii) Determinants. *Acta Paediatrica Scandinavica*, 75, 380–387.

Dahl, M. and Sundelin, C. (1987b) Early feeding problems in an affluent society: iii) Follow-up at 2 years: natural courses, health, behaviour and development. *Acta Paediatrica Scandinavica*, 76, 872–880.

Dahl, M. and Sundelin, C. (1987c) Early feeding problems in an affluent society: iv) Impact on growth up to 2 years of age. *Acta Paediatrica Scandinavica*, 76, 881–888.

Dahl, M., Rydell, A.M. and Sundelin, C. (1994) Children with early refusal to eat: follow-up during primary school. *Acta Pediatrica Scandinavica*, 83, 54–58.

Davies, D.P. (1979) Is inadequate breast feeding an important cause of failure to thrive? *Lancet*, 1, 541–542.

Davies, A.E.M. and Sandhu, B.K. (1995) Diagnosis and treatment of gastro-oesophageal reflux. *Archives of Disease in Childhood*, 73, 82–86.

Department of Health and Social Security (1979) Recommended daily amounts of food energy and nutrients for groups of people in the United Kingdom. *Report on Health and Social Subjects*, 15. London: HMSO.

Eaton-Evans, J. and Dugdale, A.E. (1987) Effects of feeding and social factors on diarrhoea and vomiting in infants. *Archives of Disease in Childhood*, 62, 445–448.

Emde, R.N. (1987) Infant mental health: clinical dilemmas, the expansion of meaning, and opportunities. In J.D. Osofsky (ed.) *Handbook of Infant Development*. New York: Wiley, 1299–1320.

Evans, T.J. and Davies, D.P. (1977) Failure to thrive at the breast: an old problem revisited. *Archives of Disease in Childhood*, 52, 974.

Evans, R.W., Allardyce, R.A., Fergusson, D.M. and Taylor, B. (1981) Maternal diet and infantile colic in breastfed infants. *Lancet*, i, 1340–1342.

Evans-Morris, S. (1977a) Interpersonal aspects of feeding problems. In J.M. Wilson (ed.) *Oral Motor Function and Dysfunction in Children*. Chapel Hill: University of North Carolina, 106–122.

Evans-Morris, S. (1977b) Oral-motor development: normal and abnormal. In J.M. Wilson (ed.) *Oral Motor Function and Dysfunction in Children*. Chapel Hill: University of North Carolina, 114–128.

Evans-Morris, S. (1985) Developmental implications for the management of feeding problems in neurologically impaired infants. *Seminars in Speech and Language*, 6, 293–314.

FAO/WHO/UNU (1985) *Report of a Joint Expert Consultation: Energy and Protein Requirements*. Technical Report Series 724. Geneva: WHO.

Fawzi, W.W., Herrera, M.G., Nestel, P., Amin, A. and Mohammed, K.A. (1998) A longitudinal study of prolonged breastfeeding in relation to child undernutrition. *International Journal of Epidemiology*, 27, 255–260.

Forsyth, B.W.C. (1989) Colic and the effect of changing formulas: a double blind, multiple crossover study. *Journal of Pediatrics*, 115, 521–526.

Forsyth, B.W., McCarthy, P.L. and Leventhal, J.M. (1985a) Problems of early infancy, formula changes and mothers' beliefs about their infants. *Journal of Pediatrics*, 106, 1012–1017.

Forsyth, B.W.C., Leventhal, J.M. and McCarthy, P.L. (1985b) Mothers' perceptions of problems of feeding and crying behaviors. *American Journal of Diseases of Children*, 139, 269–272.

Foster, K., Lader, D. and Cheesbrough, S. (1997) Infant feeding 1995. Results from a survey carried out by the social survey division of ONS on behalf of the UK health departments. Office for National Statistics. London: The Stationery Office.

Gisel, E.G. (1992) Eating assessment and efficacy of oral motor treatment in eating-impaired children with cerebral palsy. *Cerebral Palsy Today*, 2, 1–3.

Gisel, E.G. and Patrick, J. (1988) Identification of children with cerebral palsy unable to maintain a normal nutritional state. *Lancet*, 1, 283–286.

Gutbrod, T., Meier, P., Rust, L. and Wolke, D. (1999) Early maternal attachment, infant irritability and feeding in VLBW infants. Paper presented at the Biennial Meeting of the Society for Research in Child Development, Albuquerque, New Mexico, USA.

Hack, M., Eastbrook, M.M. and Robertson, S.S. (1985) Development of sucking rhythms in preterm infants. *Early Human Development*, 11, 133–140.

Hide, D.W. and Guyer, B.M. (1982) Prevalence of infant colic. *Archives of Disease in Childhood*, 57, 559–560.

Hill, A. and Volpe, J.J. (1981) Disorders of sucking and swallowing in the newborn infant: clinicopathological correlations. In *Progress in Perinatal Neurology*. Philadelphia: W.B. Saunders, 157–181.

Hirschman, C. and Butler, M. (1981) Trends and differential in breastfeeding: update. *Demography*, 18, 39–54.

Hitchcock, N.E., Gracey, M. and Owles, E.N. (1981) Growth of healthy breastfed infants in the first six months. *Lancet*, ii, 64.

Humphrey, T. (1964) Some correlations between the appearance of human fetal reflexes and the development of the CNS. *Progress in Brain Research*, 4, 93–135.

Illingworth, R.S. (1954) Three months colic. *Archives of Disease in Childhood*, 29, 165–174.

Illingworth, R.S. and Lister, J. (1964) The critical or sensitive period with special reference to certain feeding problems in infants and children. *Journal of Pediatrics*, 65, 839–848.

Jakobsson, I. and Lindberg, T. (1983) Cow's milk proteins cause infantile colic in breastfed infants: a double-blind crossover study. *Pediatrics*, 71, 268–271.

Kanner, L. (1972) *Child Psychiatry*, 4th edn. Springfield, Ill.: Charles C. Thomas.

Keane, V., Charney, E., Strauss, J. and Roberts, K. (1988) Do solids help baby sleep through the night? *American Journal of Diseases of Children*, 142, 404–405.

Kedesdy, J.H. and Budd, K.S. (1998) *Childhood feeding disorders: biobehavioural assessment and intervention*. Baltimore: Paul H. Brookes Publishing Co., Inc.

Knights, J.K. (1985) Processing and evaluation of the antigenicity of protein hydrolysates. In P. Lifshitz (ed.) *Nutrition for Special Needs in Infancy: Protein Hydrolysates*. New York: Marcel Dekker, 105–115.

Lawrence, R.A. (1989) *Breast Feeding: A Guide for the Medical Profession*. St Louis, Miss.: Mosby.

Lawrence, R. (1995) The clinician's role in teaching proper infant feeding techniques. *Journal of Pediatrics*, 126, S113–S117.

Lebenthal, E. (1985) Impact of digestion and absorption in the weaning period on infant feeding practices. *Pediatrics*, 75, 207–213.

Lewis, J.A. (1982) Oral motor assessment and treatment of feeding difficulties. In P. Accardo (ed.) *Failure to Thrive in Infancy and Early Childhood: A Multidisciplinary Team Approach*. Baltimore: University Park Press, 265–295.

Lindberg, L. (1994) *Early Feeding Problems: A Developmental Perspective*. Uppsala: Acta Universitatis Upsaliensis.

Lipsitt, L.P., Crook, C. and Booth, C.A. (1985) The transitional infant: behavioral development and feeding. *American Journal of Clinical Nutrition*, 41, 485–496.

Llewellyn-Jones, D. (1983) *Breastfeeding – How to Succeed*. London: Faber and Faber, 319–335.

Lothe, L., Lindberg, T. and Jakobsson, I. (1982) Cow's milk formula as a cause of infantile colic: a double-blind study. *Pediatrics*, 70, 7–10.

Lucas, A. and St James-Roberts, I. (1998) Crying, fussing and colic behaviour in breast- and bottle-fed infants. *Early Human Development*, 53, 9–18.

Macknin, M.L., Medendorp, S.V. and Maier, M.C. (1989) Infant sleep and bedtime cereal. *American Journal of Diseases of Children*, 143, 1066–1068.

Marchi, M. and Cohen, P. (1990) Early childhood eating behaviours and adolescent eating disorders. *Journal of the American Academy of Child and Adolescent Psychiatry*, 29, 112–117.

Martin, P.B., Surendrar-Kumar, D. and Sandhu, B.K. (1992) Oesophageal pH, barium studies and clinical symptoms in children. Proceedings of British Paediatric Association meeting. Warwick.

Mathisen, B., Skuse, D., Wolke, D. and Reilly, S. (1989) Oral-motor dysfunction and failure to thrive among inner-city infants. *Developmental Medicine and Child Neurology*, 31, 293–302.

Mayes, S.D., Humphrey, F.J., Handford, H.A. and Mitchell, J.F. (1988) Rumination disorder: differential diagnosis. *Journal of the American Academy of Child and Adolescent Psychiatry*, 27, 300–302.

Mennella, J.A. and Beauchamp, G.K. (1998) The early development of human flavour preferences. In E.D. Capaldi (ed.) *Why We Eat What We Eat: The Psychology of Eating*. Washington, DC: APA, 83–112.

Millard, C.L. and Graham, M.A. (1985) Breastfeeding in two Mexican villages: social and demographic perspectives. In V. Hull and M. Simpson (eds) *Breastfeeding, Child Health and Child Spacing: Cross Cultural Perspectives*. London: Croom Helm, pp. 55–77.

Miller, A.J. (1999) *The Neuroscientific Principles of Swallowing and Dysphagia*. San Diego and London: Singular Publishing Group Inc.

Palmer, S., Thompson, R.J. and Linscheid, T.R. (1975) Applied behavior analysis in treatment of childhood feeding problems. *Developmental Medicine and Child Neurology*, 17, 333–339.

Paton, J.Y., Nanayakkhara, C.S. and Simpson, H. (1988) Vomiting and gastro-oesophageal reflux. *Archives of Disease in Childhood*, 63, 837–856.

Patton, R.G. and Gardner, L. (1963) *Growth Failure in Maternal Deprivation.* Springfield, Ill.: Charles C. Thomas.

Ramsey, M., Gisel, E. and Boutry, M. (1993) Non-organic failure to thrive: growth failure secondary to feeding skills disorder. *Developmental Medicine and Child Neurology*, 35, 285–297.

Reilly, S., Skuse, D., Mathisen, B. and Wolke, D. (1995) The objective rating of oral motor functions during feeding. *Dysphagia*, 10, 177–191.

Reilly, S., Skuse, D., Wolke, D. and Stevenson, J. (1999) Oral motor dysfunction in children who fail to thrive: organic or non-organic? *Developmental Medicine and Child Neurology*, 41, 115–122.

Robinschon, P. (1971) Pica practice and other hand–mouth behaviour and children's developmental level. *Nursing Research*, 20, 4–16.

Rogers, B., Stratton, P., Victor, J., Kennedy, B. and Andres, M. (1992) Chronic regurgitation among persons with mental retardation: a need for combined medical and interdisciplinary strategies. *American Journal of Mental Retardation*, 96, 522–527.

Rovee-Collier, C. (1987). Learning and memory in infancy. In J.D. Osofsky (ed.) *Handbook of Infant Development.* New York: Wiley, 98–148.

Sampson, H.A. (1989) Infantile colic and food allergy: fact or fiction? *Journal of Pediatrics*, 115, 583–584.

Selley, W. and Boxall, J. (1986) A new way to treat sucking and swallowing difficulties in babies. *Lancet*, i, 1182–1184.

Sheppard, J.J. and Mysak, E.D. (1984) Ontogeny of infantile oral reflexes and emerging chewing. *Child Development*, 55, 831–843.

Singh, N.N. (1981) Rumination. In N.F. Ellis (ed.) *International Review of Research in Mental Retardation.* New York: Academic Press, 139–182.

Skuse, D. (1994) Non-organic failure to thrive: a reappraisal. *Archives of Disease in Childhood*, 60(2), 173–178.

Skuse, D., Pickles, A., Wolke, D. and Reilly, S. (1985) Postnatal growth and mental development: evidence for a sensitive period. *Journal of Child Psychology and Psychiatry and Allied Disciplines*, 35(3), 521–545.

Spitz, L., Roth, K., Kiely, E.M., Brereton, R.J., Drake, D.P. and Milla, P.J. (1993) Operation for gastro-oesophageal reflux associated with severe mental retardation. *Archives of Disease in Childhood*, 68, 347–351.

Stahlberg, M. (1984) Infantile colic: occurrence and risk factors. *European Journal of Paediatrics*, 143, 108–111.

Stevenson, R.D. and Allaire, J.H. (1991) The development of normal feeding and swallowing. *Paediatric Clinics of North America*, 38, 1439–1452.

Sullivan, S.A. and Birch, L.L. (1994) Infant dietary experience and acceptance of solid foods. *Pediatrics*, 93, 271–277.

Sullivan, P.B. and Brueton, M.J. (1991) Vomiting in infants and children. *Current Pediatrics*, 1, 13–16.

Taitz, L.S. (1974) Overfeeding in infancy. *Proceedings of the Nutrition Society*, 33, 113–118.

Tuchman, D.N. (1988) Dysfunctional swallowing in the paediatric patient: clinical considerations. *Dysphagia*, 2, 203–208.

Vuorenskoski, V., Warz-Hockert, O., Kolvisto, E. and Lind, J. (1969) The effect of cry stimulus on the temperature of the lactating breast of primiparae: a thermographic study. *Experientia*, 25, 1286.

Walloo, M.P., Petersen, S.A. and Whitaker, H. (1990) Disturbed nights and 3–4 month old infants: the effects of feeding and thermal environment. *Archives of Disease in Childhood*, 65, 499–501.

Werlin, S.L., Dodds, W.J., Hogan, W.J. and Arndorfer, R.C. (1980) Mechanisms of gastrooesophageal reflux in children. *Journal of Pediatrics*, 97, 244–249.

Wessel, M.A., Cobb, J.C., Jackson, E.B., Harris, G.S. and Detwiler, A.C. (1954) Paroxysmal fussing in infancy, sometimes called 'colic'. *Pediatrics*, 14, 421–434.

Whitehead, R.G. (1985) Infant physiology, nutritional requirements and lactational adequacy. *American Journal of Clinical Nutrition*, 41, 447–458.

Whitehead, R.G. and Paul, A.A. (1981) Infant growth and human milk requirements: a fresh approach. *Lancet*, ii, 161–163.

Whitehead, R.G., Paul, A.A. and Ahmed, E.A. (1986) Weaning practices in the UK and variance in anthropometric development. *Acta Paediatrica Scandinavica*, 323, 14–23.

Widdowson, E.M. (1973) Changes in pigs due to undernutrition before birth and for one, two and three years afterwards and the effects of rehabilitation. In A.F. Roche and F. Falkner (eds) *Nutrition and Malnutrition* New York: Plenum Press, 165–181.

Widdowson, E.M. (1985) Responses to deficits of dietary energy. In K. Blaxter and J.C. Waterlow (eds) *Nutritional Adaptation in Man*. London: Libby, 97–104.

Winton, A.S.W. and Singh, N.N. (1983) Rumination in paediatric populations: a behavioural analysis. *Journal of the American Academy of Child Psychiatry*, 22, 269–275.

Wolf, L.S. and Glass, R.P. (1992) *Feeding and Swallowing Disorders in Infancy: Assessment and Management*. Tuscon, Ariz.: Therapy Skill Builders.

Wolke, D. (1993) The treatment of problem crying behaviour. In I. St James-Roberts, G. Harris and D. Messer (eds) *Infant Crying, Feeding and Sleeping: Development, Problems and Treatments*. Hemel Hempstead: Harvester-Wheatsheaf, 47–79.

Wolke, D. (1994) Feeding and sleeping across the lifespan. In M. Rutter and D. Hay (eds) *Development Through Life: A Handbook for Clinicians*. Oxford: Blackwell Scientific Publications, 517–557.

Wolke, D. (1996) Probleme bei Neugeborenen und Kleinkindern. In J. Margraf (ed.) *Lehrbuch der Verhaltenstherapie*. Heidelberg: Springer, 363–380.

Wolke, D. and Meyer, R. (1995) The colic debate. *Pediatrics*, 96, 165–166.

Wolke, D. and Meyer, R. (1998) Excessive infant crying and later behaviour problems: findings of the Bavarian Longitudinal Study (BLS), Abstracts of papers presented at the Eleventh International Conference on Infant Studies, Atlanta, Georgia. *Infant Behavior and Development*, 21 (Special ICIS Issue), 114.

Wolke, D., Gray, P. and Meyer, R. (1994) Excessive infant crying: a controlled study of mothers helping mothers. *Pediatrics*, 94, 322–332.

Wolke, D., Meyer, R., Ohrt, B. and Riegel, K. (1995a) Co-morbidity of crying and feeding problems with sleeping problems in infancy: concurrent and predictive associations. *Early Development and Parenting*, 4, 191–207.

Wolke, D., Meyer, R., Ohrt, B. and Riegel, K. (1995b) The incidence of sleeping problems in preterm and fullterm infants discharged from neonatal special care units: an epidemiological longitudinal study. *Journal of Child Psychology and Psychiatry*, 36, 203–223.

Wolke, D., Söhne, B., Riegel, K., Ohrt, B. and Österlund, K. (1998) An epidemiological study of sleeping problems and feeding experience of preterm and fullterm children in South Finland: comparison to a south German population sample. *Journal of Pediatrics*, 133, 224–231.

Wright, P. (1981) Development of feeding behaviour in early infancy: implications for obesity. *Health Bulletin*, 39, 197–206.

Wright, P., McLeod, H.A. and Cooper, M.J. (1983) Waking at night: the effect of early feeding experience. *Child: Care, Health, and Development*, 9, 309–319.

Chapter 2

The management of infant feeding problems

Dieter Wolke, David Skuse and Sheena Reilly

Introduction

One of the major concerns of parents, from the time of their infant's birth onwards, is how to provide adequate nutrition and feed the child correctly. Those who have not previously experienced child-rearing often feel the need for professional guidance. This need for information is reflected in the fact that articles on feeding frequently form a major proportion of the content of popular magazines on parenting (Young, 1990). Furthermore, there are numerous books on 'good parenting'. Views on how best to feed infants changed dramatically during the last century (Truby-King, 1913; Spock, 1968; Leach, 1986). Unfortunately, most of the advice given to parents and professionals was, until recently, based more on beliefs and fashions than on empirical evidence (Young, 1990). In the past few years a re-awakening of interest in the feeding and nutrition of infants has provided a better understanding of feeding practices and nutritional requirements to promote normal growth and development (DHSS, 1988; McDade and Worthman, 1998; Wolke, 1994). Nevertheless, many gaps in knowledge remain and, in particular, there has been little empirical evaluation of the best way of managing feeding and eating problems (Bax, 1989; Ottenbacher *et al.*, 1983).

The biological and psychological function of feeding

Although the primary aim of feeding is to ingest sufficient nutrition to ensure survival, there are important psychological aspects to the feeding process, and these possess certain characteristics in infancy. They serve the functions both of enabling young children to eat and enjoy eating the food provided by their caregivers, and also of facilitating a reciprocal dyadic relationship from which both infants and their caregivers can derive satisfaction and pleasure (Birch and Fisher, 1996; Galef, 1996). Provided the feeding relationship is working well, the infant is delighted that his hunger is satiated, and his mother derives satisfaction from the fact that she has been able to meet the biological demands of her infant. Accordingly, infants learn both that they can rely on and trust their mothers to satisfy them, and that they can please their mothers by eating.

In the early weeks of life, infants spend between one-third and a half of the time they are awake feeding. Only a small proportion of the remainder is spent in social contacts (St James-Roberts and Wolke, 1984; Bunton *et al.*, 1987). The feeding situation thus represents a major opportunity for the parent and child to interact. Feeding interaction has frequently been observed in the course of research on child development, and the significance of the social interchanges between mother and infant during feeds for the later attachment of the mother–child relationship has been well documented (Ainsworth *et al.*, 1972).

Prevention is better than cure

Approximate milestones for the development of different oral skills, the introduction of different textures and types of food, and the development of feeding-related adaptive and social skills are shown in Table 2.1.

I to 3 months: breast- or bottlefeeding

Breastfeeding has been promoted in the professional health literature (DHSS, 1980) and popular literature (Young, 1990) for the last three decades. Breast milk has been reported as having distinct advantages over proprietary cow's milk preparations because of its nutritional value and factors that protect against disease, including immunoglobulin A and G and anti-infective agents (DHSS, 1988; Taitz and Wardley, 1989). Indeed, a British Department of Health publication states that, 'There is no better nutrition for healthy infants both at term and during the early months of life . . . and [breastfeeding] should be encouraged' (DHSS, 1988). It has also been suggested that breast-feeding helps to consolidate the mother–infant relationship, but, in contrast to the evidence which has been provided for the health benefits of breastfeed-ing (Welsh and May, 1979), there is little empirical support for the latter idea (Fergusson *et al.*, 1987). Earlier research on this subject was flawed because it failed to take into account social and other variables that were confounded with breastfeeding (Taylor and Wadsworth, 1984). The good outcome for breastfed babies could not therefore be attributed simply to the breastfeeding *per se*.

Breastfeeding is cheaper than artificial feeding in that it requires no special equipment. It is also convenient because no bottles need to be prepared. Its ready access makes the mother potentially more mobile. Unfortunately, these factors have little influence on the mother's choice of feeding. Women in lower-income families are more likely to bottlefeed (Martin and White, 1988; Grossman *et al.*, 1990). This is because they perceive a number of disadvan-tages with breastfeeding. Pain, including uterine contractions in the first few

Table 2.1 Developmental sequence of oral-motor and self-feeding skills and common feeding difficulties

Approximate age	Food types/textures	Oral skills	Adaptive/social skills	Positioning	Difficulties
0–12 weeks	Liquid breast- or bottlefeeding	Reflexes: Rooting lip closure/ opening lateral tongue movements; mouth opening; biting; babkin; gag reflex Functional: Rhythmic; sucking or sucking swallow pattern (burst–pause pattern);? nutritive (1 suck/swallow) vs non-nutritive (2 sucks/ swallows – comforting); loses some liquid during sucking or corner of mouth – rarely drools (minimal saliva production)	Begins hand to mouth; increasing control of behavioural state and alertness; responsiveness, smile; day and night rhythm shift starts	Supine with the head slightly elevated; or prone; or at an angle of less than 45 degrees or side-lying (e.g. next to caretaker)	Nipple problems; too little milk (perceived), poor suck, spitting up
12–20 weeks	May begin cereals or strained (soft)/ puréed foods (semi-solids)	Reflexes: As above Functional: Suckling/suck pattern as	Begins mouthing objects; begins reaching purposefully; begins anticipatory mouth opening for nipple;	Semi-solids fed in a supported semi-sitting position reclining at an angle of 45 to 90 degrees	Not interested, choking, refusal, spits out lumps

(continued overleaf)

Table 2.1 (Continued)

Approximate age	Food types/textures	Oral skills	Adaptive/social skills	Positioning	Difficulties
		food approaches or touches lips; upper lip does not assist food removal – primitive suckle/swallow response – intermittent gagging or choking occurs; pre-chewing movements present (i.e. moving bolus from lateral to centre, brief rhythmic, symmetrical, bilateral depressions – solids then ejected): decrease in loss of milk from corners of mouth; increase in strength of sucking	prolonged alertness and face to face play (primary) intersubjectivity – self/other distinction; conditioned reactions (e.g. happiness)		
20–28 weeks (6 months)	Strained/puréed foods: mashed in cracker/rusks; teething biscuits introduced	Reflexes: As above – generally more subtle involving fewer movements Functional: Chewing pattern with lip closure ('munching'); starts swallowing higher	Recognises spoon, opens and positions mouth for spoon insertion; transfers objects; drops objects; readiness to hold digestive biscuits etc.; consolidation self/other distinction	Approximating 90 degrees sitting position, external support (side, back, e.g. pillow) in high chair/baby chair	Excessive drooling, refusal

Age	Foods	Oral-motor/reflexes	Feeding/social skills	Positioning	Problems/behaviour
28–32 weeks (7 months)	Junior foods: mashed, cooked, canned; introduction of liquids from cup	textured foods, jaw more stabilised; moves lips in eating Reflexes: Very subtle – ? rooting, babkin disappearing Functional: Centring, processing and swallowing get established; lips remove food from spoon (upper lip)	Begins finger feeding; holding two objects and bangs together	90 degrees sitting position – some lateral support needed	Asserts himself; may want to finger feed (see above)
8–10 months	Junior mashed foods, minced fine table food, finger foods (crackers)	Closes mouth on cup rim; bites on objects; holds crackers between gums and breaks off (?phasic bite pattern – munching); still problems: suck/swallow/breathe when drinking from cup; moves food with tongue; food from centre to side mount – blows 'raspberries'	Finger feeds crackers/rusks; accepts one sip at a time from cup; holds a bottle; emerging specific emotions expressed (separation anxiety, love, attachment); secondary intersubjectivity (understands others' motivations and 'willingly' coordinates or obstructs)	Sitting infant/high chair; no additional side support	Refuses lumps, behaviour problems

(continued overleaf)

Table 2.1 (Continued)

Approximate age	Food types/textures	Oral skills	Adaptive/social skills	Positioning	Difficulties
10–12 months	Mashed to coarsely chopped table foods; finely chopped meats/dried fruits	Controlled sustained bite on biscuit, uses an intermittently elevated tongue when swallowing; no/little loss of food during swallowing – moves tongue from side to side; licks food from lower lip; rotary chewing beginning; when drinking from cup, swallowing follows sucking with no pause – some choking may occur if too fast flowing liquid from cup	Finger feeds small pieces, begins to grasp spoon and stir and lift food with spoon; accepts 4–5 continuous sips; strives for autonomy and control; picks up small objects; starts coordinated placing of objects on table	Sitting in high/infant chair	Refuses lumps; tantrums; wants to self-feed; very messy
12–18 months	Coarsely chopped foods, raw fruits and vegetables	Rotary chewing; licks all of lower lip with tongue; little loss of food or saliva during chewing; decreased drooling; spits foods	Grasps spoon; attempts to take to mouth (starts messy self-feeding); drinks from beaker independently and cup with assistance; decrease in mouthing objects; scribbles with crayon; emerging words and basic comprehension of commands; starting to drink from straw;	Infant/high chair; clip-on chair on table; seating on infant table in chair with side and back rest; feet reaching floor	Faddiness; power struggles

18–24 months	Regular table foods; some chopped fine meats	Mature rotary chewing; controlled sustained biting (grades jaw opening to bite foods of different thickness)	development of guilt, embarrassment; consolidation of attachment and at same time increasing struggle for autonomy	Self-feeding (still messy); drinks from cup and places on table; weaning off bottle completely; unscrews lids; turns pages in book; sustained attention	Infant chair/own table/booster seat (i.e. with the adults at table)	As above; wants to use knife and fork

days and nipple pains over the first few weeks of feeding, is common (Drewett *et al.*, 1987a; DHSS, 1988). A substantial number of mothers experience sore and cracked nipples or difficulty getting their infant to 'latch on'. Some women experience engorged and painful breasts; others have backpain, often due to difficulty in finding a comfortable position for feeding. In addition, breastfed babies are less likely than bottlefed babies to sleep through the night in the first half of the first year: bottlefed infants sleep through the night earlier and more consistently (Eaton-Evans and Dugdale, 1988; Wolke *et al.*, 1998; Elias *et al.*, 1986; Walloo *et al.*, 1990; Wright *et al.*, 1983) and cry less (Barr *et al.*, 1989).

Infant feeding problems in the early days after birth may include posseting after feeds and behavioural difficulties such as drowsiness (which is usually idiopathic but may be due to neonatal jaundice). Feeds can be disrupted by crying and irritability. A weak suckle is not uncommon, but disorganised suckling patterns are rare and warrant a thorough neurological investigation. Many breastfeeding mothers are concerned about whether their infant is ingesting sufficient milk and is satisfied. This is the greatest concern for mothers six weeks after hospital discharge (Martin and White, 1988; Wright, 1987a). Overall, about one in three mothers report that they have problems with breastfeeding after they have been discharged from hospital (Martin and White, 1988; Pridham, 1987).

The following general advice for the prevention of breastfeeding problems can be given:

1 No undue pressure should be exerted on women giving birth to breast-feed. Mothers who do not want to breastfeed are likely either to resist from the outset or to give it up soon after discharge from hospital (Martin and White, 1988; Stein *et al.*, 1987). These women should not be made to feel guilty.

2 Breastfeeding should be attempted as soon as possible after birth to help establishment of lactation.

3 Correct positioning on the breast should be demonstrated to the mother. The infant should be assisted to draw both the nipple and areola into her mouth for efficient suckling action. It is essential that women who have not previously breastfed are given advice and support from someone experienced in the necessary techniques.

4 Infants should be fed on demand; that is, intervals between feeds and length of feeds should not be determined by a rigid schedule in the first two months of life. Contrary to popular belief, demand feeding is not a cause of cracked/sore nipples or engorged breasts. Frequent and vigorous sucking, especially in the first days when the infant only receives colostrum, helps the production of the more nutritious breastmilk by leading to the release of oxytocin. This hormone causes contraction of myo-epithelial cells in the milk ducts which propel milk out of the breast.

Also, it provokes the production of prolactin which in turn stimulates the formation and maturation of the milk.

5   No rule should be given that both breasts need to be offered at each feed. The infant should be encouraged to finish suckling from the first breast. The 'two breast feed' which is often recommended (Nelfert and Seacat, 1986; Truswell, 1985) may provoke the 'oversupply syndrome'. That is, an infant changes breasts before having reached the high-calorie hind milk from the first breast. A point may be reached at which the infant is unable to consume sufficient calories at a feed, because the volume of fluid of relatively low caloric density milk exceeds his stomach capacity. Thus, paradoxically, 'overfeeding' may lead to a state of relative 'calorie deprivation' (Lucas *et al.*, 1980; Woolridge and Fisher, 1988).

6   Breastmilk alone should be sufficient for the nutritional needs of most babies in the first three months. Even though the volume of breastmilk reduces during a feed and across the day (Wright, 1987a), the fact that the hind milk is relatively rich in protein and energy compensates for this (Woolridge *et al.*, 1980). Vitamin D and iron supplements, which have been recommended (Fomon *et al.*, 1979), are usually not necessary if the nursing mother is on an appropriate diet (DHSS, 1988; Taitz and Wardley, 1989); nor are complementary formula feeds or semi-solid feeds in most cases. Mothers use subtle behavioural signs and sleep, wake and crying behaviours as indicators of infant satiety (McDade and Worthman, 1998; Wright, 1987a, 1987b). The decision to introduce mixed feeding should take their observations into account: there are no rigid 'age rules' that can be applied in all circumstances (Wilkinson and Davies, 1978).

7   Feeding should take place in a positive and relaxed atmosphere. Stress can interfere with the let-down reflex and lead to distraction of the infant, poor fixation to the breast and irritability. A quiet and only moderately stimulating environment is particularly important for the fragile, poorly organised or preterm infant (Wolke and Eldridge, 1998; Wolke, 1987).

Detailed advice on how to deal with sore or cracked nipples, breast engorgement, mastitis, thrush infection of nipples, maternal medication in relation to breastfeeding and other problems is given in the excellent manual of the Royal College of Midwives (1991).

Ideally, education on breastfeeding should start before the woman becomes pregnant. Maternal preferences for feeding a child are often formed before conception and are rarely altered during pregnancy, antenatal classes or by the birth experience (Martin and White, 1988).

Bottlefeeding

The problems experienced by bottlefeeding mothers are a little different from those of breastfeeding mothers. One in five bottlefed infants is reported to experience feeding difficulties (Martin and White, 1988). These include, most frequently, vomiting, spitting out, and persistent hunger. Forsyth *et al.* (1985) also reported bottlefed infants to have more frequent episodes of diarrhoea or constipation.

To prevent bottlefeeding problems the following steps should be followed:

1   Mothers should be reassured that bottlefeeding is a safe and satisfactory alternative to breastfeeding provided an approved formula is being used.
2   Expectant primiparous mothers should be shown how to make up a bottle. This should be done during antenatal classes and also demonstrated after birth. Infants should be given a quantity of formula that is appropriate for their age and weight. If the artificial milk persistently contains an excessive formula to fluid ratio (i.e. too high a density) the baby may become obese (Taitz, 1971) as a result of resetting the infant's internal sensory mechanisms (Hertherington and Rolls, 1996). On the other hand, over-diluted feeds may lead to the need for excessive volumes to be ingested in order to achieve an adequate caloric intake (McJunkin *et al.*, 1987), potentially a cause of vomiting, malnutrition and failure to thrive (Taltz and Wardley, 1989).
3   Mothers should be educated on the importance of sterilising bottles and teats. Heating in a microwave does not ensure sterility of bottles and, unless allowed to cool sufficiently, before fluid is added, carries the additional risk of causing scalding (DHSS, 1988).
4   Mothers should be discouraged from mixing glucose or rusks with the formula milk and/or enlarging the teat to satisfy an apparently very hungry baby. This is likely to lead to vomiting or diarrhoea.
5   Mothers should be discouraged from prop feeding, i.e. leaving the infant unattended, sucking from a bottle supported by pillows, etc. The importance of positioning the infant in direct bodily contact, in order to foster social interaction, should be emphasised.
6   Feeding should take place in a quiet and relaxed atmosphere. Because bottlefeeding lends itself to feeding in public places, spitting out and other problems may arise because the infant becomes distracted (Wolke and Eldridge, 1998).

3–9 months: the introduction and establishment of solid feeding

While numerous booklets and research papers exist on the subject of early breast- or bottlefeeding, much less work has been done on the introduction of mixed feeding and its attendant problems.

Mixed feeding commences when semi-solids are introduced in addition to milk. The term 'weaning' is rather ambiguous and probably best avoided. It refers sometimes to the introduction of mixed feeding and sometimes to all cessation of breast or bottle feeds. There has been a longstanding controversy about when solid foods should first be introduced, and the practice has changed considerably over the last thirty years with parents generally introducing solids later nowadays than in the 1970s (Martin and White, 1988). Advice for commencing solid feeds is usually based on either weight criteria (e.g. when the infant reaches 5.5 kg; Leach, 1986) or age criteria: for example, Spock (1968) and Leach (1986) advise beginning solid feeding at around 3 months, Fomon *et al.* (1979) suggest 5–6 months, while the often quoted paper by Illingworth and Lister (1964) recommends 6–7 months, the time of 'onset' of chewing, as a good time for introducing solids.

Research has indicated that the timing of the introduction of mixed feeding is dependent on a range of factors including maternal education, age, social class, whether the infant is bottle- or breastfed, and whether it is a boy or a girl (Hitchcock *et al.*, 1986; Underwood and Hofvander, 1982; Martin and White, 1988, Whitehead *et al.*, 1986). Furthermore, infants' growth and behaviour patterns are also important influences upon parents' decisions to introduce semi-solids. Relevant behavioural cues include demands for more frequent feeding, crying after a meal and nightwaking; these are often interpreted as signs that the infant is not satisfied with milk only and is hungry (Harris, 1988, 1993; Wilkinson and Davies, 1978; Wright, 1987a, 1993). The influence of early or late introduction of mixed feeding upon appetite development, food preferences (Harris and Booth, 1987) and feeding and growth problems (Underwood and Hofvander, 1982; Illingworth and Lister, 1964) has not been sufficiently studied in healthy infants in affluent societies. Furthermore, little information exists about feeding practices in different subcultures (e.g. among ethnic minorities in western societies).

The WHO now recommends exclusive breastfeeding for the first 6 months of life, while recognising that some mothers are unable or unwilling to follow it (Black and Victoria, 2002). The following recommendations regarding the age and time of introduction of solids can be made (McDade and Worthman, 1998):

1   Mixed feeding does not have to commence at the same age or the same weight for all infants, but 6 months of exclusive breastfeeding is desirable.
2   Mixed feeding should not commence before 3 months of age (to avoid problems such as diarrhoea; Rowland, 1986) and not later than 6–8 months of age (to avoid growth faltering and failure to thrive) (Auerbach and Eggert, 1987; Davies, 1979; Roddey *et al.*, 1981; Wolke, 1994; Kessler and Dawson, 1999).
3   There is little danger that complementary solid feeding will lead to obesity as both milk intake and sucking time are consequently reduced in

proportion to the amount of solids consumed (Drewett *et al.*, 1987b). Finney (1986) has provided an excellent account of the advice parents can be given about the introduction of solid foods.

9–24 months: learning mealtime manners and habits

The caregiver's recognition of hunger patterns and of the infant's food preferences will have an important influence on eating and mealtime behaviour and the development of appetite (Capaldi, 1996). The period between 6 and 12 months heralds important biological and behavioural changes with infants developing greater mobility, an understanding of other people's intentions, the onset of stranger anxiety, wariness (Schaffer *et al.*, 1972) and attachment behaviour (Ainsworth *et al.*, 1972). A capacity to 'intentionally' manipulate the environment is also usually acquired within the first year. Oral-motor skills develop, allowing the infant to chew (munch) solids, to feed himself using first the fingers and later feeding utensils (see Table 2.1), and to sit independently in an appropriate chair.

Mealtimes constitute a context in which conflicts between toddlers and their parents are especially likely to occur. They are also a great opportunity to acquire conventionally acceptable behaviour patterns (Birch, 1987). It is perfectly normal and healthy that a child tests limits at such times and challenges the parents. These behaviours are indicators of the infant's developmental progress. The parents' reactions, and their own and the child's flexibility of response, determine whether or not such behaviour will go on to become a problem.

Table 2.2 contains guidelines which can be given to parents to help their infant develop appropriate mealtime behaviour. These recommendations are closely adapted from Finney (1986) and incorporate other resource material (Lowenberg, 1981; Birch, 1987; Capaldi, 1996; Yoos *et al.*, 1999; Kedesdy and Budd, 1998) and principles of general learning theory (Kanfer and Goldstein, 1980).

Caloric requirements and growth

Caloric requirements to sustain adequate growth vary with age. The highest caloric requirements (per kg of child's weight) during childhood are found during the first six months of life when the infant more than doubles his/her birth weight. Table 2.3 provides rough guidelines for caloric requirements and expected weight gain and longitudinal growth during childhood. It is important to point out that these are average figures. Growth patterns and daily requirements vary between children. If there are no growth and health problems and the child eats a variety of foods (balanced diet), then there is generally no need for supplementation with other nutrients such as vitamins or minerals (Wolke, 1994).

Table 2.2 Management of mealtime behaviour (12–24 months)

1 Establish sit-down, family-style meals, where everyone sits down together to eat. Turn off the television.

2 Set a reasonable time limit for each meal (for example, from twenty to thirty minutes).

3 Establish a set of mealtime rules for your child. Some examples are: (1) You must remain seated; (2) You are to use your spoon or fork, not your fingers; (3) Don't throw food; (4) Close your mouth when you chew, etc. The rules should be reasonable, based on the age of your child. Don't expect a young child to learn all the rules quickly. Start with two or three rules. After your child has learned to follow them, add a few more rules at a time, until gradually you have introduced all the rules.

4 Tell your child the rules (using a nice tone of voice) once at the beginning of each meal until the child has learned to follow them consistently. Do not nag your child about the rules.

5 Give your child small portions of preferred foods – an amount you are sure the child will eat. You can always give more. At first, give a small amount which your child must eat to succeed, and then praise your child for eating it. Then gradually increase the quantity you require the child to eat and the types of food you want the child to try. Do not make your child 'clean the plate'.

6 Do not carry on conversations with another adult for longer than a few minutes at a time. Include your child in conversations and talk about things that you know interest your child. Make sure you do not nag, threaten, or warn during mealtimes. Use mealtimes as an opportunity to praise your child for appropriate behaviours throughout the day and to teach your child how to behave in a social situation.

7 Be sure to praise your child for appropriate behaviours (such as using utensils, sitting quietly, talking nicely) whenever they occur throughout the meal. You cannot praise too often. Praise is how you teach your child what behaviour pleases you.

8 If your child breaks a rule, have the child practise the correct behaviour. The third time your child breaks any rule, use discipline. 'Time-out' is one good way to teach your child the rules at meals. Put the child in time-out for misbehaviours as many times as necessary until the time limit for the meal is up.

9 When the time for the meal is up, clear the table, regardless of whether your child has finished. Do not say anything to your child beyond announcing that the meal is over.

10 If your child did not finish the last meal, do not offer dessert and do not allow your child to eat or drink anything except water until the next meal. If your child whines and constantly asks for snacks, place the child in time-out.

11 Even under normal circumstances, limit snacks. If you allow your child to fill up on snacks, the child will not be hungry at mealtimes. Give snacks that have nutritional value (such as carrot sticks, raisins, fruit) rather than 'junk' food. You will also be teaching your child good eating habits.

12 When your child has learned to follow your mealtime rules consistently, you no longer need to go over them at the beginning of each meal. However, it is still a good idea to review the rules from time to time. The best way to do this is to 'catch 'em being good': remind your child of a rule by praising the child for following it.

Table 2.3 Caloric requirements and growth

Age	Average caloric requirements (kcal/kg/day)[a]	Average protein requirements (grams/kg/day)[a]	Median daily weight gain (grams)	Median height gain (cm/month)
Birth to 3 months	108	2.2	24–30	3.4
3–6 months	108	2.2	20	2.2
6–9 months	98	1.6	14–15	1.5
9–12 months	98	1.6	11	1.3
1–3 years	102	1.2	6	0.9
3–6 years	90	1.1	5	0.5
6–10 years	70	1.0	7–8[b]	0.5

Source: Needleman, Adair and Bresnahan, 1998.

Notes
[a] Source: National Academy of Sciences, National Research Council, Food and Nutrition Board, 1989.
[b] Data elevated by inclusion of pubertal growth spurts in some children.

Treatment of feeding problems

Common problems of orally fed infants

The most frequent feeding problems reported in community surveys are faddy or 'picky' styles of eating (Richman *et al.*, 1982). Behaviour patterns that lead to referral for professional advice and which are of particular concern include refusal to eat, extreme faddiness and related behaviour problems (i.e. not sitting at mealtimes etc.), rumination and failure to thrive (Richman, 1988; Woolston, 1983; Skuse *et al.*, 1994b; Wolke, 1994).

A four-step treatment approach

The treatment of feeding problems in our approach follows four steps (see Wolke, 1996a, 1999):

1 *Observe* (learn about the child and family).
2 *Formulate hypotheses* about the factors that maintain inadequate feeding behaviour and discuss these with the parents, often using video-feedback.
3 *Design a problem hierarchy and specific intervention measures* (the goals should be clearly defined and the changes in the feeding situation clearly stated, with the parents using explorations of their own behaviour).
4 *Follow-up* the families to receive feedback about success and failure.

Initial assessment

Decisions on the extent of diagnostic assessment and treatment required should be based on two key factors:

1   Is there any growth failure in the infant?
2   Does the infant appear neglected or abused, or is he at risk for future abuse?

A medical screening, an interview with the caretaker about the problem and, importantly, the observation of a feed usually suffice for diagnostic purposes when there is no growth failure and the risk of abuse is low. The treatment may consist of a short series of consultations about behaviour management (Roberts, 1986; Kedesdy and Budd, 1998) and advice along the lines of the suggestions made in Table 2.3. In contrast, if the problem produces exceptional strains for the family (and may lead to an increased risk of abuse), or when a restricted food intake compromises the growth or development of the infant, comprehensive medical and psychological–behavioural evaluations are needed (Wolke, 1994; Kessler and Dawson, 1999). The assessments aim to establish the aetiology of somatic symptoms (e.g. oesophageal reflux and neurological problems), behavioural problems (parents' feeding technique, infant's temper tantrums), and nutritional problems (inadequate restricted diets, prolonged breastfeeding). Environmental and family characteristics (social or housing problems, family stresses, level of social support) may also contribute to the feeding problem.

A comprehensive diagnostic and treatment system has been developed in our clinic, based on several years of research with failure to thrive infants (Heptinstall *et al.*, 1987; Mathisen *et al.*, 1989; Wolke *et al.*, 1990a; Skuse *et al.*, 1992, 1994a, 1994b; Reilly *et al.*, Chapter 1 in this book; Wolke, 1994). This system is outlined below.

Assessments are carried out by a mixture of interviews and direct observation techniques. The aim is to gain a comprehensive picture of the child's characteristics, the caretakers' characteristics and the mother–infant joint behaviour. Full dietary histories and family assessments are obtained if regarded as essential to diagnosis or treatment (e.g. the child is failing to thrive or the family presents with social difficulties or family discord). A rough guide to caloric requirements and growth is shown in Table 2.3.

The team

A team approach to the diagnosis and management of problems is essential. The core team consists of a child psychiatrist/paediatrician, a developmental/paediatric psychologist and a speech/dysphagia therapist. Additional consultations are provided by a senior dietician and advice is available from a variety of specialists ranging from social workers to a paediatric gastroenterologist. Before any therapy is attempted a structured assessment of the problem and of the precipitating and maintaining factors is carried out. Once assessments are completed, the team meets to formulate a management plan.

Child characteristics

All infants receive a standard pediatric and neurological assessment as outlined by Berkowitz (1985) and Frank and Zeisel (1988). A full perinatal and medical history is obtained, with specific enquiry about frequent infections, eczema, rashes, asthma, and other allergic reactions (Rider and Bithoney, 1999). It is often a wise precaution to determine whether there is any degree of iron deficiency by obtaining a full blood count and serum ferritin (Schwartz *et al.*, 1986). The physical and neurological examination, in conjunction with the history taking, should identify most chronic diseases. Chronic illnesses and growth disturbances are usually closely interlinked (Goldson, 1999). Certain physical or medical disabilities provide barriers to adequate nutrition because of structural problems (e.g. cleft palate, micrognathy), oral-motor dysfunction (e.g. cerebral palsy) or mechanical difficulties (e.g. tonsillar-adenoidal hypertrophy). Other chronic disorders may compromise the infant's nutritional state because of malabsorption (e.g. coeliac disease, cystic fibrosis) or problems in retaining food (e.g. gastro-oesophageal reflux). Infants who have a history of vomiting, rumination or repeated diarrhoea are also seen by a pediatric gastroenterologist (Krebs, 1999).

Chronic illnesses may contribute to growth failure because the process of feeding itself is exhausting and physiologically taxing for the infant (Reilly *et al.*, Chapter 1 in this book). Insufficient calories are ingested to provide for both physical activity and growth, as for example in those suffering cardio-respiratory disease. A feeding problem may be the first indication of such a disorder. However, it needs to be emphasised that impaired growth and nutrition in chronically ill infants and those who were preterm may also reflect behavioural, psychosocial and nutritional difficulties (Bauchner *et al.*, 1988).

Laboratory assessments should be kept to a minimum because of the stress they may cause to the infant, their cost and the negligible contribution they make to the diagnosis in most cases (Berwick *et al.*, 1982). Stool examinations and cultures may be useful in infants with a history of diarrhea or malodorous stools (e.g. giardiasis) (Gupta and Urrutia, 1982). Tests for HIV antibodies should be considered when the mother is an intravenous drug user or the partner of an intravenous drug user or bisexual man, or when the mother has a history of receiving blood transfusions (Frank and Zeisel, 1988).

Full anthropometric assessments including weight, height, head circumference and skinfold thickness are carried out routinely.

All infants have a developmental assessment consisting of the administration of the Bayley Scales of Infant Development (Bayley, 1993). This is helpful in determining whether interaction patterns and oral-motor functioning are appropriate for the child's developmental age. A standard procedure for evaluating oral-motor functioning, the Schedule for Oral Motor Assessment (SOMA), is administered (Reilly et al., 1995; Mathisen et al., 1989). The infant is presented with different types and textures of foods, and oral-motor behaviour is video-recorded in close-up. The assessment also includes an examination for oral hypersensitivity to touch, and for any structural problems in the intra-oral area, such as a high arched palate, in which food may become impacted (Reilly et al., 1995).

The behaviour of the infant during the Bayley Scales administration and the SOMA procedure is rated using the Tester's Rating of Infant Behaviour (Wolke et al., 1990a). These ratings provide information on how the infant behaves with a stranger and whether behaviour problems are specific to the feeding situation or generalise across situations (i.e. are pervasive).

Caretaker characteristics

No special psychological assessments are carried out, unless the interview with the mother regarding the feeding problem and its history and observations of her behaviour raise issues that warrant further investigation. Mothers are interviewed regarding their attributions about, and perceptions of, their child's behaviour. They are asked about their own childhood and family history. A formal psychological and psychiatric assessment is usually not undertaken, to avoid the implication of 'blame' for the problem (Skuse, 1985).

Some mothers do, however, require a psychiatric screening to determine their emotional state (e.g. depression). Also, if the preliminary interview has led to suspicions of unconventional eating habits these are enquired about in more detail; in such cases it may be enlightening to ask about preferences regarding their own and the infant's body shape (e.g. slim, chubby). In 1994, Wolke reported that mothers of failure to thrive infants, in particular those who are overweight, prefer leaner infants. A mother's own eating problems may contribute to the way she feeds her infant (Stein, et al., 1994). Her behaviour towards her infant during the interviews is assessed using the HOME-R (Caldwell and Bradley, 1984).

Caretaker–infant interaction

The caretaker–infant interaction during a main meal is filmed in the family's home. Our experience indicates the importance of obtaining this information in its natural setting (Werle et al., 1998). During observations made at a clinic, appropriate feeding utensils such as a high chair and appropriate food are often provided (Kedesdy and Budd, 1998). Our research has shown that, in a substantial number of cases, the organisation of the feeding environment at home is quite different (Reilly et al., Chapter 1 in this book).

To learn whether possible problems in the interaction are confined to the feeding situation, mother–child interactions are also observed during a structured play situation (see Lindberg *et al.*, 1996). Both feeding and play behaviour are analysed, using standardised coding instruments, i.e. the Feeding Interaction Scale (FIS; Wolke, 1986a) and the Play Observation Scheme and Emotion Rating (POSER; Wolke, 1986b; Wolke *et al.*, 1990a). The Nursing Child Assessment Teaching Scale (NCATS; Barnard, 1978) is used for infants of less than 9 months of age. These scales not only record the mother's and infant's social behaviour but also how food is transferred to the infant and whether it is accepted or rejected.

Family growth patterns

The height and weight of both the parents and the index child's siblings are determined. Berkowitz (1985) reported that 15 per cent of parents of infants seen in her feeding clinic have 'constitutional' short stature. We are cautious in drawing the conclusion that infants may be growing poorly because their parents are relatively small. These parents may have suffered growth failure in their own childhoods, because of environmental deprivation.

Feeding history and nutritional intake

A detailed feeding interview is carried out with all caregivers. The interview comprises different sections enquiring about early feeding methods, when and how solids were introduced, how mealtimes are managed, etc. Additional questions ask about the caregiver's perceptions of infant cues for hunger, pacing and termination of mealtimes (Mathisen *et al.*, 1989; Reilly and Skuse, 1992). A detailed twenty-four-hour recall dietary assessment is obtained (Heptinstall *et al.*, 1987), although this information may be unreliable because mothers may be unable to judge how much food was offered to the infant and also how much was actually swallowed (Cunningham and McLaughlin, 1999). If a mealtime has been video-recorded it is possible to make a count of the teaspoons of food offered and consumed. By combining this information, a detailed record of the type and amount of food offered and lost can be made (e.g. drooling, spitting out, throwing, etc.). From such analysis it can be demonstrated that infants who are growing poorly actually consume significantly less energy than appears to be the case from the dietary recall or behavioural observation of the interaction.

A behavioural feeding intervention approach

Psychodynamic, family therapy and behavioural interventions have all been suggested as ways to treat infant feeding problems. However, the range of associated disorders usually justifies an eclectic approach. We propose an

approach that is primarily behavioural, but which incorporates other therapeutic strategies where necessary. The focus of the intervention is primarily
the feeding situation, but factors outside this setting are also taken into
account.

The initial assessments determine whether a feeding problem or disorder
exists (Wolke, 1994). However, the decision to proceed is not automatic as an
ill-timed or poorly conducted intervention (lacking resources and knowledge)
may itself have adverse iatrogenic effects – for example, make the problem
worse or turn the parents off from seeking any advice in the future. The
decision to proceed should thus rest on answering the following questions
(Kedesdy and Budd, 1998):

1   Is feeding intervention necessary for medical reasons? What will happen
    in the longer term if no intervention is initiated?
2   Are the caregivers receptive to environmental intervention at the present
    time?
3   Are sufficient resources available to support the family and implement
    the intervention with a reasonable chance of success?

If the consequences for the child are severe (e.g. severe undernutrition or risk
of abuse and severe family problems), then an intervention is indicated
independent of questions 2 and 3. However, the success will depend on the
motivation of the parents and the readiness for intervention and the resources
available to carry out the intervention, and this needs to be discussed with the
parents and written into a therapy contract.

Feeding intervention parameters

A checklist of possible problem behaviours and associated contextual features
provides help in pinpointing areas that require modification (see Table 2.4).
Mealtimes may occur at irregular intervals, the child may be fed on the
sofa with the television on, the mother may walk in and out of the room
leaving the infant to self-feed. On the basis of information gathered by interview and observation, modifications are suggested and explained to the
mother to rectify the environmental and social context of meals. Guided by
these feeding intervention parameters, the aim is to establish organised mealtimes that occur at regular times and that are predictable to the infant and
other family members. The infant should be placed in an appropriate seat
with good back and side support. The caretaker should be present during the
mealtimes and should ideally sit facing the infant on the same level (i.e. eye to
eye). The television should be switched off and, ideally, other family members
should be present and eating too, to provide a model of eating behaviour
(Budd *et al.*, 1998; Yoos *et al.*, 1999; Werle *et al.*, 1998; Whitehouse and
Harris, 1998).

Table 2.4 Feeding intervention parameters – a brief checklist of problems and actions

Item	Problem	Action
Mealtime environment		
Lighting	room too dark/too glaring light	lighten/dim room
Noise	room too noisy (e.g. radio, TV)	reduce noise
Distraction	too many distractions – people – pets – toys	reduce distractions
Feeding site	inappropriate place (e.g. bedroom)	appropriate place (e.g. kitchen)
	inconsistent place	consistent places for meals
	child inflexible	alternate places, e.g. restaurants, friends' houses (slow approximation/exposure)
Utensils	inappropriate equipment	provision of equipment appropriate to infant's needs (e.g. for toddler spoon, knife, bib, own bowl, cup, bottle, toothbrush)
Seating	inappropriate – no particular equipment	provide e.g. highchair, low chair, infant table
Positioning		
Symmetry/support of infant in chair	no trunk/head/feet support	stabilise infant in chair
Mother at eye level	mother too high or out of room – no eye-to-eye contact	mother present and appropriate eye level
Proximity of food	food too close to infant or kept out of reach	place close enough to allow food exploration
Mealtime/household organisation		
Mealtime routine	no fixed times for meals	establish a routine
	hunger/appetite poor (e.g. snacking)	increase appetite/hunger (spacing meals)
Cooking	no planning, no menus	plan menu
	no cooking – packet/convenience food only	learn recipes for simple dishes
	plain, boring presentation of food	attractive presentation, colourful
Budgeting	costs of pre-packaged food prohibitive – run out of money	better use of finances available – planning
Nutrition	amount given too little/too large	increase/reduce amount offered
	variety of foods poor	increase variety

Item	Problem	Action
	textures of foods poor/limited	increase variety of textures
	novelty very restricted	new food encouraged
	diet lacking micronutrients	supplement (e.g. iron)
	cult diet/muesli belt	introduce diet supplementation – careful discussions
Infant problems		
Adaptive skills coordination	poor eye–hand	practise eye–hand coordination games
	poor grasp of spoon/fork	practise for better grasp
	no opportunity for finger feeding	allow finger feeding
	poor management of cup drinking	better placement of hands/lips
Oral-motor skills sensitivity	hypersensitivity to touch	reduction of aversion to touch
Oral reflexes	gag reflex persistent	hypersensitive gag
	rooting present	inhibition, etc.
	bite reflex present	non-metallic spoon desensitisation
Spoon feeding	lip closure on spoon poor	facilitate better lip closure
	self-feeding not experienced	opportunity given for use with spoon
Chewing	no-biting skills	encourage biting – toys/food
	no munching	alternate side placement of food/type of food (bite-dissolves) e.g. prawn crackers
	no rotary movement of tongue	model, bolus placement alternate sides of tongue
Drinking	no lip closure on cup	facilitate better closure
	poor sucking	encourage sucking then gradually reduce dummy/bottle, encourage trainer cup usage
Maternal problems		
Emotional status	depressed, mood disorder, etc., low self-concept	appropriate treatment/referral (individual therapy, systemic)
Eating/food	overeating, excessive dieting, bingeing, laxative abuse, etc.	see above – discuss – individual therapy

(continued overleaf)

Table 2.4 (Continued)

Item	Problem	Action
Caretaker's behaviour		
Control	over-controlling, force-feeding	introduce positive reinforcement, control techniques, ignore negative infant behaviour
	under-controlling, *laissez-faire*	introduce concept of limit setting
Stimulation	over-stimulating, hasty, introducing too many foods, talking constantly	reduce stimulation, relax mother
	under-stimulating, uninvolved	encourage appropriate talking or food games
Emotional expression	negative, irritable	teach self-control techniques
Sensitivity	not attuned to infant's cues (including hunger, satiety cues)	learn cue reading (e.g. by video feedback)
Timing	parent feeds too slow/fast	use video feedback slow/speed up feed
Infant behaviour		
Food refusal	refuses most/all food	deconditioning/operant methods (in conjunction with family-centred techniques)
	faddy/picky	expose different tastes, present in conjunction with (mixed) preferred food
	eats no lumps	shaping/slow approximation
General behaviour	overactive	behavioural management (reward scheme)
	tantrums	time-out, extinction
	passive/withdrawn, poor communication	introduce play, increased stimulation (teach mother), increase infant's expressive repertoire through communication games
Joint behaviour		
Harmony	frequent conflict	reduce by clear rule setting, introduce behavioural management techniques for conflict resolution

Behavioural intervention: a home intervention approach

The first treatment visit

The treatment, if time and distance allow it, should be carried out in the family's home. Alternatively, an outpatient approach may be used, where parents are asked to bring in what they need for a mealtime (i.e. the food, feeding utensils) (Schmitt and Mauro, 1989). However, as discussed earlier, in some cases of severe failure to thrive hospitalisation of the infant may be necessary.

During the first treatment visit medical aspects of the previous assessment visits are discussed and explained by the physician – otherwise the parents are assured that no medical problems have been found. Nutritional aspects of the treatment are not discussed at the beginning of the first visit but postponed to the end of the subsequent treatment visit. Raising issues such as incorrect feeding and providing the wrong sort of food often undermines a mother's self-confidence if introduced at too early a stage.

After the general feedback from the diagnostic sessions, the first treatment session starts by filming a main meal. The therapist makes notes during the filming about critical situations (e.g. infant refusing to eat, mother shouting, infant throwing food, etc.) (Sanders et al., 1993). The therapist and caretaker then sit down and watch the video-recording of the mealtime. The setting of the mealtime and the various critical situations are explored in discussion with the mother. For example, for each critical event the mother is asked, after she has watched the episode, whether she remembers the episode and how she felt at the time; how she explains the occurrence of the situation and what she could do to deal with it. This method provides insight into the mother's thinking (Goodnow, 1988) and helps her to reflect on her actions and feelings. Rather than adopting an educational-directive approach, telling the mother how to rectify her behaviour, we use a non-directive approach helping the mother to find solutions herself (Wolke, 1996b, 1999, 2003). This approach avoids the antagonism that might be caused by giving direct advice, and it also provides the mother with a feeling of confidence in her own abilities to find solutions. Using video-material, the situation can be replayed numerous times thus providing visual cues that assist exploration of the feeding interaction. It is successful even in mothers with intellectual abilities below the normal range.

Mother and therapist then together compile a list of those problems, as seen by them on the video-recording, which cause most difficulty for the mother (i.e. a problem hierarchy is established). We then explain that it will take time and considerable effort for all involved to rectify the problem – there is no miracle cure. The therapist subsequently produces an itemised list of the agreed therapeutic goals and sends it to the mother with practical suggestions on how to achieve them. It is often important for the parents to have a written record to remind them of what to do. This written treatment plan also includes nutritional advice.

Subsequent interventions

Subsequent visits start by reviewing the behavioural progress made since the last consultation and any specific problems encountered. At each visit, another mealtime is filmed and reviewed with the mother. New goals are set and those reached are ticked off. After each visit a short written report is given to the mother for feedback purposes stressing the positive aspects of the achievements made.

Many of these discussions, focusing primarily on feeding the infant, lead to reflections on other family relationships, including that with the partner, problems with grandparents, and the mother's own difficulties and eating problems. These broader issues are taken up and a flexible treatment approach is used, which may incorporate elements from cognitive behavioural therapy or family therapy, if indicated (Iwaniec et al., 1985; Hanks et al., 1988).

Some sessions also include basic advice on child care outside the feeding situation, such as the management of crying and sleeping problems (Gray, 1987; Douglas and Richman, 1984; Wolke, 1993, 1996c, 1999). Many of the infants who are referred for treatment come from low-income families (Pollitt et al., 1975). Ways to provide help with housing and financial problems should be explored, and the assistance of a social worker may be necessary. Some education on the family's budgeting, home cooking and healthy eating is often necessary. Advice given is taken from publications such as those from the London Food Commission (1985), Francis (1987) and Taitz and Wardley (1989).

Food preparation is a particular difficulty for mothers who are limited in their intellectual abilities (Sheridan, 1956) and also for recent immigrants with a poor knowledge of English who may buy inappropriate pre-packaged foods that are limited in variety (e.g. egg custard/baby rice), being unaware of their nutritional inadequacy (Frank and Zeisel, 1988; Wolke, 1994). Understanding cultural diversity in diets, variations due to religious beliefs or cults, and obsessions with healthy eating that include an emphasis on high-fibre and low-fat diets, is important. Occasionally such dietary eccentricities may point to the reason for an infant's poor nutritional intake ('Muesli belt syndrome'). In such cases, it is important to introduce the idea of dietary changes and nutritional supplementation without threatening the family's belief systems or religious beliefs. Suggestions on how to do so are described by Taitz and Wardley (1989, pp. 47–56).

Test weighing and nutritional advice

The infant is not usually weighed at each visit. An undue focus on weight gain is counterproductive. Instead, the aim is to work on aspects of behaviour – feeding and eating have to become fun and an enjoyable experience again. Only after this is accomplished and the infant accepts age-appropriate amounts of food can the focus shift to weight gain. The daily caloric needs for catch-up growth in calories per kilogram (Kcal/Kgm) in children who are seriously under-weight for their length are estimated as follows (MacLean *et al.*, 1980):

Kcal/kg = 120 Kcal/kg × median weight for current height (kg)/current weight (kg)

For example, if a male child's length is 75 cm the median (50th centile) weight for length would be 9.8 Kgm. A child whose actual weight is 8.0 Kgm would require (9.8 ÷ 8.0) × 120 Kcal/gm = 147 Kcal/Kgm – i.e. a total intake of 1176 Kcal per twenty-four hours.

According to this calculation, most infants will require 1.5 to 2.0 times the expected intake for their age to achieve optimal catch-up growth (Frank and Zeisel, 1988). Attempting to achieve this intake in an infant who has food refusal problems, faddiness or poor appetite by using either fortified foods, additional tube feeding or force-feeding of the child is likely to be counter-productive. Fortification of feeds is justified in young infants where the mother may have made errors in formula preparation or fed exclusively from the breast for prolonged periods (McJunkin *et al.*, 1987; Roddey *et al.*, 1981; Schmitt and Mauro, 1989). We advise that tube or force-feeding should usually be avoided in non-organic failure to thrive cases, and only be used under exceptional circumstances (Kessler and Dawson, 1999). Nasogastric feeding can interfere with normal oral-motor development. Continuous feeding regimens (e.g. overnight) can compromise the acquisition of hunger and satiety rhythms, eating consequently becoming completely subject to external control (Evans-Morris, 1989). The procedure may thereby inadvertently reinforce the very problem it is intended to alleviate. Furthermore, high volumes administered at 'mealtimes' via nasogastric tubes, with the aim of promoting catch-up growth, may lead to vomiting and diarrhoea in those infants with moderate to severe malnourishment.

Emphasis should be placed on the infant's need for micronutrients. Whenever indicated, a multivitamin supplement containing iron and zinc should be prescribed for children with failure to thrive, during treatment and nutritional rehabilitation. Iron deficiency, with or without associated anaemia, is often seen in failure to thrive infants (Cutts and Geppert, 1999; Taitz and Wardley, 1989) and can be associated with irritability and short attention span (Aukett *et al.*, 1986). Hence, alleviation of the deficiency can facilitate behavioural management.

Basic behavioural intervention techniques

In the following a range of behavioural techniques are briefly introduced. They, by themselves, do not make up the treatment. However, within an individualised treatment approach some of these procedures are often applied to help modify behaviour. Apart from providing an overview of techniques, brief examples of the use of the techniques in feeding situations are given.

Behavioural intervention procedures are a body of techniques that are rooted in learning theory and that can be applied to socially relevant problems to strengthen adaptive behaviours and to reduce maladaptive behaviours. Of particular interest in clinical feeding interventions are: (1) aspects of the feeder's responses that have an inadvertent impact on feeding patterns (e.g. food refusal and only offering limited preferred food); and (2) planned techniques for 'unlearning' or modifying maladaptive feeding patterns (e.g. spitting out food and receiving a lot of attention from parents) by rearranging social and environmental concomitants to feeding (Kedesdy and Budd, 1998). There is a range of adapted techniques that can be used in infants from 6 months of age onwards. An overview of the behaviour intervention strategies and examples of application to the feeding situation are given in Table 2.5 and are briefly described. It is important to point out that the briefly reviewed techniques are usually effective if part of an individualised package of strategies that parents can apply. Some of the individual techniques are also not acceptable to some parents. Other important ingredients of a treatment programme include parental modelling, changes in the physical and social feeding environment (see checklist in Table 2.4), exposure to different tastes and textures and emotional support of the parents.

Operant methods: reinforcement and reinforcement withdrawal

The major techniques used in behavioural interventions are operant or respondent conditioning principles. The frequency of a behaviour is increased by providing reinforcement, and decreased by providing punishment (Karoly, 1980). Positive reinforcement is the delivery of a desired stimulus (e.g. praise, preferred food), contingent on performance of a target behaviour (accepting less preferred food), which strengthens the probability that the target behaviour will occur in future. The preferred positive reinforcer in the feeding situation is social attention. This includes providing attention for desired behaviour such as praise ('good girl', 'well done', clapping for the child, 'you did it all by yourself'). In older toddlers and children specific feedback labelling the specific behaviour is helpful (instead of just 'good boy' indicating 'you ate all your dinner, well done'). Training in positive reinforcement emphasises precise delivery of attention while the child is cooperating, rather than the 'natural' tendency to respond to the child's inappropriate or disruptive behaviour. In many feeding situations parents pay (falsely) a lot of attention to refusal of food, jumping around at the table, etc., and ignore any positive (desired) behaviour such as eating. This needs to be re-learned. It is important to find the adequate positive reinforcer for each individual child. Social reinforcement such as praise and attention is highly effective. This can be supplemented by further (delayed) reinforcers such as tokens and star

Table 2.5 Overview of behaviour management principles and applications to feeding interventions

Underlying principle	Description of application	Examples
	To increase desired behaviours	
Positive reinforcement	Provide positive consequences for desired behaviour	Give praise, physical affection, or tangible rewards (tokens)
Negative reinforcement	Terminate aversive stimulus contingent on desired behaviour	Release physical restraint (for food expulsion) when child accepts food
Discrimination	Reinforce target behaviour in presence of defined stimulus	Praise modelled behaviour of eating
		Reward cooperation with feeding requests
Shaping	Reinforce successive approximations toward desired response	Praise (1) looking at food, then (2) allowing food to touch lips, then (3) opening mouth, then (4) accepting food
Fading	Gradually remove assistance and reinforcement needed to maintain behaviour	Decrease extent of guidance and rewards as child gains self-feeding skills
Exposure/flooding (stimulus-response)	Provide food stimuli to reduce aversion	Expose to different tastes and textures (e.g. applied to toys)
	To decrease undesired behaviours	
Extinction	Withhold rewarding stimulus contingent on target response	Ignore mild inappropriate behaviour
		Continue prompts during escape behaviour
Satiation	Continually present desired stimulus until it loses its reinforcing value	Offer unlimited portions of food to reduce rumination
Punishment	Present aversive stimulus or remove rewarding stimulus contingent on undesired behaviour	Use time-out
		Give verbal reprimand
		Restrict toys
		Use over-correction
Desensitisation	Pair conditioned aversive stimulus with absence of aversive events or with presence of positive events	Distract child during fearful procedure
		Use gentle massage to promote acceptance of touch

Source: Kedesdy and Budd, 1998.

charts to obtain a valued object or activity (e.g. going to the zoo) after a week or two of adequate behaviour (e.g. food acceptance and adequate mealtime behaviour lead to a certain number of tokens) in preschool and school children. According to the Premack (1959) principle, a high probability behaviour (e.g. eating preferred food) can be used to reinforce a low probability behaviour (eating new or non-preferred food). However, in preschool and school children promising a preferred food (e.g. ice-cream) when the child eats a non-preferred food (e.g. spinach) can lead to the attribution that the non-preferred food 'is really pretty awful that mum has to coach me with my most preferred desert' (Birch, 1990). Thus social reinforcement should be the reinforcing stimulus of choice in feeding interventions.

Extinction can be considered as the opposite of reinforcement – it is the systematic discontinuance of a reward following an inadequate response to decrease the probability of the response occurring in future. For example, parents often start coaching an infant when refusing food or react with shouting and providing attention. This should be discontinued, i.e. the child should be ignored, during feeding situations. Parents may turn their face away from the child, or stop talking when the defined undesired behaviour occurs. In a treatment plan positive reinforcement and extinction are combined in a method called differential social attention: desired behaviour is reinforced and the child briefly ignored on misbehaviour, which aids the child to learn the behaviours that are desired by the feeder. A number of feeding interventions have also applied Differential Reinforcement of Other Behaviour (DRO) where rewarding stimuli contingent on any response except the target behaviour one wishes to decrease are delivered (e.g. Stark et al., 1993). Although extinction procedures are usually very effective they are often difficult for parents to accept or difficult to apply in children who show a high rate of disruptive behaviour (Linscheid, 1992).

Negative reinforcement and punishment are disciplinary strategies. Negative reinforcement is the withholding of an aversive stimulus contingent on performance of a desired behaviour. This strengthens the probability that the desired behaviour will occur in the future. An example of negative reinforcement is if a child fails to accept offered food after a few seconds, the feeder inserts the food in the child's mouth and holds the jaw until the child accepts the food. Termination of holding the jaw (the aversive stimulus) when the child accepts the food (the desired behaviour) is assumed to reinforce food acceptance (Riordan et al., 1984).

Punishment is either the delivery of an aversive stimulus or the removal of a rewarding stimulus. In children a technique used to weaken the probability that the inadequate response will occur is mainly time-out from reinforcement. It is a commonly used disciplinary measure in situations where inadequate behaviour occurs, such as temper tantrums. For example, if food is thrown, the child may be turned from the table and no interaction is directed at the child. The child may also be asked to leave the table or the food is removed for a predefined short period of time. It has also been used to reduce rumination, by the parents indicating a firm 'No' and then withdrawing any attention for ten seconds. Time-out should always be combined with guidance for clear alternatives for the child, i.e. reinforcement of behaviours to access favoured social stimuli or foods. In our treatment approach punishment and negative reinforcement have no place. It has been suggested that they should only be used if more positive strategies have failed and the target behaviour is damaging to the child. It also requires good professional monitoring such as in hospital (Kedesdy and Budd, 1998).

Graded approaches

The progressive training technique is often necessary as there is initially no desired behaviour observed that is reinforceable. Thus the criteria for the delivery of (shaping) reinforcement in relation to the child behaviour have to be progressively changed.

The difficulty with food refusers is that they rarely or never show the desired behaviour that is to be reinforced. The new behaviour thus needs to be developed on some variation of an old behaviour. In other words, a series of responses that approximates to the desired behavioural response is reinforced, whereas undesirable responses are ignored and attention is withdrawn. Reinforcement for any step in the right direction (i.e. acceptance of food) should be immediate. For example, reinforcement for any response that approximates to opening the mouth and taking in a foodstuff should be social attention such as praise, smiles, clapping hands, etc. For older children who achieve a predefined target (e.g. eating a small portion of food) it may be appropriate to employ a reinforcer such as allowing play with a favourite toy after the meal, reading a story, etc. It is probably best to avoid giving desired food or liquid as a reward because their usage can lead to the difficulty that foods the child does not want are thereby implicitly categorised as even less desirable (Birch, 1990; Harris, 1993). Shaping is one of the most useful behavioural tools in the treatment of child behaviour problems or feeding disorders because it provides a strategy for producing new response combinations from an existing (often limited) behavioural repertoire (Bijou, 1993).

Fading is the gradual removal of prompts, assistance or reinforcement to allow the independent execution of the behaviour. While at the beginning of a programme working with food refusers consistent reinforcement and cueing are necessary this will be changed to intermittent reinforcement (e.g. every third bite taken) and slowly faded out. Thus the behaviour is not dependent on external stimuli but the child maintains it by executing it her/himself. Shaping and fading are useful in many feeding interventions and are often applied with children with physical handicaps, allowing them to learn within successive small steps a chain of behaviours such as spoon feeding (Sullivan and Rosenbloom, 1996a).

Observation learning: modelling

Observational learning accounts for a large amount of cultural practices in children. It is also one of the predominant forms of learning in the feeding situation and for the acquisition of food preferences (Birch, 1980, 1987; Birch and Fisher, 1996). In modelling, the discriminative stimulus is the behaviour of another person (e.g. parent, peer or sibling) and imitation of the behaviour leads to vicarious reinforcement (Bandura, 1969). The natural tendency to model people who are highly regarded by the child is useful in many ways during feeding. For example, parents and siblings eat together with the child, indicate that they accept new foods and show that the food has positive consequences for them. In contrast, parents who do not sit down for a meal, eat in front of the television and use frequent snacking and at other times excessive dieting and food selection can provide a negative model for the child.

Food refusal and classical conditioning

Within the classical learning paradigm, an (unconditioned) neutral stimulus acquires the property of a negative event by being paired with this event (stimulus-response learning). Aversive conditioning is such an example. For example, when a person is unwell and eats a certain food and has to vomit subsequently, s/he is likely to consider the food as aversive and is less likely to eat it again (Mennella and Beauchamp, 1996). Conversely, if the person is recovering from an illness and is offered certain food, this food may become associated with feeling well. Many food preferences are learned by stimulus-response learning (Capaldi, 1996). Aversive conditioning in infants often occurs when particular foods or textures of foods have led to choking or vomiting and thus take on an aversive quality. This can occur within 'normal' feeding if certain types of foods are introduced too early or force-fed (Harris, 1993). Food phobia, food aversion, conditioned dysphagia, or the more recently labelled post-traumatic feeding disorder (PTFD; Benoit and Coolbear, 1998; Chatoor et al., 1988) appear to have become more common because a growing number of infants undergo intrusive medical procedures involving mouth, nose, and throat.

The mechanism postulated is that the infant associates stimulation in and around the mouth with pain, discomfort, or fear. Such experiences occur in relation to intrusive medical treatment such as intubation, suctioning, repeated insertion and removal of nasogastric feeding or medical problems associated with oesophagitis/heartburn associated with gastro-oesophagaeal reflux (Benoit and Coolbear, 1998; Di Scipio et al., 1978) or aversive feeding techniques such as force-feeding, choking and gagging (Harris, 1993).

A second postulated mechanism to explain PTFD is visceral hyperalgesia, a neuropathic condition in which prior experience (e.g. heartburn or oesophagitis) changes sensory nerves (e.g. in the oesophagus) so that previously innocuous stimuli (e.g. swallowing solids) are perceived as painful (Hyman, 1994). Refusal can be directed towards certain 'feared' textures (e.g. chunky textures that have made the infant gag) or total refusal of all solids and liquids (requiring tube feeding). Good history-taking of the feeding experience and medical interventions soon reveals the onset of, and stimuli involved in, the aversive conditioning. More detailed observation of the feeding situation and history-taking of the feeding development (e.g. introduction of different textured foods, feeding situation) are usually necessary to delineate the learning process that has taken place in food refusers who have no medical condition, and to determine the factors maintaining food refusal (Lindberg et al., 1996; Sanders et al., 1993).

Linscheid and Rasnake (1985) have proposed a classical conditioning paradigm to explain the origins of food refusal in such circumstances. In this model, an example is given of maternal anxiety as the unconditioned stimulus, and infant anxiety, engendered by mother's attitude, the unconditioned response (this is analogous to Pavlov's dogs, who salivated at the sight and smell of food). Now, if maternal anxiety is paired with the presentation of food (analogous in Pavlov's experiment to the sound of a bell) because the mother herself is anxious about whether or not her child will eat properly, the infant may become conditioned to feel distressed, not simply by exposure to maternal anxiety, but also by the presentation of food itself, which now becomes a conditioned stimulus. Infant distress is the conditioned response.

It is important to keep in mind that feeding behaviours resulting from classical conditioning (stimulus-response learning) are only to a small degree influenced by consequences (e.g. reward or punishment) after the behaviours occur. To reverse the effects of aversive conditioning two behavioural techniques are most successful (in addition to changes to mealtimes as outlined in the feeding checklist): flooding (or implosion) and desensitisation.

Desensitisation is carried out by repeatedly pairing the conditioned aversive stimulus with the absence of aversive events or with the delivery of positive reinforcement for an alternative, adaptive response (Kedesdy and Budd, 1998). Adults usually learn relaxation techniques and apply relaxation in anxiety-provoking situations. Systematic desensitisation provides slow and gradual exposure to the source of fear (e.g. food) (Benoit and Coolbear, 1998). Thus, graduated exposure in a relaxing atmosphere such as playing or watching a video is often used in young children. Toddlers who are particularly sensitive to touch in the oral region are touched gently in the region while playing and socially interacting. This is gradually followed by intra-oral stimulation (e.g. toothbrush) and then the presence of food is slowly introduced. Certain tastes can be introduced, for example, by applying these to the surface of toys, and the infant then sucks on these toys and becomes exposed to the food.

Siegel (1982) described a case of treatment of a 6-year-old boy who refused solid food. The boy showed anticipatory nausea, anxiety and gagging when presented with solid food (the conditioned aversive stimulus), presumably secondary to illness following an overdose of medication. Television viewing was used as a way of relaxing the child while gradually the food smell, taste and tasting were introduced. In smaller children, social interaction with people or play rather than television should be utilised. An advantage of desensitisation is that the infant rarely becomes upset during the treatment – the approach is adapted to the reactions of the child.

In contrast, flooding provides rapid and intense exposure to the source of fear (e.g. spiders or food), with the therapist largely controlling the rate and intensity of exposure (Benoit and Coolbear, 1998). The therapist provides in the sessions active anxiety control. The refused food is placed on the lips or into the mouth while the feeder tries to reduce the infant's distress in the first sessions by stroking, talking or singing to the infant. Five to ten seconds after the first exposure to the food, the feeder places another small amount of food on the lips or inside the mouth and reassures the infant again (if the child has not swallowed the previously inserted food an empty spoon is inserted into the mouth). The feeder repeats this sequence for the predetermined mealtime of fifteen to thirty minutes every five to ten seconds. Many infants cry, gag or retch when the spoon is inserted (flight-like behaviours) – this should not interrupt the preset feeding pace of five to ten seconds. The feeder should always positively reassure according to Benoit and Coolbear (1998). Flooding needs to be repeated during three to four meals per day.

Flooding is not applicable for children with a high risk for aspiration or who have neurological swallowing difficulties. The approach has been shown in a pre-post-test treatment study to be highly successful. However, it does not lead to full recovery where children do not chew or move the food in the mouth when inserted, refuse swallowing and spit it out. These infants may cooperate less because of neurological problems or because they have the highest levels of fear (Benoit and Coolbear, 1998). Gradual approximation may be more appropriate in these cases. Flooding may also be very disturbing to parents due to the intense distress experienced by the infants in the first sessions.

Failure to thrive

Failure to thrive (FTT) has been described under many different names, including maternal deprivation syndrome (Field, 1987; Wolke, 1996a), reactive attachment disorder (Minde and Minde, 1986), anorexia nervosa of infancy (Chatoor, 1989), or hospitalism syndrome (Spitz, 1945), and has been defined using clinical and behavioural criteria (e.g. Drotar et al., 1990), although there is now growing consensus that it should be defined on growth parameters alone (Bithoney and Dubowitz, 1985; Skuse, 1993). However, definitions referring to weight for age, height for age, weight for height, or indices of the velocity of growth lead to quite diverse prevalence estimates (Lancet –

Editorial, 1990a; Wright *et al.*, 1994; Drewett *et al.*, 1999). We have proposed that a minimum criterion should be weight below the third centile for population standards in normal birth-weight infants that has persisted for more than three months (Skuse *et al.*, 1994b; Wilensky *et al.*, 1996). This criterion detects infants having a very low weight for age. FTT is thus a symptom rather than a disorder (Ramsay, 1995).

The onset of FTT is usually in the first year of life and has to be distinguished from nutritional or stress-induced hyperphagia (psychosocial dwarfism), which usually begins after the second year and is most frequently associated with major family disruption (Oates, 1984; Skuse, 1993; Kessler and Dawson, 1999; Gilmour and Skuse, 1999). Recent community surveys in Britain and Israel found a prevalence of FTT of 3–4 per cent in full-term, appropriate for gestational age 1-year-olds (Skuse *et al.*, 1992; Wilensky *et al.*, 1996). About 2.9 per cent of children on community child abuse registers are included with FTT as primary diagnosis (Creighton, 1985).

The prognosis for infants who fail to thrive is mixed, with 22–60 per cent achieving no long-term catch-up growth (Wolke, 1994; Drewett *et al.*, 1999), and FTT children as a group have been reported to have cognitive abilities 1–1.5 standard deviations below population or control group means (see Wolke, 1994, for a review). Around 20–40 per cent have mild to moderate learning disabilities (IQ <70), and FTT infants are much more likely than their peers to be seriously delayed in reading (Oates *et al.*, 1985) and to fail in school (Glaser *et al.*, 1968; Dowdney *et al.*, 1998). About 28–50 per cent show other behavioural problems in middle to later childhood (Oates *et al.*, 1985), with eating problems persisting in many children (Heptinstall *et al.*, 1987; Dowdney *et al.*, 1998). These adverse effects are mainly found in children in referred clinical samples (Oates *et al.*, 1985) or NOFT community samples, with the children also stunted and head growth being subnormal (Dowdney *et al.*, 1998). Recent evidence indicates that the adverse effects on cognitive development may be limited to the first few years of life and catch-up in cognitive abilities occurs in most NOFT children by middle childhood (Boddy, 1997; Drewett *et al.*, 1999).

Traditionally, failure to thrive has been thought of as due either to organic factors or to an insufficient nurturing environment that leads to reactive attachment disorder and poor growth despite adequate food intake (Spitz, 1945; Field, 1987; Provence and Lipton, 1962). The latter is referred to as non-organic failure to thrive (NOFT). Often the distinction has been drawn on the basis of improved weight gain during hospitalisation (Ellerstein and Ostrov, 1985), with those showing weight gain with adequate caloric intake considered NOFT cases. However, several studies have shown that FTT infants with treatable organic diseases are often more likely to show improved growth than NOFT infants (Kristiansson and Fällström, 1987). More recently it has been proposed that many organic diseases, including congenital heart failure and cerebral palsy, only in interaction with poor feeding and nutritional provision lead to FTT (Lancet – Editorial, 1990b; Menon and Poskitt, 1985; Reilly et al., Chapter 1 in this book), and these cases should be considered mixed cases. Although organic illness is implicated in roughly 20–40 per cent of infants in hospital samples (Frank and Zeisel, 1988), organic FTT is rarely found in the community; it accounts for less than 10 per cent of cases (Skuse et al., 1992; Wilensky et al., 1996).

Traditionally, NOFT has been considered as due to maternal psychiatric illness, social deprivation, lack of stimulation and poor caretaking (Spitz, 1951; Provence and Lipton, 1962; McJunkin et al., 1987; Drotar et al., 1990; Hess et al., 1977; Singer et al., 1990). However, emotional deprivation per se is not the major cause of non-organic failure to thrive; for example, no differences in psychiatric or family dysfunction or mother–infant interaction have been reported in community samples compared to normal growing controls (Wolke, 1996a; Skuse et al., 1992; Wilensky et al., 1996). Any inadequate interactions between infant and mother in clinical samples are as likely to be the consequence of persistent feeding problems and parental anxiety about getting food into the infant, as to be the cause of NOFT (Ramsay, 1995; Duniz et al., 1996). Only in a small minority of NOFT cases (9 per cent) is neglect or abuse the reason for the infant's placement on the at risk register (Skuse et al., 1995a).

For the diagnosis and treatment it is important to consider that FTT is usually primarily due neither to organic disease nor to deficient social environments. It is a result of the interaction of characteristics of the individual infant and environmental features that maintain poor weight gain and contribute to the developmental problems. Undernutrition occurs because the infant is not offered enough food, refuses food, or cannot take in sufficient nutrition for growth (Field, 1984; Skuse, 1985; Wolke, 1994). NOFT infants receive inadequate nutrition for quite heterogeneous reasons. A small number of NOFT infants are neglected, others experience irregular, insufficient and disorganised meals (e.g. Heptinstall et al., 1987). Others have insufficient diets because of prolonged exclusive breastfeeding or errors in the preparation of bottle feeds (Reilly et al., Chapter 1 in this book; Schmitt and Mauro, 1989; Wright, 1993), or because the mother has an eating disorder (Smith and Hanson, 1972; van Wezel-Meijler and Wit, 1989) or distorted perceptions about infant slimness (Wolke, 1994; Birch, 1990), or there are religious or cultural reasons (Pugliese et al., 1987) for providing low-calorie or low amounts of food. Furthermore, infants may be malnourished because of subtle oral-motor problems, making the intake of higher-textured and denser food difficult (Mathisen et al., 1989; Reilly et al., 1999).

Some infants have a history of being very easy and insufficiently demanding (e.g. they miss feeds from the first weeks of life by sleeping through them; Carey, 1985; Wolke, 1994; Skuse et al., 1994b; Habbick and Gerrard, 1984), while others are temperamentally difficult (Wolke et al., 1990a), difficult to feed or food refusers (Harris and Booth, 1992; Dahl and Sundelin, 1986).

Often factors such as disorganised mealtimes (e.g. missing meals, frequent snacking), oral-motor problems and parental provision of nutritionally inadequate diets occur in conjunction.

Furthermore, ethnic differences need to be considered. For example, while 3–5 per cent of white, Chinese Asian, Carribbean and mixed race infants suffered NOFT, 14.9 per cent of Indian Asian and none of the African infants all residing in the same London health region did so (Skuse et al., 1992). Within the Indian Asian community, genetic factors, the late introduction of solids of low caloric density (see Underwood and Hofvander, 1982), as well as the frequent social isolation of the mothers (Fenton et al., 1989), are likely contributors to the high rates of failure to thrive. In sum, cultural, parental and infant characteristics, most likely in interaction, lead to a resetting of the internal nutrient demand of NOFT infants and provide them with different oral-motor experiences (e.g. provision of low-textured foods). Little appetite and interest in food leads to further caloric deprivation, with important health implications, such as recurrent infections and anaemia, which in turn are associated with lower exploratory behaviour and motivation (Frank and Zeisel, 1988).

The DSM-IV (American Psychiatric Association, 1997) does not classify FTT as a reactive attachment disorder any more but includes FTT as a symptom of Feeding Disorder in Infancy and Childhood while still maintaining the fuzzy dichotomy of organic versus non-organic FTT (Ramsay, 1995). However, compared to other conditions discussed, many FTT infants have no obvious feeding problems (e.g. no general food refusal, no vomiting), but the problems are subtle (e.g. little appetite, subtle oral-motor problems) (Skuse et al., 1995b; Reilly et al., 1995; Wolke, 1996a). Diagnosis requires a broad approach to identify factors contributing to and maintaining poor growth. These should include, apart from the usual components outlined previously in this chapter (e.g. oral-motor assessment, feeding interaction assessment), a good history-taking of early temperament (e.g. sleeping through feeds), investigation of indications of neglect or abuse and parental eating patterns (e.g. vicarious dieting of infant). Multidisciplinary and home intervention, advocated here, can be successful, as recent trials indicate. For example, a multidisciplinary team approach leads to better catch-up growth than standard paediatric care (Bithoney et al., 1991). Furthermore, additional home visiting by lay visitors to promote parenting and child development knowledge leads to improved interactive competence during feeding and improved language scores compared to care in the paediatric clinic alone (Black et al., 1995), thus reducing some secondary consequences of NOFT.

Special problems: organic disorders in infants

Feeding problems are relatively frequently encountered in infants with chronic organic disorders, ranging from cerebral palsy (Polnay and Hill,

1985) to a diversity of congenital malformations, such as those associated with the Pierre Robin syndrome (Lewis and Pashayan, 1980), Noonan's syndrome (Ranke *et al.*, 1988), cleft palate, and oesophageal atresia (Puntis *et al.*, 1990). Some of these problems require long-term intensive treatment, such as the use of tube feeding or the fitting of a gastrostomy to prevent severe stunting and marasmus (Sullivan and Rosenbloom, 1996a). There is now a growing realisation that in some cases poor growth rates associated with conditions such as cerebral palsy may be in part due to low nutritional intakes which could be improved with appropriate behavioural, occupational and oral-motor treatment. The list of possible varieties of treatments appropriate for individual problems is very large indeed. However, two of the most commonly encountered difficulties will be discussed below: namely, how to manage oral-motor problems in cerebral palsy infants, and how to introduce or re-introduce oral feeding in children who have been fed for prolonged periods by the nasogastric route, by a gastrostomy or by total parenteral nutrition.

Treatment of feeding difficulties in cerebral palsy

For reasons that are not fully understood, most infants with cerebral palsy – whether full-term (Pryor and Thelander, 1967) or preterm (Brothwood *et al.*, 1988) – are small. Those with a greater degree of neurological impairment have a more pronounced growth disorder (Sullivan and Rosenbloom, 1996b). A number of reasons for the associated impaired growth have been proposed including the poorer ability of these infants to communicate food preferences, their impairment in adaptive skills (e.g. self-feeding is difficult or impossible), oral-motor dysfunction and gastro-oesophageal reflux (Reilly *et al.*, Chapter 1 in this book; Sullivan and Rosenbloom, 1996a). In the child with cerebral palsy and pharyngeal involvement these problems may be so severe that oral feeding leads to vomiting and aspiration (Griggs *et al.*, 1989; Helfrich-Miller *et al.*, 1986). Consequently, a normal diet cannot be maintained; single feeds may last hours, exhausting both infant and mother (Gisel and Patrick, 1988). Some such infants may require nasogastric or gastrostomy feeding (Patrick *et al.*, 1986; Rempel *et al.*, 1988), but unfortunately there are several potential complications associated with these procedures (for medical side-effects, see Cowen, 1987; Haws *et al.*, 1986; McClead and Menke, 1987; Moore and Greene, 1985). These include the lack of any social setting for feeding, withdrawal of any hedonic aspects of eating (Birch, 1987; Lipsiett *et al.*, 1985), and the loss of an opportunity to learn oral-motor skills (Alexander, 1987; Evans-Morris, 1989; Monahan *et al.*, 1988).

A standardised assessment of oral-motor functioning for cerebral palsy and other feeding problem children is now available (Reilly *et al.*, 1995; Skuse *et al.*, 1995b). The Schedule of Oral Motor Assessment (SOMA) is a full diagnostic instrument which points to areas of abnormal or delayed functioning that can be addressed in the intervention.

The approach to the treatment of feeding difficulties in infants with cerebral palsy who do not require tube feeding is similar to that for other feeding problems. The treatment starts with a full diagnostic assessment, together with measures of the feeding environment and of the interaction between the child and caregiver. However, special emphasis should be placed on an assessment of general motor functioning (e.g. tonicity, movement restrictions, body posture, etc.) and, specifically, oral-motor skills. Abnormal movement patterns include jaw clenching, jaw thrusting, lip pursing, lip retraction, tongue retraction, tongue thrust and tonic biting (Alexander, 1987; Evans-Morris and Klein, 1987). Motor integration problems include poorly coordinated breathing with eating, difficulties associated with swallowing or sucking, and a hypo- or hypersensitive gag reflux. Infants with cerebral palsy are often hypersensitive to touch in the oral region, but it is not clear to what extent this is an indication of a neurological abnormality and to what extent it is a conditioned response (Di Scipio et al., 1978).

Currently, there are many theories and beliefs regarding the treatment of associated oral-motor dysfunction but few have been systematically evaluated (Fischer-Brandies et al., 1987; Ottenbacher et al., 1983; Carroll and Reilly, 1996). They include surgery, orthodontic appliances, behavioural and social interaction approaches (see review by Ottenbacher et al., 1983). Emphasis should be placed on the correct positioning of the infant, as an appropriate position can inhibit abnormal muscle tone and reflexes, reducing compensatory movements involving the neck and thereby facilitating normal oral-motor functioning (Alexander 1987; Evans-Morris and Klein, 1987; Evans-Morris, 1989; Lewis, 1982; Sheppard, 1987). A physiotherapist or occupational therapist can often help to design a suitable chair which will adequately support the infant's head, neck and trunk. Benefits may also result from slight changes in the angle of presentation of food (e.g. to the midline), or in the texture of food given.

The development of oral-motor skills can also be enhanced by using suitable objects, toys or toothbrush training sets which the infant can use for mouthing. Exposure to oral stimulation using very small quantities of foodstuff (e.g. sham feeding) is also helpful in reducing oral hypersensitivity (Evans-Morris, 1989).

A detailed outline of treatment programmes for the management of oral and pharyngeal dysfunction in cerebral palsy children is provided by Carroll and Reilly (1996).

Artificially fed infants: the (re)establishment of oral feeding

Tube feeding via the nasal route is often undertaken in infants with acute problems, where the introduction or reinstitution of oral feeding is expected soon. In contrast, gastrostomy is used where oral feeding is not expected for many months (Lloyd and Pierro, 1996). Parents often find nasogastric and gastrostomy feeding worrying at first, but usually these feeding regimens eventually become established and accepted. Parents often then become anxious when reinstitution of oral feeding is attempted (Blackman and Nelson, 1985). The majority of parents have significant difficulties orally feeding infants who have had repair of oesophageal atresia (Puntis *et al.*, 1990). They state that feeding difficulties dominate their lives and many express feelings of isolation and helplessness; yet only 11 per cent of these parents seek professional advice. The following recommendations about reinstating feeding by the oral route are based on a review of the available treatment literature (Blackman and Nelson, 1985; Evans-Morris and Klein, 1987; Evans-Morris, 1989; Handen *et al.*, 1986; Illingworth, 1969; Lloyd and Pierro, 1996).

General prevention (support for rudimentary oral-motor skills)

Whenever tube feeding is necessary for a prolonged period or a gastrostomy is fitted, a suitably qualified specialist should work with the child to provide concurrent oral-motor therapy. Attention should also be paid to the potential oral hypersensitivity that can result from aversive conditioning to associated unpleasant oral experiences, including hygiene, auctioning and associated medical examinations.

Review

Are the conditions for the reestablishment of oral feeding met? The following conditions should be fulfilled:

1   The infant's medical condition which led to the introduction of the artificial route must be corrected (e.g. cardiac surgery). Nutritional status should be stabilised (infant's rate of weight gain adequate; not failing to thrive).
2   There should be no serious anatomic or functional impediment to swallowing. Clinical signs of swallowing problems (e.g. a delayed or absent swallow reflex, excessive coughing, choking, suspected aspiration) should be evaluated using videofluoroscopy or ultrasound (Loveday, 1996).
3   The infant should be functioning at an adequate developmental level (6 months or more) to benefit from behavioural treatment aimed at introducing solid or semi-solid food.
4   The child's caregivers should be sufficiently stable and committed to maintain oral feeding once established.

Preparation stage (getting ready to start treatment)

A relaxed period of preparation is most important to prepare the child and parents for the difficult treatment period.

1 The tube or gastrostomy feeding schedule should approximate to a normal diurnal pattern – i.e. only three to five feedings should be administered in twenty-four hours at times when family mealtimes occur (three large volume feeds and maybe two 'snack' feeds). This helps to set a pattern of regular 'mealtimes' and assists the establishment of hunger feelings.
2 The duration of the feed should be increased to approximately 20–30 minutes.
3 A standard formula or liquidised and diluted normal meal for gastrostomy or tube feeds should be used.
4 Supervision of feeds should be provided by a small number of people who can start to get to know the parents well and build up their confidence that the child will eventually eat orally.

Treatment

Young children who have been fed non-orally for many months will find oral stimulation, by taste or texture, to be unpleasant. The first goal is to overcome resistance to oral stimulation, and then to encourage the child to swallow food. Apply the different behavioural modification techniques discussed in other sections in this chapter:

(a) Develop a hierarchy of problems that should be addressed first and those functions that should be facilitated first.
(b) By shaping, through positive reinforcement and ignoring undesirable behaviour, try to build an association between feelings of hunger, oral feeding, and satiation.
(c) Create a positive, relaxed environment.
(d) Provide good positioning for feeding.
(e) Use modelling (e.g. encourage the parents/siblings to eat with the child).
(f) Use slow approximation, by thickening food very slowly over days.
(g) Support the parents in persisting with oral feeding as the progress may be slow and difficult.
(h) It is not generally advisable, although proposed by some (Blackman and Nelson, 1985), to use force-feeding. Parents usually consider force-feeding to be unacceptable and extremely distressing (Puntis et al., 1990). It may well exacerbate food refusal by leading to a conditioned association between oral feeding and an aversive stimulus.

Conclusions

Feeding problems can dominate the lives of those who feel helpless when denied one of their important parenting roles by a young child who is unable or unwilling to eat. Many feeding problems challenge the diagnostic and treatment skills of the most experienced paediatrician, psychologist or speech therapist. To make progress in treating feeding problems, we have to put more effort and resources into the development and evaluation of comprehensive treatment programmes involving a team of diverse specialists, who have worked together on these problems, and can bring a range of expertise to bear on the subject. Illingworth (1969), stated that 'part of the difficulty [in treating dysphagia] may lie in the fact that affected children may be referred to any of a variety of specialists . . . so that few have adequate experience of the problem' (p. 655). Thirty years on, we know more about aetiological and maintaining factors. There are also some hospitals and clinics with feeding specialists and teamwork; however, they are still few and far between. Considering that efficient eating is a primary need and feeding problems affect the child and whole family adversely, it is concerning that the adequate diagnosis and management of feeding disorders in young children, both in hospital and in the community, still leave much to be desired.

References

Ahearn, W. H., Kerwin, M. E., Eicher, P. S., Shantz, J. and Swearingin, W. (1996) An alternating treatment comparison of two interventions for food refusal. *Journal of Applied Behavior Analysis*, 29, 321–332.

Ainsworth, M. D. S., Bell, S. M. and Stayton, D. J. (1972) Individual differences in the development of some attachment behaviours. *Merrill Palmer Quarterly*, 18, 123–143.

Alexander, R. (1987) Prespeech and feeding development. In E. T. McDonald (ed.) *Treating Cerebral Palsy for Clinicians*. Austin, Tex.: PRO-ED Inc., pp. 133–152.

American Psychiatric Association (1997) *Diagnostic and Statistical Manual of Mental Disorders*, 3rd edn (revised). Washington, DC: APA.

Auerbach, K. G. and Eggert, L. D. (1987) The importance of infant suckling patterns when a breast-fed baby fails to thrive (letter). *Journal of Tropical Pediatrics*, 33, 156–157.

Aukett, M. A., Parks, Y. A., Scott, P. H. and Wharton, B. A. (1986) Treatment with iron increases weight gain and psychomotor development. *Archives of Disease in Childhood*, 61, 849–857.

Bandura, A. (1969) Modelling and vicarious processes. In A. Bandura (ed.) *Principles of Behavior Modification*. New York: Holt, Rinehart and Winston, pp. 118–126.

Barnard, K. (1978) *Nursing Child Assessment Teaching Scale (NCATS)*. Seattle: University of Washington.

Barr, R. G., Kramer, M. S., Pless, I. B., Boisjoly, C. and Leduc, D. (1989) Feeding and temperament as determinants of early infant crying/fussing behavior. *Pediatrics*, 84(3), 514–521.

Bauchner, H., Brown, E. and Peskin, J. (1988) Premature graduates of the newborn intensive care unit: a guide to follow-up. *Pediatric Clinics of North America*, 35, 1207–1225.

Bax, M. (1989) Editorial: Eating is important. *Developmental Medicine and Child Neurology*, 31, 285–286.

Bayley, N. (1993) *Bayley Scales of Infant Development – Second Edition, Assessment focus – people products quality*. The Psychological Corporation, Order Service Center, P.O. Box 839954, San Antonio.

Benoit, D. and Coolbear, J. (1998) Post-traumatic feeding disorders in infancy: behaviors predicting treatment outcome. *Infant Mental Health Journal*, 19(4), 409–421.

Berkowitz, C. (1985) Comprehensive pediatric management of failure to thrive: an interdisciplinary approach. In D. Drotar (ed.) *New Directions in Failure to Thrive: Implications for Research, and Practice*. New York: Plenum Press, pp. 193–210.

Berwick, D. M., Levy, J. C. and Kleinerman, R. (1982) Failure to thrive: diagnostic yield of hospitalization. *Archives of Disease in Childhood*, 57, 347–351.

Bijou, S. W. (1993) *Behavior Analysis of Child Development* (2nd edn). Englewood Cliffs, NJ: Prentice-Hall.

Birch, L. L. (1980) Effects of peer models' food choices and eating behaviors on preschoolers' food preferences. *Child Development*, 51, 489–496.

Birch, L. L. (1987) The acquisition of food acceptance patterns in children. In R. A. Boakes, D. A. Poppiewell and M. J. Burton (eds) *Eating Habits: Food Physiology and Learned Behaviour*. New York: John Wiley and Sons, pp. 107–130.

Birch, L. L. (1990) Development of food acceptance patterns. *Developmental Psychology*, 26(4), 515–519.

Birch, M. (1999) Psychological issues and infant–parent psychotherapy. In D. B. Kessler and P. Dawson (eds.) *Failure to Thrive and Pediatric Undernutrition*. Baltimore: Paul H. Brookes Publishing Co. Inc., pp. 395–410.

Birch, L. L. and Fisher, J. A. (1996) The role of experience in the development of children's eating behavior. In E. D. Capaldi (ed.) *Why We Eat What We Eat. The Psychology of Eating*. Washington, DC: American Psychological Association, pp. 113–141.

Bithoney, W. G. and Dubowitz, A. (1985) Organic concomitants of nonorganic failure to thrive: implications for research. In D. Drotar (ed.) *New Directions in Failure to Thrive: Implications for Research and Practice*. London: Plenum Press, pp. 47–68.

Bithoney, W. G., McJunkin, J., Michalek, J., Snyder, J., Egan, H. and Epstein, D. (1991). The effect of a multidisciplinary team approach on weight gain in non-organic failure to thrive children. *Journal of Developmental and Behavioral Pediatrics*, 12, 254–258.

Black, M. M., Dubowitz, H., Hutcheson, J., Berenson-Howard, J. and Starr, R. H. (1995) A randomized trial of home intervention for children with failure to thrive. *Pediatrics*, 95(6), 807–814.

Black, R. E. and Victoria, C. G. (2002) Optimal duration of exclusive breastfeeding in low income countries. *British Medical Journal*, 325, 1252–1253.

Blackman, J. A. and Nelson, C. L. A. (1985) Reinstituting oral feedings in children fed by gastrostomy tube. *Clinical Pediatrics*, 24, 434–438.

Boddy, J. M. (1997) Maternal characteristics and development of children who failed to thrive. Unpublished Ph.D. thesis, University of London.

Brothwood, M., Wolke, D., Gamsu, H. and Cooper, D. (1988) Mortality, morbidity, growth and development of babies weighing 501–1000 grams and 1001–1500 grams at birth. *Acta Paediatrica Scandinavica*, 77, 10–18.

Budd, K. S., Chugh, C. S. and Berry, S. L. (1998) Parents as therapists for children's food refusal problems. In J. M. Briesmeister and C. E. Schaefer (eds) *Handbook of Parent Training* (2nd edn). New York: John Wiley and Sons, pp. 418–440.

Bunton, J., Bisset, E. and Harvey, D. (1987) The social experience of newborn babies in hospital. In D. Harvey (ed.) *Parent–Infant Relationships* (*Perinatal Practice: Vol. 4*). New York: John Wiley and Sons, pp. 43–70.

Caldwell, B. and Bradley, R. (1984) *Home Observation for the Measurement of the Environment – Revised*. Little Rock: University of Arkansas at Little Rock.

Capaldi, E. D. (ed.) (1996) *Why We Eat What We Eat* (1st edn). Washington, DC: American Psychological Association.

Carey, W. B. (1985) Temperament and increased weight gain in infants. *Developmental and Behavioral Pediatrics*, 6(3), 128–131.

Carroll, L. and Reilly, S. (1996) The therapeutic approach to the child with feeding difficulty: II. management and treatment. In P. B. Sullivan and L. Rosenbloom (eds) *Feeding the Disabled Child*. London: Mac Keith Press.

Chatoor, I. (1989) Infantile anorexia nervosa: a developmental disorder of separation and individuation. *Journal of the American Academy of Psychoanalysis*, 17, 43–64.

Chatoor, I., Conley, C. and Dickson, L. (1988) Food refusal after an incident of choking: a post-traumatic eating disorder. *Journal of the American Academy of Child and Adolescent Psychiatry*, 27, 105–110.

Cowen, S. L. (1987) Feeding gastrostomy: nutritional management of the infant or young child. *Journal of Pediatric and Perinatal Nutrition*, 1, 51–60.

Creighton, S. J. (1985) An epidemiological study of abused children and their families in the United Kingdom between 1977 and 1982. *Child Abuse and Neglect*, 9, 441–448.

Cunningham, C. E. and Linscheid, T. R. (1976) Elimination of chronic infant rumination by electric shock. *Behavior Therapy*, 7, 231–234.

Cunningham, K. F. and McLaughlin, M. (1999) Nutrition. In D. B. Kessler and P. Dawson (eds) *Failure to Thrive and Pediatric Undernutrition*. Baltimore: Paul H. Brookes Publishing Co. Inc., pp. 99–120.

Cutts, D. B. and Geppert, J. (1999) Anemia, lead exposure, renal disease, and dental caries. In D. B. Kessler and P. Dawson (eds) *Failure to Thrive and Pediatric Undernutrition*. Baltimore: Paul H. Brookes Publishing Co Inc., pp. 269–274.

Dahl, M. and Sundelin, C. (1986) Early feeding problems in an affluent society: categories and clinical signs. *Acta Paediatrica Scandinavica*, 75, 370–375.

Davies, D. P. (1979) Is inadequate breast-feeding an important cause of failure to thrive? *The Lancet*, 1, 541–542.

DHSS (Department of Health and Social Security) (1980) *Present Day Practice in Infant Feeding: 1980*. London: Her Majesty's Stationery Office.

DHSS (Department of Health and Social Security) (1988) *Present Day Practice in Infant Feeding: Third Report*. London: Her Majesty's Stationery Office.

Di Scipio, W. J., Kaslon, K. and Ruben, R. J. (1978) Traumatically acquired conditioned dysphagia in children. *Annals of Otology*, 87, 509–514.

Douglas, J. and Richman, N. (1984) *My Child Won't Sleep*. Harmondsworth: Penguin.

Dowdney, L., Skuse, D., Morris, K. and Pickles, A. (1998) Short normal children and environmental disadvantage: a longitudinal study of growth and cognitive development from 4 to 11 years. *Journal of Child Psychology and Psychiatry*, 39(7), 1017–1030.

Drewett, R., Kahn, S., Parkhurst, S. and Whiteley, S. (1987a) Pain during breast-feeding: the first three months postpartum. *Journal of Reproductive and Infant Psychology*, 5, 183–186.

Drewett, R. F., Payman, B. C. and Whiteley, S. (1987b) Effect of complementary feeds on sucking and milk intake in breastfed babies: an experimental study. *Journal of Reproductive and Infant Psychology*, 5, 133–143.

Drewett, R. F., Corbett, S. S. and Wright, C. M. (1999) Cognitive and educational attainments at school age of children who failed to thrive in infancy: a population-based study. *Journal of Child Psychology and Psychiatry*, 40(4), 551–561.

Drotar, D., Eckerle, D., Satola, J., Pallotta, J. and Wyatt, B. (1990) Maternal interactional behaviour with nonorganic failure to thrive infants: a case comparison study. *Child Abuse and Neglect*, 14, 41–51.

Duniz, M., Scheer, P. J., Trojovsky, A., Kaschnitz, W., Kvas, E. and Macari, S. (1996) Changes in psychopathology of parents of NOFT (non-organic failure to thrive) infants during treatment. *European Child and Adolescent Psychiatry*, 5, 93–100.

Eaton-Evans, J. and Dugdale, A. E. (1988) Sleep patterns of infants in the first year of life. *Archives of Disease in Childhood*, 63, 647–649.

Elias, M. J., Nicolson, N. A., Bora, C. and Johnston, J. (1986) Sleep/wake patterns of breast-fed infants in the first 2 years of life. *Pediatrics*, 77, 322–329.

Ellerstein, N. S. and Ostrov, B. E. (1985) Growth patterns in children hospitalized because of caloric-deprivation failure to thrive. *American Journal of Diseases of Children*, 139, 164–166.

Evans-Morris, S. (1989) Development of oral-motor skills in the neurologically impaired child receiving non-oral feedings. *Dysphagia*, 3, 135–154.

Evans-Morris, S. and Klein, M. D. (1987) *Pre-Feeding Skills: A Comprehensive Resource for Feeding Development*. Tucson, Ariz.: Therapy Skill Builders.

Fenton, T. R., Bhat, R., Davies, A. and West, R. (1989) Maternal insecurity and failure to thrive in Asian children. *Archives of Disease in Childhood*, 64, 369–372.

Fergusson, D. M., Horwood, L. J. and Channon, F. T. (1987) Breast feeding and subsequent social adjustment in 6 to 8 year old children. *Journal of Child Psychology and Psychiatry*, 28, 378–386.

Field, M. (1984) Follow up developmental status of infants hospitalized for nonorganic failure to thrive. *Journal of Paediatric Psychology*, 9, 241–256.

Field, T. (1987) Interaction and attachment in normal and atypical infants. *Journal of Consulting and Clinical Psychology*, 55(6), 853–859.

Finney, J. W. (1986) Preventing common feeding problems in infants and young children. *Pediatric Clinics of North America*, 33, 775–788.

Fischer-Brandies, H., Avalle, C. and Limbrock, G. J. (1987) Therapy of orofacial dysfunctions in cerebral palsy according to Castillo-Morales: first results of a new treatment concept. *European Journal of Orthodontics*, 9, 139–143.

Fomon, S. J., Filer, L. J., Anderson, T. A. and Ziegler, E. E. (1979) Recommendations for feeding normal infants. *Pediatrics*, 63, 52–59.

Forsyth, B. W. C., McCarthy, P. L. and Leventhal, J. M. (1985) Problems of early infancy, formula changes, and mothers' beliefs about their infants. *Journal of Pediatrics*, 106, 1012–1017.

Francis, D. E. M. (1987) *Diets for Sick Children*. Oxford: Blackwell.

Frank, D. A. and Zeisel, S. H. (1988) Failure to thrive. *Pediatric Clinics of North America*, 35(6), 1187–1205.

Galef, B. G. (1996) Social influences on food preferences and feeding behaviors of vertebrates. In E. D. Capaldi (ed.) *Why We Eat What We Eat. The Psychology of Eating*. Washington, DC: American Psychological Association, pp. 207–231.

Gilmour, J. and Skuse, D. (1999) A case-comparison study of the characteristics of children with short stature syndrome induced by stress (hyperphagic short stature) and a consecutive series of unaffected 'stressed' children. *Journal of Child Psychology and Psychiatry*, 40(6), 969–978.

Gisel, E. G. and Patrick, J. (1988) Identification of children with cerebral palsy unable to maintain normal nutritional state. *The Lancet*, 1, 283–286.

Glaser, H., Heagarty, M., Bullard, D. and Pivchik, E. (1968) Physical and psychological development of children with early failure to thrive. *Journal of Pediatrics*, 73(5), 690–698.

Goldson, E. (1999) Neurological and genetic disorders. In D. B. Kessler and P. Dawson (eds) *Failure to Thrive and Pediatric Undernutrition*. Baltimore: Paul H. Brookes Publishing Co. Inc., pp. 245–254.

Goodnow, J. J. (1988) Parents' ideas, actions and feelings: models and methods from developmental and social psychology. *Child Development*, 59, 286–320.

Gray, P. (1987) *Crying Baby – How to Cope*. London: Wisebuy Publications.

Griggs, C. A., Jones, P. M. and Leigh, R. E. (1989) Video-fluoroscopic investigation of feeding disorders of children with multiple handicap. *Developmental Medicine and Child Neurology*, 31, 303–308.

Grossman, L. K., Fitzsimmons, S. M., Larsen-Alexander, J. B., Sachs, L. and Harter, C. (1990) The infant feeding decision in low and upper income women. *Clinical Pediatrics*, 29, 30–37.

Gupta, M. C. and Urrutia, J. J. (1982) Effect of periodic antlascaris and antigiardia treatment on nutritional status of preschool children. *American Journal of Clinical Nutrition*, 36, 79–86.

Habbick, B. F. and Gerrard, J. W. (1984) Failure to thrive in the contented breast-fed baby. *Canadian Medical Association Journal*, 131, 765–768.

Handen, B. L., Mandell, F. and Russo, D. C. (1986) Feeding induction in children who refuse to eat. *American Journal of Diseases of Children*, 140, 52–54.

Hanks, H. G. I., Hobbs, C. I., Seymour, D. and Stratton, P. (1988) Infants who fail to thrive: an intervention for poor feeding practices. *Journal of Reproductive and Infant Psychology*, 6, 101–111.

Harris, G. (1988) Determinants of the introduction of solid food. *Journal of Reproductive and Infant Psychology*, 6, 241–249.

Harris, G. (1993) Feeding problems and their treatment. In I. St.James-Roberts, G. Harris and D. Messer (eds) *Infant Crying, Feeding and Sleeping: Development, Problems and Treatments*. London: Harvester Wheatsheaf, pp. 118–132.

Harris, G. and Booth, D. A. (1987) Infants' preference for salt in food: its dependence upon recent dietary experience. *Journal of Reproductive and Infant Psychology*, 5, 97–104.

Harris, G. and Booth, I. W. (1992) The nature and management of eating problems in preschool children. In P. J. Cooper and A. Stein (eds) *Feeding Problems and Eating Disorders in Children and Adolescents*. New York: Harwood Academic Publishers, pp. 61–84.

Haws, E. B., Sieber, W. K. and Kiesewetter, W. B. (1986) Complications of tube gastrostomy in infants and children. *Annals of Surgery*, 164, 284–290.

Helfrich-Miller, K. R., Rector, K. L. and Straka, J. A. (1986) Dysphagia: its treatment in the profoundly retarded patient with cerebral palsy. *Archives of Physical and Medical Rehabilitation*, 67, 520–525.

Heptinstall, E., Puckering, C., Skuse, D., Dowdney, L. and Zur-Szplro, L. (1987) Nutrition and mealtime behaviour in families of growth retarded children. *Human Nutrition: Applied Nutrition*, 41a, 390–402.

Hess, A., Hess, K. and Hard, H. (1977) Intellectual characteristics of mothers of failure to thrive syndrome children. *Child: Care, Health and Development*, 3, 377–387.

Hetherington, M. H. and Rolls, B. J. (1996) Sensory-specific satiety: theoretical frameworks and central characteristics. In E. D. Capaldi (ed.), *Why We Eat What We Eat. The Psychology of Eating*. Washington, DC: American Psychological Association, pp. 267–290.

Hitchcock, N. E., Gracey, N., Gilmour, A. I. and Owles. E. N. (1986) Nutrition and growth in infancy and early childhood. *Monographs in Pediatrics*, Vol. 19 (ed. F. Falkner, N. Kretchmer and E. Rossi). Basel: S. Karger and Co.

Homer, C. and Ludwig, S. (1981) Categorisation of etiology of failure to thrive. *American Journal of Diseases of Children*, 135, 848–851.

Hyman, P. E. (1994) Gastroesophageal reflux: one reason why baby won't eat. *Journal of Pediatrics*, 125, 103–109.

Illingworth, R. S. (1969) Sucking and swallowing difficulties in infancy: diagnostic problem of dysphagia. *Archives of Disease in Childhood*, 44, 655–665.

Illingworth, R. S. (1985) Infantile colic revisited. *Archives of Disease in Childhood*, 60, 981–985.

Illingworth, R. S. and Lister, J. (1964) The critical or sensitive period, with special reference to certain feeding problems in infants and children. *Journal of Pediatrics*, 65(6), 839–848.

Iwaniec, D., Herbert, M. and McNeish, A. S. (1985) Social work with failure-to-thrive children and their families. Part I: Psychosocial factors. *British Journal of Social Work*, 15, 243–259.

Kanfer, F. H. and Goldstein, A. P. (eds) (1980) *Helping People Change*. Oxford: Pergamon Press.

Karoly, P. (1980) Operant methods. In F. H. Kanfer and A. P. Goldstein (eds) *Helping People Change*. Oxford: Pergamon Press, pp. 210–247.

Kedesdy, J. H. and Budd, K. S. (1998) *Childhood Feeding Disorders*. Baltimore: Paul H. Brookes Publishing Co. Inc.

Kessler, D. B. and Dawson, P. (1999) *Failure to Thrive and Pediatric Undernutrition*. Baltimore: Paul H. Brookes Publishing Co. Inc.

Krebs, N. F. (1999) Gastrointestinal problems and disorders. In D. B. Kessler and P. Dawson (eds), *Failure to Thrive and Pediatric Undernutrition*. Baltimore: Paul H. Brookes Publishing Co. Inc, pp. 215–226.

Kristiansson, B. and Fällström, S. P. (1987) Growth at the age of four years subsequent to early failure to thrive. *Child Abuse and Neglect*, 11, 35–40.

Lancet – Editorial (1990a) Failure to thrive revisited. *The Lancet*, 335, 662–663.

Lancet – Editorial (1990b) Growth and nutrition in children with cerebral palsy. *The Lancet*, 335, 1253–1254.

Leach, P. (1986) *Baby and Child*. London: Dorling Kindersley.

Lewis, J. A. (1982) Oral motor assessment and treatment of feeding difficulties. In P. A. Accardo (ed.) *Failure to Thrive in Infancy and Early Childhood*. Baltimore: University Park Press, pp. 265–295.

Lewis, M. B. and Pashayan, H. M. (1980) Management of infants with Robin Anomaly. *Clinical Pediatrics*, 19, 519–528.

Lindberg, L., Bohlin, G., Hagekull, B. and Palmerus, K. (1996) Interactions between mothers and infants showing food refusal. *Infant Mental Health Journal*, 17(4), 334–347.

Linscheid, T. R. (1992) Eating problems in children. In C. E. Walker and M. C. Roberts (eds) *Handbook of Clinical Child Psychology* (2nd edn). New York: John Wiley and Sons, pp. 451–473.

Linscheid, T. R. and Rasnake, L. K. (1985) Behavioral approaches to the treatment of failure to thrive. In D. Drotar (ed.) *New Directions in Failure to Thrive: Implications for Research and Practice*. New York: Plenum Press, pp. 279–294.

Lipsitt, L. P., Crook, C. and Booth, C. A. (1985) The transitional infant: behavioral development and feeding. *American Journal of Clinical Nutrition*, 41, 485–496.

Lloyd, D. A. and Pierro, A. (1996) The therapeutic approach to the child with feeding difficulty: III. Enteral feeding. In P. B. Sullivan and L. Rosenbloom (eds) *Feeding the Disabled Child*. London: Mac Keith Press, pp. 132–150.

London Food Commission (1985) *Food and Drink for the Under Fives* (dietary information for those working in day care). Available from Box 291, London N5 IDV.

Loveday, E. (1996) Diagnostic imaging and special investigations in the assessment of the disabled child. In P. B. Sullivan and L. Rosenbloom (eds) *Feeding the Disabled Child*. London: Mac Keith Press, pp. 77–91.

Lowenberg, M. E. (1981) The development of food patterns in young children. In C. B. S. Wood and J. A. Walker-Smith (eds) *MacKeith's Infant Feeding and Feeding Difficulties* (6th edn). Edinburgh: Churchill Livingstone, pp. 85–100.

Lucas, A., Drewett, R. B., and Mitchell, M. D. (1980) Breast-feeding and plasma oxytocin concentrations. *British Medical Journal*, 281, 834–835.

McClead, R. E. and Menke, J. A. (1987) Neonatal Iatrogenesis. In L. A. Barness, A. M. Bonglovanni, G. Morrow, F. Oski and A. M. Rudolph (eds) *Advances in Pediatrics* (Vol. 34). Chicago: Year Book Medical Publishers, Inc., pp. 335–356.

McDade, T. W. and Worthman, C. M. (1998) The weanling's dilemma reconsidered: a biocultural analysis of breastfeeding ecology. *Journal of Developmental and Behavioral Pediatrics*, 19, 286–299.

McJunkin, J. E., Bithoney, W. G. and McCormick, M. C. (1987) Errors in formula concentration in an outpatient population. *Journal of Pediatrics*, 111, 848–850.

MacLean, W. C., Lopez De Romana, G., Massa, E. and Graham, G. G. (1980) Nutritional management of chronic diarrhea and malnutrition: primary reliance on oral feeding. *Journal of Pediatrics*, 97, 316–323.

Martin, J. and White, A. (1988) *Infant Feeding 1985*. London: Her Majesty's Stationery Office.

Mathisen, B., Skuse, D., Wolke, D. and Reilly, S. (1989) Oral-motor dysfunction and failure to thrive among inner-city infants. *Developmental Medicine and Child Neurology*, 31, 293–302.

Mennella, J. A. and Beauchamp, G. K. (1996) The early development of human flavor preferences. In E. D. Capaldi (ed.) *Why We Eat What We Eat. The Psychology of Eating* Washington, DC: American Psychological Association, pp. 83–112

Menon, G. and Poskitt, E. M. E. (1985) Why does congenital heart disease cause failure to thrive? *Archives of Disease in Childhood*, 60, 1134–1139.

Minde, K. and Minde, R. (1986) *Infant Psychiatry. An Introductory Textbook*. London: Sage Publications.

Monahan, P., Shapiro, B. and Fox, C. (1988) Effect of tube feeding on oral function. *Developmental Medicine and Child Neurology*, 57, Abstract 12.

Moore, M. C. and Greene, H. L. (1985) Tube feeding of infants and children. *Pediatric Clinics of North America*, 32, 401–417.

National Academy of Sciences, National Research Council, Food and Nutrition Board (1989) *Recommended Dietary Allowances* (10th edn). Washington, DC: National Academy Press.

Nelfert, M. R. and Seacat, J. M. (1986) Medical management of successful breast-feeding. *Pediatric Clinics of North America*, 33, 743–762.

Oates, R. (1984) Similarities and differences between nonorganic failure to thrive and deprivation dwarfism. *Child Abuse and Neglect*, 8, 439–445.

Oates, K., Peacock, A. and Forrest, D. (1985) Long term effects of nonorganic failure to thrive. *Pediatrics*, 75(1), 36–39.

Ottenbacher, K., Bundy, A. and Short, M. A. (1983) The development and treatment of oral-motor dysfunction: a review of clinical research. *Physical and Occupational Therapy in Pediatrics*, 3, 1–13.

Patrick, J., Boland, M., Stoski, D. and Murray, G. E. (1986) Rapid correction of wasting in children with cerebral palsy. *Developmental Medicine and Child Neurology*, 28, 734–739.

Pollitt, E., Eichler, A. W. and Chan, C. K. (1975) Psychosocial development and behavior of mothers of failure to thrive children. *American Journal of Orthopsychiatry*, 45, 525–537.

Polnay, L. and Hill, D. (1985) *Community Paediatrics*. Edinburgh: Churchill Livingstone.

Premack, D. (1959) Toward empirical behavior laws: I. Positive reinforcement. *Psychological Review*, 66, 219–233.

Pridham, K. (1987) Meaning of infant feeding issues and mothers' use of help. *Journal of Reproductive and Infant Psychology*, 5, 145–152.

Provence, S. and Lipton, R. C. (1962) *Infants in Institutions*. New York: International Universities Press.

Pryor, H. B. and Thelander, A. G. (1967) Growth deviations in handicapped children. *Clinical Pediatrics*, 6, 501–512.

Pugliese, M., Weyman-Daum, M., Moses, N. and Lifshitz, F. (1987) Parental health beliefs as a cause of NOFT. *Pediatrics*, 80(2), 175–182.

Puntis, J. W. L., Ritson, D. G., Holden, C. E. and Buick, R. G. (1990) Growth and feeding problems after repair of oesophageal atresia. *Archives of Disease in Childhood*, 65, 84–88.

Ramsay, M. (1995) Feeding disorder and failure to thrive. *Child and Adolescent Psychiatric Clinics of North America*, 4(3), 605–616.

Ranke, M. B., Heidemann, P., Knupfer, C., Enders, H., Schmaltz, A. A. and Bierich, J. R. (1988) Noonan syndrome: growth and clinical manifestations in 144 cases. *European Journal of Pediatrics*, 148, 220–227.

Reilly, S. and Skuse, D. (1992) Characteristics and management of feeding problems of young children with cerebral palsy. *Developmental Medicine and Child Neurology*, 43, 379–388.

Reilly, S., Skuse, D., Mathisen, B. and Wolke, D. (1995) The objective rating of oral-motor functions during feeding. *Dysphagia*, 10, 177–191.

Reilly, S. M., Skuse, D. H., Wolke, D. and Stevenson, J. (1999) Oral-motor dysfunction in children who fail to thrive: organic or non-organic? *Developmental Medicine and Child Neurology*, 41(2), 115–122.

Rempel, G. R., Colwell, O. and Nelson, R. P. (1988) Growth in children with cerebral palsy fed via gastrostomy. *Pediatrics*, 82, 852–862.

Richman, N. (1988) Feeding problems. In J. Douglas (ed.) *Emotional and Behavioural Problems in Young Children: A Multi-Disciplinary Approach to Identification and Management*. Windsor: NFER-Nelson, pp. 11–17.

Richman, N., Stevenson, J. and Graham, P. J. (1982) *Preschool to School: A Behavioural Study*. London: Academic Press.

Rider, E. A. and Bithoney, W. G. (1999) Medical assessment and management and the organization of medical services. In D. B. Kessler and P. Dawson (eds) *Failure to Thrive and Pediatric Undernutrition*. Baltimore: Paul H. Brookes Publishing Co. Inc., pp. 173–194.

Riordan, M. M., Iwata, B. A., Finney, J. W., Wohl, M. K. and Stanley, A. E. (1984) Behavioral assessment and treatment of chronic food refusal in handicapped children. *Journal of Applied Behavior Analysis*, 17, 327–341.

Roberts, M. C. (1986) *Paediatric Psychology: Psychological Intervention and Strategies for Paediatric Problems*. Oxford: Pergamon Press.

Roddey, D. F., Martin, E. S. and Swetenburg, R. L. (1981) Critical weight loss and malnutrition in breast-fed infants. *American Journal of Diseases of Children*, 135, 597–599.

Rowland, M. G. M. (1986) The weanling's dilemma: are we making progress? *Acta Paediatrica Scandinavica*, Supplement 323, 33–42.

Royal College of Midwives (1991) *Successful Breastfeeding: A Practical Guide for Midwives*. London.

St James-Roberts, I. and Wolke, D. (1984) Comparison of mothers' with observers' reports of neonatal behavioural style. *Infant Behaviour and Development*, 7, 299–310.

Sanders, M., Patel, R., Le Grice, B. and Shepherd, R. (1993) Children with persistent feeding difficulties: an observational analysis of the feeding interactions of problem and non problem eaters. *Health Psychology*, 12(1), 64–73.

Schaffer, H. R., Greenwood, A. and Parry, M. H. (1972) The onset of wariness. *Child Development*, 43, 165–175.

Schmitt, B. D. and Mauro, R. D. (1989) Nonorganic failure to thrive: an outpatient approach. *Child Abuse and Neglect*, 13, 235–248.

Schwartz, J., Engel, C. and Pitcher, A. (1986) Relationship between childhood lead blood levels and stature. *Pediatrics*, 77, 281–288.

Sheppard, J. J. (1987) Assessment of oral motor behaviors in cerebral palsy. In E. D. Mysak (ed.) *Communication Disorders of the Cerebral-Palsied: Assessment and Treatment* (Seminars in Speech and Language, Vol. 8, No. 1). New York: Thieme Medical Publishers, Inc., pp. 57–69.

Sheridan, M. D. (1956) The intelligence of 100 neglectful mothers. *British Medical Journal*, i, 91–93.

Siegel, L. J. (1982) Classical and operant procedures in the treatment of a case of food aversion in a young child. *Journal of Clinical Child Psychology*, 11, 167–172.

Singer, L., Song, L., Hill, B. and Jaffe, A. (1990) Stress and depression in mothers of failure to thrive children. *Journal of Pediatric Psychology*, 15(6), 700–720.

Skuse, D. (1985) Non-organic failure to thrive: a reappraisal. *Archives of Disease in Childhood*, 60, 173–178.

Skuse, D. (1993) Epidemiologic and definitional issues in failure to thrive. *Child and Adolescent Psychiatric Clinics of North America*, 2(1), 37–59.

Skuse, D., Wolke, D. and Reilly, S. (1992) Failure to thrive. Clinical and developmental aspects. In H. Remschmidt and M. Schmidt (eds), *Child and Youth Psychiatry. European Perspectives. Vol. II: Developmental Psychopathology*. Stuttgart: Hans Huber, pp. 46–71.

Skuse, D., Pickles, A., Wolke, D. and Reilly, S. (1994a) Postnatal growth and mental development: evidence for a sensitive period. *Journal of Child Psychology and Psychiatry*, 35(3), 521–545.

Skuse, D., Reilly, S. and Wolke, D. (1994b) Psychological adversity and growth during infancy. *European Journal of Clinical Nutrition*, 48, 113–130.

Skuse, D., Gill, D. G., Reilly, S., Lynch, M. and Wolke, D. (1995a) Failure to thrive and the risk of child abuse: a prospective population study. *Journal of Medical Screening*, 2, 145–150.

Skuse, D., Stevenson, J., Reilly, S. and Mathisen, B. (1995b) Schedule for oral-motor assessment (SOMA): methods of validation. *Dysphagia*, 10, 192–202.

Smith, S. M. and Hanson, R. (1972) Failure to thrive and anorexia nervosa. *Postgraduate Medical Journal*, 48, 382–384.

Spitz, R. (1945) Hospitalism; an enquiry into the psychiatric conditions of early childhood. *Psychoanalytic Study of the Child*, 1, 53–74.

Spitz, R. A. (1951) The psychogenic diseases in infancy: an attempt at their etiologic classification. *Psychoanalytic Study of the Child*, 6, 255–275.

Spock, B. (1968) *Baby and Child Care* (3rd edn). Boston: New English Library.

Stark, L. J., Knapp, L. G., Bowen, A. M., Powers, S. W., Jelalian, E., Evans, S., Passero, M. A., Mulvihill, M. M. and Howell, M. (1993) Increasing calorie consumption in children with cystic fibrosis: replication with 2-year follow-up. *Journal of Applied Behavior Analysis*, 26, 435–450.

Stein, A., Cooper, P. J., Day, A. and Bond, A. (1987) Social and psychiatric factors associated with the intention to breastfeed. *Journal of Reproductive and Infant Psychology*, 5, 165–171.

Stein, A., Wooley, H., Cooper, S. D. and Fairburn, C. G. (2004) An observational study of mothers with eating disorders and their infants. *Journal of Child Psychology and Psychiatry*, 35, 733–748.

Sullivan, P. and Rosenbloom, L. (eds) (1996a) *Feeding the Disabled Child*. London: Mac Keith Press.

Sullivan, P. B. and Rosenbloom, L. (1996b) The causes of feeding difficulties in disabled children. In P. B. Sullivan and L. Rosenbloom (eds) *Feeding the Disabled Child*. London: Mac Keith Press.

Taitz, L. S. (1971) Infant over-nutrition among artificially fed infants in the Sheffield region. *British Medical Journal*, i, 3115–3116.

Taitz, L. S. and Wardley, B. L. (1989) *Handbook of Child Nutrition*. Oxford: Oxford University Press.

Taylor, B. and Wadsworth, J. (1984) Breast feeding and child development at five years. *Developmental Medicine and Child Neurology*, 26, 73–80.

Truby-King, F. (1913) *Feeding and Care of the Baby*. London: Society for the Health of Women and Children.

Truswell, A. S. (1985) ABC of nutrition: infant feeding. *British Medical Journal*, 291, 333–337.

Underwood, B. A. and Hofvander, Y. (1982) Appropriate timing for complementary feeding of the breast-fed infant. *Acta Paediatrica Scandinavica*, Supplement 294, 1–32.

Van Wezel-Meijler, G. and Wit, J. (1989) The offspring of mothers with anorexia nervosa: a high risk group for undernutrition and stunting. *European Journal of Pediatrics*, 149, 130–135.

Walloo, M. P., Petersen, S. A. and Whitaker, H. (1990) Disturbed nights and 3–4 month old infants: the effects of feeding and thermal environment. *Archives of Disease in Childhood*, 65, 499–501.

Welsh, J. K. and May, J. T. (1979) Anti-infective properties of breast milk. *Journal of Pediatrics*, 94, 1–9.

Werle, M., Murphy, T. and Budd, K. (1993) Treating chronic food refusal in young children: home based parent training. *Journal of Applied Behaviour Analysis*, 26, 421–433.

Werle, M. A., Murphy, T. B. and Budd, K. S. (1998) Broadening the parameters of investigation in treating young children's chronic food refusal. *Behavior Therapy*, 29, 87–105.

Whitehead, R. G., Paul, A. A. and Ahmed, E. A. (1986) Weaning practices in the United Kingdom and variations in anthropometric development. *Acta Paediatrica Scandinavica*, Supplement 323, 14–23.

Whitehouse, P. J. and Harris, G. (1998) The inter-generational transmission of eating disorders. *European Eating Disorders Review*, 6, 238–254.

Wilensky, D. S., Ginsberg, G., Altman, M., Tulchinsky, T. H., Yishay, F. B. and Auerbach, J. (1996) A community based study of failure to thrive in Israel. *Archives of Disease in Childhood*, 75, 145–148.

Wilkinson, P. W. and Davies, D. P. (1978) When and why are babies weaned? *British Medical Journal*, 1, 1682–1683.

Wolke, D. (1986a) The Feeding Interaction Scale (FIS)-Manual. Unpublished manuscript, University of Hertfordshire.

Wolke, D. (1986b) Play Observation Scheme and Emotion Ratings (POSER). Unpublished manuscript, University of Hertfordshire.

Wolke, D. (1987) Environmental and developmental neonatology. *Journal of Reproductive and Infant Psychology*, 5, 17–42.

Wolke, D. (1993) The treatment of problem crying behaviour. In I. St James-Roberts, G. Harris and D. Messer (eds) *Infant Crying, Feeding and Sleeping: Development, Problems and Treatments*. London: Harvester Wheatsheaf, pp. 47–79.

Wolke, D. (1994) Feeding and sleeping across the lifespan. In M. Rutter and D. Hay (eds) *Development Through Life: A Handbook for Clinicians*. Oxford: Blackwell Scientific Publications, pp. 517–557.

Wolke, D. (1996a) Failure to thrive, epidemiological findings: approaches to diagnosis and treatment. Paper presented at the The Menninger Foundation, Topeka (USA), 22–23 March.

Wolke, D. (1996b) Failure to thrive: the myth of maternal deprivation syndrome. *The Signal: Newsletter of the World Association for Infant Mental Health*, 4, 1–6.

Wolke, D. (1996c) Probleme bei Neugeborenen und Kleinkindern. In J. Margraf (ed.) *Lehrbuch der Verhaltenstherapie* (Vol. 2). Heidelberg: Springer, pp. 363–380.

Wolke, D. (1999) Interventionen bei Regulationsstoerungen. In R. Oerter, C. von Hagen and G. Röper (eds) *Klinische Entwicklungspsychologie*. Weinheim: Beltz PVU, pp. 351–380.

Wolke, D. (2003) Frequent problems in infancy and toddler years: excessive crying, sleeping and feeding difficulties. In K. E. Bergman and R. L. Bergman (eds) *Health Promotion and Disease Prevention in the Family*. Berlin: DeGruyter, pp. 44–88.

Wolke, D. and Eldridge, T. (1998) The environment of care. In A. G. M. Campbell and N. McIntosh (eds) *Forfar and Arneil's Textbook of Paediatrics* (5th edn). Edinburgh: Churchill Livingstone.

Wolke, D., Skuse, D. and Mathisen, B. (1990a) Behavioural style in failure-to-thrive infants – a preliminary communication. *Journal of Pediatric Psychology*, 15(2), 237–254.

Wolke, D., Skuse, D., Reilly, S. and Sumner, M. (1990b) Socioemotional development, diet and feeding behaviour of non-organic failure to thrive infants: a whole population survey. Paper presented at the 4th European Conference on Developmental Psychology, University of Stirling, Scotland, 27–31 August.

Wolke, D., Söhne, B., Riegel, K., Ohrt, B. and Österlund, K. (1998) An epidemiological study of sleeping problems and feeding experience of preterm and fullterm children in South Finland: comparison to a South German population sample. *Journal of Pediatrics*, 133, 224–231.

Woolridge, M. and Fisher, C. (1988) Colic, 'overfeeding', and symptoms of lactose malabsorption in the breast-fed baby: a possible artifact of feed management? *The Lancet*, 2, 382–384.

Woolridge, M. W., Baum, J. D. and Drewett, R. F. (1980) Does a change in the composition of human milk affect sucking patterns and milk intake? *The Lancet*, 2, 1292–1294.

Woolston, J. L. (1983) Eating disorders in infancy and early childhood. *Journal of the American Academy of Child Psychiatry*, 22(2), 114–121.

Wright, P. (1987a) Hunger, satiety, and feeding behaviour in early infancy. In R. A. Boakes, D. O. Poppiewell, and M. J. Burton (eds) *Eating Habits, Food, Physiology, and Learned Behaviour*. London: John Wiley and Sons, pp. 26–41.

Wright. P. (1987b) Mothers' assessment of hunger in relation to meal size in breastfed infants. *Journal of Reproductive and Infant Psychology*, 5, 173–181.

Wright, P. (1993) Mothers' ideas about feeding in early infancy. In I. St James-Roberts, G. Harris and D. Messer (eds) *Infant Crying, Feeding and Sleeping. Development, Problems and Treatment*. London: Harvester Wheatsheaf, pp. 99–117.

Wright, P., Macleod, H. A. and Cooper, M. J. (1983) Waking at night: the effect of early feeding experience. *Child: Care, Health and Development*, 9, 309–319.

Wright, C., Matthews, J., Waterston, A. and Aynsley-Green, A. (1994) What is a normal rate of weight gain in infancy? *Acta Paediatrica Scandinavica*, 83, 351–356.

Yoos, H. L., Kitzman, H. and Cole, R. (1999) Family routines and the feeding process. In D. B. Kessler and P. Dawson (eds) *Failure to Thrive and Pediatric Undernutrition*. Baltimore: Paul H. Brookes Publishing Co. Inc., pp. 375–384.

Young, K. T. (1990) American conceptions of infant development from 1955 to 1984: what the experts are telling parents. *Child Development*, 61, 17–28.

Chapter 3

The nature and management of eating problems in pre-school children

Gillian Harris and Ian W. Booth

Incidence

The most frequent problem encountered in feeding the pre-school child is that of refusal to eat. Indeed, most pre-school children will refuse to eat some foods at some time during the first five years of life. In a survey of parents of pre-school children, 75 per cent of the parents reported refusal to eat at mealtimes as a problem (Eppright *et al.*, 1969). For some children, however, the problem is more extreme and of longer duration. The range of foods accepted by these children is severely limited, or the overall daily intake extremely low. In a recent pilot study that we carried out with children with diabetes, the control group of pre-school children ate a mean number of thirty-five different foods during a seven-day observation period. One child within the diabetic group, however, who was described as a problem feeder, ate only two different foods during this same period.

At present, the nutritional impact of these apparently aberrant behaviours is difficult to assess. However, the observation that 16 per cent of randomly selected children are thin, with an inappropriate low weight for height (Crisp *et al.*, 1970), would be consistent with at least some of the reported feeding difficulties being nutritionally important. Moreover, children from whose diets foods have been excluded by their parents on the basis of presumed food allergy are significantly shorter than controls between the ages of 5 and 11 (Price *et al.*, 1988). In the case of feeding problems in Asian toddlers, a nutritional impact is highly likely. One recent study of a Bangladeshi community in London (Jones, 1987) found that a high incidence of late weaning, the use of sweet convenience foods, low in iron and protein, the prolonged predominance of milk feeding and a very late progression onto family foods are common. This diet is reflected in impaired growth between 1 and 3 years of age, and a high incidence of iron deficiency anaemia (Harris *et al.*, 1983; Aukett *et al.*, 1986). It is of note that iron deficiency appears to be a readily correctable cause of developmental delay in these children (Aukett *et al.*, 1986).

The true incidence of chronic food refusal in early childhood has never been adequately established and, as with many syndromes whose incidence and definition are unclear, there is no consensus on appropriate treatment.

Definition

In attempting to define chronic food refusal we immediately encounter difficulties. We expect, of course, some long-term history of feeding problems, and would therefore exclude from our definition short-term problems, such as anorexia following inter-current infection. Frequently the child will have been quite difficult to feed from birth. Parents will often report that the infant was slow to feed, had poor sucking strength, or frequently vomited. It is important to remember, however, that the parents' description of the infant as being slow to feed is subjective. We have often noted that a rate of feeding regarded by one parent as slow is perfectly acceptable to another parent.

The onset of the problem in its extreme form usually comes with the introduction of solid foods to the infant. This introduction may be delayed until well after the age of 6 months. This may be either because the infant shows no behavioural signals that the parent might interpret as need for a greater intake than that provided by the milk diet, or because difficulties were experienced when attempting to introduce solid foods at an earlier age. There is now some evidence of a link between the late introduction of solids, and subsequent feeding problems in the child (Northstone, Emmett and Nethersole, 2001). Alternatively, chronic food refusal may have its origins in the onset of an illness which may, or may not, be related to a diminished appetite or to gastrointestinal disease. Onset therefore cannot be well defined; the infant may have a history of poor feeding, and may have an additional organic problem (past or current), but neither of these is always present.

The relationship between feeding problems and non-organic failure to thrive

While the infant may be under the recommended weight and height for age, or may show growth faltering, growth may be adequate if the feeding problem is mainly one of limited dietary range. Infants who are reported as difficult to feed and in whom there is weight faltering have been described as showing non-organic failure to thrive. However, infants with early non-organic failure to thrive are not always reported as being difficult to feed, even though their intake may be low.

Skuse (1990), in his study of a large sample of children with failure to thrive, found that mothers of infants whose weight was faltering did not report a greater incidence of feeding problems than did the mothers in the matched control group. It may be that non-organic failure to thrive and chronic food refusal are merely the two ends of a continuum in an interactional model of child feeding problems; the resolution of the child's problem is dependent upon parental response. Children with chronic food refusal typically give strong, clear signals of dislike and refusal; whereas infants with a typical pattern of failure to thrive are described as showing 'a lack of competence in communicating clearly and unambiguously their needs during mealtimes' (Skuse, 1990), or as having 'a lack of social responsiveness' (Derivan, 1982).

In the literature, chronic food refusal has been described as a type of non-organic failure to thrive, as a behavioural feeding problem (Bernal, 1972), or even as a food aversion (Handen et al., 1986). The way in which chronic food refusal is defined, therefore, is closely related to the approach being proposed for its treatment. Linscheid and Rasnake (1986), who take a behavioural approach, describe food refusal as one of two forms of non-organic failure to thrive due to 'ineffective behavioural interactions between parent and child'. In Type I non-organic failure to thrive, which is of early onset, there is pervasive disturbance in the parent–child relationship; whereas in the Type II form, which is of later onset, the disturbance in the parent–child interaction is confined to the feeding situation. In contrast, Chatoor et al. (1985) describe chronic food refusal as a separation disorder, indicative of a struggle for autonomy between parent and child. This struggle for autonomy is centred around the feeding situation, although chronic malnutrition is not seen as an inevitable outcome for the child. Chatoor et al. also stress the importance of parental anxiety about the child's health or weight gain in the maintenance of this disorder. There is, therefore, often an attempt to describe the behaviour of children who show chronic food refusal in terms of a non-organic failure to thrive model; that is, of a dysfunction within the relationship between parent and child.

It seems more sensible, however, to differentiate failure to thrive from chronic food refusal and to describe the latter in operational terms: the child has a reduced intake and exhibits negative behaviours during feeding. Such a child may behave appropriately outside the feeding situation and is unlikely to have general behaviour problems. The child's weight may be faltering or it may be within acceptable limits. The child is, however, usually securely attached to the mother, and the mother is usually extremely anxious about the child's feeding behaviour. It is this anxiety that causes the mother to adopt maladaptive behavioural strategies when feeding the child. Consideration of a reported case study shows how such maladaptive strategies emerge.

Herbert (1987) cites a case of a 2-year-old boy whose height and weight were below the third percentile. The boy was described as being difficult to feed from birth. He suffered from pyloric stenosis and frequently vomited during the first few months of life. Solid foods were unsuccessfully introduced at 5 months of age, and, from this time, feeding 'became a battle'. The child persistently refused to eat, the mother became angry and force-fed him. The infant subsequently screamed and vomited at any attempts to feed him, and eventually at the sight of the mother.

This pattern is typical of a child with chronic food refusal, with or without associated weight faltering. The course of learned food aversions in the child, and of interactional problems with the mother, is easy to follow. The definition of such a condition where there is no weight faltering, however, is problematic. The child must eat less than is thought to be adequate for a child of that weight or height, or must eat such a limited range of foods that recommended daily allowances of certain nutrients are not reached. Usually, therefore, a child whose growth is adequate is deemed as having a feeding problem if the feeding behaviour is adversely affecting parents or care-staff. That is, parents who cannot accept their child's poor or limited appetite will seek help because they feel that there is a related underlying organic problem, or because they themselves have contributed to the situation developing into a behavioural, or interactional, problem. If there is, in addition to the food refusal, an associated organic problem, then the parent might seek help because of increased anxiety about the child, or because of the importance to the child's health of maintaining an adequate, or specific, food intake. An example of this is children who are diagnosed as having diabetes and must maintain a specific dietary regimen. Such children who consistently refuse to take foods necessary to their diet are clearly at risk.

In summary, chronic food refusal may be regarded as present when there is a severely limited or restricted diet which gives rise to anxiety in the parent or referring agent, with or without associated growth faltering. There are also usually associated behavioural problems specific to the feeding process. These are learned from past feeding experiences, either of adverse consequences of ingesting food, or of interactions with others during the feeding process. The difference between chronic food refusal and non-organic failure to thrive is that, in the latter, there is always growth faltering, the parents are less likely to report that feeding the child is a problem, and the course of development of the feeding problem is less easy to describe. However, the difference between these two syndromes may only be a difference of parental reaction to an innate response to food within the child.

Similar feeding and behavioural patterns to those observed in children with chronic food refusal may also be seen in children where the onset of the problem has been physically determined, such as infants who have been nasogastrically fed for long periods, or children with cancer anorexia.

Aetiology

Difficulties in defining feeding problems are reflected in the difficulties in trying to classify the causes. A rigid differentiation into organic and non-organic causes, as has happened to some extent in the case of failure to thrive, is particularly unhelpful. Whilst some children with feeding problems may have started with a purely organic problem, they will have a mixture of organic and non-organic components by the time of referral. For example, infants who have been fed for prolonged periods by nasogastric tube, with little or no oral feeding or sucking, will commonly fail to feed orally when tube feeding is stopped (Mason, Harris and Blissett, 2005). Problems are often then compounded by attempts at force-feeding. Such children may no longer have any definable organic disease but their problem cannot be considered in purely non-organic or psychological terms. This often perplexing mixture of organic and non-organic factors is also central to management, and effective treatment will commonly depend upon the availability of a multidisciplinary assessment and management team.

Primary organic causes

In association with cerebral palsy and other causes of neurodevelopmental delay

Low calorie intake and protein energy malnutrition are important problems in children with cerebral palsy (Krick and Van Duyn, 1984). Poor chewing and increased requirements due to seizures or abnormal movements are thought to be important causal factors. Children with cerebral palsy are very slow to feed and this is associated with markedly defective oro-motor function (Gisel and Patrick, 1988). In general, even substantial prolongation and increased frequency of mealtimes cannot compensate for the defective energy intake of these children.

In association with structural defects of the oro-pharynx

Gross congenital anatomical defects such as cleft palate, macroglossia and Pierre–Robin syndrome are usually self-evident on examination (Illingworth, 1969). However, one congenital abnormality, submucous cleft palate, may be missed if the palate is not palpated at the time of the original assessment, or if the associated nasal regurgitation and nasal speech pass unnoticed (Moss et al., 1990).

Following prolonged supplementary feeding

Feeding problems following prolonged parenteral nutrition or enteral feeding in infancy are well recognised (Geertsma et al., 1985) but little studied. The prolonged absence of an oral experience and the introduction of solids after the so-called 'sensitive period' may be important factors in the aetiology of subsequent food refusal. Many children who have been delayed in the introduction of solid textured foods show an inability to cope with those foods in the mouth, hypersensitivity in the mouth, and an extreme gag response. This secondary oro-motor dysfunction may present as a seemingly 'behavioural problem'; the child refuses or accepts food in a seemingly idiosyncratic fashion.

Following oesophageal surgery

Feeding difficulties are common following surgical correction of congenital atresia (Puntis *et al.*, 1989) and gastro-oesophageal reflux (Harnsberger *et al.*, 1983), and may be associated with growth retardation.

Oesophageal dysmotility and continuing gastro-oesophageal reflux, particularly in the oesophageal atresia group, may be important in the aetiology of long-standing symptoms.

In association with disordered gastrointestinal motility

It is well recognised that disorders of gut motility may occur in association with abnormal feeding (Milla, 1986). In recent years a number of new techniques for investigating oesophageal and small intestinal motility, gastro-oesophageal reflux and gastric emptying have become available for use in children (Milla, 1986; Harnsberger *et al.*, 1983; Smith *et al.*, 1989; Sondheimer, 1988; Cucchlara *et al.*, 1990). The use of these techniques has already indicated that there may be a group of children who present with what is predominantly a feeding problem but with subtle anomalies in gut motility.

For example, one child was recently referred at the age of 2 with a history of poor feeding beginning at birth, vomiting and constipation. Considerable parental anxiety had been generated, and there had been attempts at force-feeding. The child had already been seen by many professionals in many disciplines. On investigation, he was found to have gastro-oesophageal reflux (twenty-four-hour ambulatory oesophageal pH recording), delayed gastric emptying (epigastric impedance technique), abnormal oesophageal peristalsis on a barium swallow, and abnormal small bowel motility (jejunal manometry). He responded promptly to a pro-kinetic drug (cisapride) which enhances gut motility.

Secondary to organic disease

Anorexia is a prominent symptom in several pediatric disorders, notably coeliac disease, Crohn's disease, chronic renal failure, congenital heart disease and advanced cystic fibrosis. Appetite improves with successful treatment of the primary disease.

Children with growth disorders (poor growth)

Appetite in early childhood and infancy is a function of growth velocity and energy expenditure; only in later childhood and adulthood do extrinsic factors, such as the need to finish up what is on the plate, come into play. Children with growth disorders are therefore likely to have small appetites appropriate for their growth velocity. Where the growth disorder is more easily diagnosed (bone dysplasia), then interactive feeding problems are less likely to occur between parent and child. However, where the syndrome is less easily recognised (Turners, Russell-Silver), and may in fact not be identified until later childhood, interactive feeding problems are common (Blissett, Harris and Kirk, 2001). Children with Russell-Silver, or IUGR without catch-up growth, are primarily identified by their poor feeding and poor growth. If a correct diagnosis is not made, then the parents are often given inappropriate advice from health professionals which may lead to coercive feeding practices. There is also a high incidence of oro-motor disorder in children with Russell-Silver, Turners and IUGR, which often goes undiagnosed, and can lead to poor feeding and food refusal (Blissett, Harris and Kirk, 2001).

Primary non-organic causes

Constitutional factors

The first and most obvious part of our explanation might be that some children have small appetites because they are constitutionally or genetically small. In either case the child will need less food than the parent expects the child to consume for optimal health. These expectations may be based on the usual daily intake of other siblings, the usual daily intake of the parents themselves, the expectations of health workers such as health visitors or dieticians, or even information in booklets circulated to new mothers by commercial baby food manufacturers. These booklets often give examples of daily diets which are based on what most infants will eat at any specific age. The parent has, therefore, an unrealistic expectation of what the infant should be eating, and becomes anxious when the infant refuses to eat the expected amount. This anxiety may also be increased if the infant has, or has had in the past, a non-related physiological problem which has already raised parental anxiety about the child and increased their desire to keep the child in optimal physical health. It is often difficult for parents to understand that, at least by the time solid food is introduced, a healthy child is able to regulate its own intake to accord with its own caloric needs. (The child cannot, however, regulate its own intake to provide a nutritionally balanced diet.) If the child's weight is progressing at the expected rate, then any problems with feeding behaviour have usually begun with parental anxiety about infant intake (Bernal, 1972). This anxiety often decreases as the number of offspring increases, but this is not always true. If older children have all had 'good' appetites, then a later-born child with a small appetite will be perceived as problematic by comparison. If the child's weight is faltering, then parental anxiety will be a contributory factor to the feeding problem, but will not usually have been so critical to its onset.

Most children with small appetites will eat a wide range of foods, even though dietary range does decrease with appetite (Harris, 1997). A small group of children, mainly boys, do, however, seem to have a feeding problem which means that the range of foods that they eat is severely limited, even though growth may not be compromised. This feeding problem does not seem to be a function of poor early experience, or of parental management style, but seems to reflect a perseverant style of eating within the children. Foods are rejected if they are not of a normally accepted brand or flavour, if they are different in texture, or burnt or discoloured in any way. The children tend to adhere to a diet comprising very few foods, and will not improve their diet by imitating family or peer group. The children tend to show more sensory reactivity, responding strongly to food smells, to be more rule-bound, and to have more problems with social interactions (Harris *et al.*, 2000). These children have a type of feeding problem that can commonly be observed in children with autism and Asperger's syndrome, although the children themselves may not meet the criteria for inclusion in these diagnostic groups. It could be, however, that the children have some subclinical disability, in common with children with autism, which manifests as perseverant feeding behaviour in both groups. It certainly seems that such perseverant feeding problems do occur more frequently in some families, and this could mean that the disorder is genetically determined. The restricted diet observed in these children is not usually a problem to the child until they reach later childhood and care about peer group opinion. Such eating behaviour is often, however, a source of extreme anxiety to parents, who may exacerbate the problem by attempting to force the child to eat new foods; the child may then become more fearful around food and mealtimes.

Parental expectations about the child's daily intake, and consequent anxiety when these expectations are not met, are therefore usually involved in the maintenance of chronic food refusal.

Past learning

A further important contributory factor to food refusal is that of learned food aversion. Rozin (1986) has pointed out that the single most common precursor to the dislike of a specific food in adulthood is that the food has, in the past, been associated with vomiting. It is also interesting to note that these aversions were usually instances of one-trial learning; that is, it has taken only one association between ingestion of the food and vomiting for an aversion to be acquired. Such vomiting does not have to have been caused by the food, but only paired with the food in temporal contiguity. This rapid learning would have been a strong survival mechanism in primitive mankind. In more recent times, however, it often merely produces some rather idiosyncratic omissions in otherwise broadly ranging diets. Or, in the case of children receiving chemotherapy with associated vomiting, such learning exacerbates the problem of a reduced appetite in a child with cancer. This one-trial learning might also be the explanation for breast refusal apparent in a small percentage of children in studies investigating cultural patterns in infant weaning practice (Harris, 1988). Certainly in all of a series of studies on the precursors to food refusal in pre-school children, gastric pain and vomiting were often the best predictors (Johnson, 1999).

In addition to specific learned aversions, we may also include in our explanation of the ontogeny of chronic food refusal the lack of positive learning experiences with certain tastes. The preference for sweet foods in many children is innate (Crook, 1978), although this preference may be modified by subsequent dietary experience (Beauchamp and Moran, 1984). For other tastes, however, preference would seem to be based upon dietary experience, in infants of 6 months (Harris and Booth, 1987), and dietary exposure, in infants as young as 3 months (Johnson, 1999). The foods we eat and the tastes we prefer are, therefore, largely culturally determined. Experience with and exposure to a taste or food will eventually induce a preference. Birch, in her work with pre-school children, has even suggested the number of exposures to a taste which might be needed before a preference is induced: fourteen (Birch and Marlin, 1982). In some children, therefore, the refusal to eat a wide range of foods may merely reflect a dearth of experience with a range of tastes. There are even data which suggest that there may be a sensitive stage during which taste preferences are more rapidly acquired: infants exclusively breastfed until 5 or 6 months of age showed less preference for cereal with an added tastant than did exclusively breastfed infants at 3 to 4 months of age who were tested at that time. The prolonged experience with the relatively bland taste of breast milk in the period between 4 and 6 months had induced a preference for a low level of tastant in the test food. Infants are often observed who, when offered new appropriate foods, will refuse them, possibly because their experience of solid foods for the first months after introduction has been confined to those with a predominantly sweet taste (Harris *et al.*, 1990).

A second period of 'sensitivity' is also just beginning to be identified. Those children who have not had food of a more solid texture than purée or mash introduced to them by about 14 months are likely to show an inability to manage such foods in the mouth. This induced secondary oro-motor dysfunction manifests as an inability to move more solid textured foods around the mouth, to chew and place them appropriately for swallowing. The mouth is therefore more hypersensitive to tactile stimulation, and the gag response is more extreme than would be normally observed. Children with secondary oro-motor dysfunction therefore gag, choke and vomit when attempting to eat solid textured foods; these foods are usually avoided after the first attempt to eat them (Mason, Harris and Blissett, 2005).

Developmental stage

If we accept that there is a developmental stage at which a range of tastes might be introduced with optimal acceptance, then it might also be wise to consider other developmental stages which may affect food acceptance. At the age of approximately 12 months, the infant's attitude to feeding can often be observed to change. This marks the beginning of the age of autonomy. The child will want to feed him- or herself, and will often refuse to be spoon-fed. At this age also the child has learned to prefer, not specific tastes, but specific foods with the sum of tastes, textures and consistency with which they are familiar (Harris and Booth, 1987). This means that home-made versions of a well-liked commercial baby-food will be refused because of slight differences in recipe. The second year of life also shows the onset of neophobia (the fear of tasting new foods), which once might have had a socio-biological function in protecting the infant from poisoning as greater mobility was attained. At this age children will start to be identified as 'fussy' by their parents as they refuse new foods on sight alone (Birch and Marlin, 1982). As there is also a decline in growth velocity after the first year (Williamson et al., 1988), and an increase in the child's own need for auton-omy, the second year of life is therefore often a time at which more parents identify their children as difficult to feed.

A child's food preferences are learned during the first years of life; neo-phobia also increases during these first years. This means that, as the child gets older, it becomes increasingly more difficult to introduce new foods to a child with a limited diet, and oral feeding to a child who has never taken food by mouth (Harris, 2000). For children with secondary oro-motor dysfunc-tion, the fear of eating foods which may, because of their texture, cause the child to choke or vomit will increase the longer the child avoids them.

Intervention programmes should therefore be put into place as soon as it is feasible, even with a child with concurrent organic problems, rather than leaving the feeding programme until organic problems have been resolved.

Maladaptive parent–child interactions

It is probable that physiological factors, experience with food, and develop-mental stage all contribute to the incidence of chronic food refusal; however, it has also been proposed that the perception of a child's feeding behaviour as problematic may be dependent upon parental anxiety. This suggests that many feeding problems may have an interactional component; that is, a predisposition in the child which interacts with a set of expectancies or coping strategies in the parent, to present as chronic food refusal.

Let us first consider the predisposing factors within the child. It is fre-quently reported anecdotally that children with chronic food refusal are strong-willed and 'uncuddly'. Such children often fit the Thomas et al. (1968)

description of a 'difficult' child, arhythmic and responding negatively to new stimuli. Lindberg *et al.* (1994) found that 'difficultness' in an infant was a predisposing factor in failure to thrive; and it is probable that children who are described as 'difficult' and who usually gain a high score on emotionality components of temperament questionnaires are difficult because of their refusal to try new foods (Pliner and Loewen, 1997). The core characteristic that contributes to the 'difficultness' of a child is the need to control incoming stimuli. We may explain this characteristic at different levels. First, we might describe it as a strong need for autonomy, a need not to have one's behaviour controlled by others. Secondly, it could be a heightened sensitivity to stimuli, which might make aversive anything new or extreme. Thirdly, it could be dependent upon the strength or awareness of internal signals of satiety. Finally, it could merely be due to the strength of the infant's behavioural signals of satiety. It is, of course, difficult to differentiate between these hypotheses merely by observation. However, children, usually boys, who adhere rigidly to very limited diets do also score very highly on measures of reactivity to sensory stimuli, as well as scoring highly on the 'emotional' component of a temperament measure (Harris, 2000). It has also been shown that infants as young as 3 months can use behavioural signals, when spoon-fed, which reliably signal both satiety and preference (Harris *et al.*, 1990). However, the strength and conviction with which these signals are given, that is the clarity of the signal, seems to vary from child to child. This could be a function of the child, as we have already suggested, or it could be a function of the interaction between child and parent. It is most probable that it is both.

We have discussed the ways in which factors within the child may contribute to the feeding problem, but it must also be clear that factors within the parent also contribute. The parent may not appropriately accede control of the feeding process to the child, either because of insensitivity to the infant's behavioural signals or because of a conscious decision to override them. If the parent is anxious about the child's growth, then this conscious decision is more likely to be made. If a child's behavioural signals of satiety are consistently ignored then we may expect that the expression of these signals will become stronger, or so extreme, that they can no longer be ignored. It might be, therefore, that children scream, throw food, struggle, spit or even vomit, because these are the only behaviours which are effective in regaining control of their intake.

However, behavioural extremes are not always the function of the interaction with the parent. One child observed by us over a period of two years, whose feeding was sensitively handled by the mother and whose weight gain and general health were both excellent, nevertheless always showed extreme negative behavioural responses to food. While still being spoon-fed, the spoon was frequently knocked away, however gently it was proffered, and food was often spat from the mouth after being accepted. This child was also reported to have an extreme response to any new stimuli, and had, for example, screamed when she first stood on sand with bare feet. It is also of interest to note that this child was a breast-refuser. The child was therefore one of the small group of children with high sensory reactivity and high arousal who always present as difficult to feed.

On the other hand, we have also observed a child, over a similar two-year period, who never seemed to show any behavioural signals of satiety. This child would open his mouth for food whenever, and for as long as, it was offered to him. By the end of his first year his weight was far greater than would have been predicted by his height. The weight gain decreased, however, during the second year as we would expect, when the child began to feed himself.

For these children, both the one who was difficult to feed and the one who was easy to feed, the maintenance of appropriate growth was dependent upon the sensitivity of the parent when feeding the child. Anxious parents tend to be less sensitive when managing feeding interactions, and this in turn leads to food refusal by the child (Blissett and Harris, 2002).

In summary, then, we can say that the ontogenesis of chronic food refusal is dependent upon many factors which may operate singly or in interaction. Food refusal might be caused by constitutional factors, past learning, developmental stage, infant temperament, or maladaptive interactions with the parent.

Assessing the child

There is a lack of consensus about the appropriate place for referral for children who are refusing to eat. In the UK children may be referred to a pediatric gastroenterologist if there is associated vomiting, constipation, diarrhoea or weight faltering. Some of these symptoms, in conjunction with reduced appetite, may indeed indicate an organic problem, but not invariably. Weight faltering and constipation can be the result of a limited or restricted diet, whereas vomiting can be induced at will, and indeed be functional in stopping force-feeding. Food refusal, without concomitant physiological symptoms, might be referred to a health visitor, dietician or speech therapist, all of whom would take a different approach in treatment. Occasionally, if the problem is extreme, or the parent sufficiently desperate, the child will be referred to a psychologist. Many parents, however, have difficulty in getting any specialist help because their first point of referral, the general practitioner or physician, is apt to view the problem as self-limiting; that is, that the child will grow out of the problem without any treatment and without any ill effects. For children without weight faltering this is, of course, often true, except in the case of extremely perseverant children, for whom the problem will endure until adulthood (Harris, 2000). However, the stress on parents and siblings can often be extreme, possibly more so than with other behavioural management problems, because the health of the child is seen to be at risk. Both referral and treatment of chronic food refusal are therefore often idiosyncratic, and attempts to quantify incidence or monitor intervention schedules have proved difficult because of the perceived self-limiting nature of the problem.

Establishing a diagnosis: the role of the multi-disciplinary team

On reviewing the potential causes of feeding problems in pre-school children, it becomes clear that accurate diagnosis and management lie outside the expertise of any single professional group. Consequently, it is our practice to work as part of a multi-disciplinary feeding team, comprising a clinical psychologist, pediatrician, dietician, speech therapist and clinical nurse specialist in nutrition. The presenting symptoms in a child whose poor feeding results exclusively from non-organic causes may be indistinguishable from those of a child whose problems arise from, for example, an oro-motor dysfunction. It is crucial therefore to distinguish between the two. Thus, one important task of a multi-disciplinary team is to make an accurate diagnosis and, in particular, avoid overlooking organic disease such as mild cerebral palsy, growth 'syndromes' or other disorders leading to impaired oro-motor function, or disorders of gut motility and other anatomical abnormalities.

Clearly, a system whereby each patient was routinely assessed by four or maybe five professional colleagues would be hopelessly impractical and time consuming. Equally, there is no place for every patient undergoing a 'routine' series of invasive investigations. However, the judicious use of radiological contrast studies, oesophageal pH monitoring and motility studies may occasionally be therapeutically enlightening. So, in patients with a history of structural abnormalities of their gastrointestinal tract, particularly the foregut, and in those children with histories of vomiting, choking, constipation, recurrent pulmonary diseases (suggesting aspiration), or severe failure to thrive, some investigation is usually essential.

In practice, patients are referred to any member of the feeding team, who completes an assessment questionnaire (see Appendix 1). The results of the questionnaire are then discussed at a meeting of the team, at which appropriate investigations (if any) are planned together with an intervention strategy. All patients undergo a clinical assessment of nutritional status (weight, length/height, skin-fold thicknesses, mid upper arm circumference) and a dietary assessment, to establish the severity of any nutritional sequelae. If it is suspected that there is any oro-motor dysfunction, or an interactional component to the child's feeding problem, then an observation will be made of the child being fed by the primary caregiving parent. This observation is usually carried out by the psychologist and the speech and language therapist. The extent to which the child has control of the feeding process is assessed, as well as antecedents and consequences of problematic behaviour.

Management

Introduction

Clearly, it is important that management should be tailored to the individual needs of each patient, taking into account not only diagnosis, but also nutritional status and the long-term natural history of the disorder. This is particularly important in the case of handicapped children with severe oro-motor dysfunction. These children may be suffering from severe protein-energy malnutrition (Patrick *et al.*, 1986), and despite a number of techniques to improve feeding (Crane, 1987), efforts to improve oro-motor function have not been successful (Ottenbacher *et al.*, 1981). Early recourse to long-term enteral nutrition may therefore be the best option.

Approaches to behavioural treatment

It is difficult to predict reliably which children without organic impairment might show long-term behavioural feeding problems, because the indices used to make such predictions have been derived from retrospective enquiry. It is clearly the case that not all infants who are slow to feed from birth, have a small appetite, frequently vomit, or have solid foods introduced to them relatively late in the first year, exhibit a subsequent dislike of the feeding process. We have much, as yet unpublished, data from other research studies on feeding in infancy where many or all of these problems were present from or after birth and yet feeding behaviour in the second year of life was perfectly acceptable. However, from work carried out with children referred for psychological intervention at a children's hospital, some models have emerged of the aetiology of chronic food refusal on which intervention strategies may be based. The key to the problem is, perhaps, suggested by the fact that early predisposing factors occur in some children in whom the chronic syndrome does not arise. It is the behavioural management, or mismanagement, of specific children that gives rise to a chronic feeding problem. It must be stressed, however, that this does not apply to those children whose disability or illness, in itself, causes problems with appetite or ability to feed. Children who have been tube fed for long periods because of organic problems may exhibit a refusal to feed orally. Subsequent feeding behaviour, especially in an infant following prolonged tube feeding, may be similar to that of a child who is physically unimpaired but has a learned fear of feeding. The presenting problem may be similar but the interventions must differ, with account taken of the particular disease process.

Intervention strategies must be based on a detailed analysis of each individual case of food refusal, for not only is there little data available on the incidence and treatment of cases in general, but also differing aetiologies will produce the same outcome, namely limited or restricted food intake.

Intervention

Reducing parental anxiety

Our strategies for intervention with the child who shows chronic food refusal are based partly upon our aetiological model, and partly upon research studies which have looked at the phenomenology of appetite increase, or changes in food preference, in normal samples of children. In each case, intervention must be based on the child's individual history of feeding problems. Every intervention, however, is usually based on three components: reducing anxiety in the parent, acceding control of feeding to the child, and educating the parent in the management of the child's feeding behaviour. A similar approach is taken by Herbert (1987), with somewhat more emphasis placed upon improving overall the relationship between mother and child, and rather less emphasis placed specifically upon improving child feeding behaviour.

Reducing parental anxiety is important as a first stage for intervention, for subsequent stages are based upon re-educating the parent. The parent needs to be reassured that there is no physiological cause for loss of appetite and subsequent food refusal in the child. If the child's weight is faltering then the parents may have difficulty in accepting that there is no appropriate medical intervention. If the child does have some organic problem, then parents will need to understand that, although appetite may be small due to the disease process, different feeding management programmes may give rise to different outcomes in terms of food acceptance and growth. Also, an even greater problem for the therapist, the parents will have to accept that the intervention may result in short-term weight loss (Linscheid et al., 1987).

Acceding control to the child

When acceding control of feeding to the child it is important for the parent to accept that all coaxing, force-feeding and lengthy distraction techniques should be dropped from mealtimes. This will be extremely anxiety-provoking for many parents, and their co-operation will be dependent upon their faith in the therapist. It is therefore always wise to spend as much time as possible explaining to the parents the rationale behind the intervention programme. It is especially difficult for anxious parents to accept that a child might be able adequately to regulate intake. In order to help parents relinquish lengthy feeding techniques it is useful to set a time limit on feed-times, usually of approximately twenty minutes. When starting the intervention programme, the range of foods offered to the child should also be confined to those few that the child readily accepts, or will sometimes accept. This may pose problems for children who, of necessity, are on a specific diet, but for all others attention to the balance of nutrient intake should be waived for the first part of the intervention programme. If the child is still being spoon-fed then a further step is for the parents to be shown how to regulate the feeding process by using the child's behavioural signals of hunger, preference or satiety (Harris *et al.*, 1990). By these means, control of the feeding process, in terms of both how much is eaten and what is eaten, will be given to the child. Mealtimes should therefore become less aversive for both child and parent.

It must be remembered, however, that if a child is to try a new food, then that child must be motivated in some way to try it. Children do not eat foods, as adults might, because someone else thinks that they should change their diet.

Social reinforcement

The third phase of the intervention programme is to educate the parent in techniques that will enhance either appetite in general or the specific consumption of certain foods. The most powerful technique for attaining the child's compliance during feeding is the use of social reinforcement. The child is rewarded for 'good' feeding behaviour by positive facial regard or positive verbal reinforcement by the parent. All aberrant feeding behaviour is responded to by facial aversion. To begin with, 'good' feeding behaviour may only be sitting appropriately in a high chair; if this is so then a shaping procedure must be implemented. Mealtimes should be closely spaced to maximise the opportunities for practice, and to reduce the pressure to eat at any one meal. The model here is of classical conditioning rather than of operant conditioning; the child should be reinforced when eating, not after eating. The use of social reinforcement in this way can have so strong an effect that the child's internal signals of satiety may be overridden. It is also important when using this technique to point out to parents the reinforcing properties, to most children, of any kind of attention. The parent must remember to take uneaten food away without comment, and to refrain from discussing the child's odd eating habits in front of others. We have observed pre-school children who take quite a pride in their limited intake or faddish diet. (We have also heard a parent take pride in telling others that her child would only eat one, rather, exotic, food, as if this were indicative of her child's fastidiously good taste.) One of the maintaining factors of a feeding problem for the child is the attention gained from others and the power that this gives them to control others within their environment (Handen *et al.*, 1986).

In order for positive affect and eating to be paired, it is important to ensure that the child's social environment, when eating, is pleasant. This may mean that the child should be fed with the rest of the family, if family mealtimes are not tense. It may also mean that the parent who usually feeds the child may have to relinquish the task whenever possible to someone else. Some parents are extremely tense, anxious or depressed by the time they find appropriate help with their feeding problem, and because of this are not best able to implement a programme of social reinforcement. Also, when considering the social environment of mealtimes, the parent should be asked to note whether the child eats more in certain situations than in others, and this information should be utilised in the intervention programme. Many children have been observed to eat more in certain social situations (e.g. parties, visits to restaurants) than they usually eat. This is because of the reinforcing nature of social situations on eating behaviour (Birch *et al.*, 1980).

Modelling and imitation

Young children and infants will most readily imitate the adults who are feeding them, and will want to try the foods that adults are eating, or eat exclusively from a parent's plate (Harper and Sanders, 1975). This need to imitate adult models can be used to start a feeding programme, in that, at the beginning of the programme, it is important to get the child to try any new food, no matter what the source. Some of the food tried in this way may not be useful in the long term but the freedom to imitate should be encouraged; parents are sometimes shocked to find that a food-refusing child will drink beer from their father's glass.

Pre-school children have also been noticed to increase their intake and modify their food preferences when eating with groups of similar aged children (Birch, 1980). Children of this age prefer to be 'like' their peers and will imitate their behaviour. Birch (1980) even noted that the child's intake, modified to accord with that of other children, was still maintained some weeks later.

Our first aim has been to increase the child's overall intake; however, for some children with a severely restricted range of foods, the task is to introduce specific foods into the diet. Birch's (1980) method of peer group modelling can be used to increase both intake and the range of foods accepted by the child, although it does not work with the severely food phobic child. Nevertheless, we often suggest, as part of our intervention programme, that food-refusing children should eat with their peer group whenever possible. It is important, however, that the child should not be reinforced by the supervisor of the meal for not eating, and that other children within the group should be reinforced for their good eating behaviour.

Exposure to new foods

A less time-consuming method of introducing new foods, especially with an infant who may still be spoon-fed, is to offer a very small amount of the target food along with preferred foods at a number of mealtimes. Since food preference is a function of exposure (Birch and Marlin, 1982; Harris and Booth, 1987), if a child can be motivated by social reinforcement repeatedly to taste a food, then a preference for that food may be induced. This will be a far more difficult process, however, if the child has a strong aversion to the taste of the food, and is therefore more easily attempted with neutral foods. The target food should, however, never be 'hidden' in an accepted food; this will usually serve to condition an aversion to the accepted food.

When attempting to increase the range of foods of children with secondary oro-motor dysfunction, it must be remembered that care has to be taken with the texture of the foods being introduced. Oral skill should be encouraged by starting with bite and dissolve foods before progressing to the slightly firmer textures. 'Difficult' foods such as bread and meat should be introduced last in the programme.

It should also be remembered that, whichever method is used to attempt to get a child to try new foods, a preference for a novel taste or food can only be induced after repeated exposures. The child not only has to be motivated to try the food, they also have to be motivated to try the food many times before they feel that they like it.

Reward food

Similar behavioural intervention strategies to those outlined above have been suggested by different research groups. Frequently, however, the rationale underlying the intervention strategies is not made clear. For example, Chatoor *et al.* (1985) suggest as part of their intervention strategy that food should not be given as a reward; whereas both Linscheid and Rasnake (1986) and Bernal (1972) outline programmes in which preferred food is used as a reinforcer for consumption of non-preferred food. However, research carried out with pre-school children (Birch and Marlin, 1984; Lepper *et al.*, 1982) shows that if there is a contingent pairing between the consumption of two foods, then the 'instrumental food' will be cognitively devalued and its consumption decrease, whereas the value of the 'reward' food will be enhanced and its consumption increased. These data show that using food as a reward enhances its desirability in the mind of the child. However, the effect of using one food, especially a preferred food, as a reward for the consumption of another, non-preferred food, is to decrease the desirability of the non-preferred food and increase the desirability of the preferred food. Thus, in the long term, if a non-preferred food is used as an 'instrumental food' then its desirability will decrease. If we are concerned, as we must be, about the child's cognitions about the food that is to be eaten, then it is safe to use food as a reward (Birch *et al.*, 1980) but not as an instrumental task. Parents often ask whether a food-refusing child should be offered a second course within a meal, if the first course has not been eaten. It might appear that, by so doing, the child is being rewarded for not eating the less desirable (because not sweet) first course. However, this is not the case; pre-school children can differentiate between contingent tasks and those which merely follow in temporal contiguity.

We have also observed in our own intervention programmes that these cognitions about food also affect those foods that are deemed special (i.e. forbidden) and those foods that are made too freely available. Children on high calorie diets happily eat cucumber instead of chocolate, and most fussy children eat crisps. For these children, cucumber and crisps are withheld foods, and therefore are more likely to be seen as desirable.

Conclusion

We have defined children presenting with behavioural feeding problems which restrict or limit their dietary intake as showing chronic food refusal. We have made a case for such a syndrome not to be categorised with early non-organic failure to thrive, although children showing chronic food refusal may also show weight faltering. The behaviour of children with chronic food refusal but with no organic disease is similar to that of children who have been ill and tube fed for the first months of life. This refusal to feed is caused by negative learning experiences about food or feeding, oro-motor dysfunction, 'difficult' temperament, or high sensory reactivity combined with sub-clinical features of Asperger's syndrome. In some cases there has also been a dearth of positive early experience. The strong behavioural signals of refusal are developed in order that the child might control the feeding process. These behaviours may protect the child from the aversive consequences of feeding which may in the past have resulted in pain or vomiting. In the child with no organic impairment the behaviours are strong signals of satiety; weaker signals may have hitherto been ignored by the parent because of parental anxiety about the child's health or unrealistic expectations about the child's intake.

The intervention programme suggested for all children showing chronic food refusal, whether physiologically impaired or not, is behaviourally based. There is, however, strong emphasis upon educating the parent in the underlying rationale of the treatment and attending to, and analysing, feeding interactions between parent and child. We also see the need to understand the child's cognitions about feeding and food preferences.

Appendix 1

Feeding assessment form

Name	
Consultant	
Ward	
Reg. no.	
Completed by	
Date of birth	

1	What problem is your child having?
(a)	Has a poor appetite
(b)	Eats a limited variety of foods
(c)	Prefers drinks rather than food
(d)	Is slow to feed
(e)	Cannot chew food
(f)	Other, please specify

2	Does your child have any of the following problems?
(a)	Vomiting
(b)	Constipation
(c)	Diarrhoea
(d)	Abdominal pain and colic

Management

3	Feeding position at home?	
	Lap	Standing
	Baby bouncer	Cot
	High chair	Other, please specify
	Table/chair	
	Settee/armchair	

4	In what room do you feed your child?	
	Living room	Bedroom
	Dining room	Playroom
	Kitchen	Other

5	Who mainly feeds or supervises feeding?	
	Name:	
	Mother	Grandparent
	Father	Sister/brother
	Friend	Child minder
	Home helper	Other, please specify

6	Does the child usually eat with other people?	
	Parents	Child's friends
	Brothers/sisters	Neighbour
	All family	Grandparents
	By self	Other, please specify

7	What are the usual times of:		
		(a) meals?	**(b) drinks?**
	Breakfast		
	Mid-morning snack		
	Midday		
	Mid-afternoon snack		
	Evening meal		
	Bedtime snack		

8	Are feeding times (put a mark on the scale showing how you feel):	
(a)	Relaxed	Stressful
(b)	Noisy	Quiet
(c)	Unrushed	Hectic
(d)	Tearful for parents	Happy for parents
(e)	Happy for child	Tearful for child

9	Is your child's appetite:	
	Poor	Good

10	Do you think your child eats enough?	
	Yes	No

11	Is your child difficult to feed?	
	Not difficult	Difficult

Feeding behaviour/appetite

12	Does the amount of food taken by your child fluctuate from day to day?			
	Yes	No	Sometimes	Don't know

13	Does your child accept food one day but reject it on another?			
	Yes	No	Sometimes	Don't know

14	Does your child accept new foods?			
	Yes	No	Sometimes	Don't know

15	Please indicate the average duration of time to eat in the evening meal/tea
	0–10 minutes
	10–20 minutes
	20–30 minutes
	30–60 minutes
	Over 60 minutes

16	Duration of time to eat snack (e.g. biscuit)
	0–10 minutes
	10–20 minutes
	20–30 minutes
	30–60 minutes
	Over 60 minutes

17	Does your child exhibit any of the following when given food?					
		No	Yes	If yes, how often?		
				Each meal	Once a day	Once a week
(a)	Throws food/pushes food away					
(b)	Spits food					
(c)	Chews food, but will not swallow					
(d)	Turns head away repeatedly					
(e)	Closes mouth when offered food					
(f)	Knocks spoon away					
(g)	Cries/screams at the beginning of the feeds					
(h)	Cries/screams at the end of the feeds					
(i)	Vomits after or during meal					
(j)	Dribbles food out of mouth					

18	If your child doesn't finish a course or part of a meal, what do you do?
	Take it away
	Attempt to make child eat food
	Distract the child to eat
	Offer next course
	Offer child reward for eating

19	If your child is a messy eater, does it bother you?		
	Yes	No	Don't know

20	How many people does it take to feed the child?
	Feeds self
	One
	Two
	Three
	Other

21	Do you need to distract your child when eating?	
	Yes	No
	If yes, please indicate how this is achieved	
	Television	Games of aeroplanes
	Toys	Other children playing
	Reading	Other, please specify
	Singing	

22	What type of food is offered?					
		Does eat	Can eat	Never tried	Can't or won't eat	What happens when they refuse?
	Stage 1 baby-food					
	Adult purée food					
	Stage 2 baby-food					
	Adult mashed food					
	Finger foods					
	Normal adult consistency					
	Fluids only					

23	**Current feeding skills**	
	Spoon-fed by parent	Drinks from cup/glass
	Finger foods fed by parent	Drinks from straw
	Feeds self with fingers	Pours own drink
	Feeds self with spoon	Prepares own snacks
	Feeds self with fork	Other
	Uses knife	Has child ever self-fed?

24	**Which of the following foods are currently refused?**	
	Meats	Vegetables
	Fish	Potatoes/rice/spaghetti
	Eggs	Bread/chapatti
	Cheese	Breakfast cereal
	Milk	Fruit
	Yoghurt	Puddings
	Sweets/chocolate	Crisps
	Soups	Squash/lemonade
	State reason for refusal of foods	

25	**Temperature: child's reaction to:**		
		Likes	Dislikes
	Hot food		
	Cold food (ice cream/lollies)		
	Warm food		

26	**Flavour: child's reaction to:**		
		Likes	Dislikes
	Sour		
	Salty		
	Savoury		
	Sweet		
	Highly flavoured		

27	**Food intolerances**
	Please list:

28	**Vitamin supplements**
	Please list:

29	**Mineral supplements**
	Please list:

30	Dietary supplements	
		Quantity per day
	Glucose polymer	
	Hycal/fortical	
	Fresubin	
	Build up	
	Fortisip	
	Liquisorb	
	Other	

31	Is there a physical handicap affecting feeding?		
	Yes	No	Don't know

32	Has the child ever seen a speech therapist?	
	Yes	No

33	Do you think your child's speech is delayed?	
	Yes	No

Do you have any other problems with feeding your child that are not covered here?

Source: Adapted from a feeding problem questionnaire written by Jean Guest and Dr D. Kelly, University of Nebraska, Medical Centre, Omaha, USA.

References

Accardo, P. J. (1982) Growth and development: an interactional context for failure to thrive. In P. J. Accardo (ed.) *Failure to Thrive in Infancy and Early Childhood: A Multi-disciplinary Approach*. Baltimore: University Park Press.

Aukett, M. A., Parks, Y. A., Scott, P. H. and Wharton, B. A. (1986) Treatment with iron increases weight gain and psychomotor development. *Archives of Disease in Childhood*, 61, 849–857.

Beauchamp, G. K. and Moran, M. (1984) Acceptance of sweet and salty tastes in 2-year-old children. *Appetite*, 5, 291–305.

Bernal, M. (1972) Behavioural treatment of a child's eating problem. *Journal of Behavioural Therapy and Experimental Psychiatry*, 3, 43–50.

Birch, L. L. (1980) Effects of peer models' food choice and eating behaviors on preschoolers' food preferences. *Child Development*, 51, 489–496.

Birch, L. L. and Marlin, D. W. (1982) I don't like it, I never tried it: effects of exposure to food on two-year-old children's food preferences. *Appetite*, 3, 353–360.

Birch, L. L. and Marlin, D. W. (1984) Eating as a 'means' activity in a contingency: effects on young children's food preference. *Child Development*, 55, 431–439.

Birch, L. L., Zimmerman, S. I. and Hind, H. (1980) The influence of social-effective context on the formation of children's food preference. *Child Development*, 50, 856–861.

Blackman, J. A. and Nelson, C. L. (1985) Reinstituting oral feedings in children fed by gastrostomy tube. *Clinical Pediatrics*, 24, 8, 434–438.

Blissett, J. and Harris G. (2002) A behavioural intervention in a child with feeding problems. *Journal of Human Nutrition and Dietetics*, 15, 1–7.

Blissett, J., Harris, G. and Kirk, J. (2001) Feeding problems in children with Silver-Russell Syndrome. *Developmental Medicine and Child Neurology*. 43, 39–44.

Chatoor, I., Dickson, L., Schaefer, S. and Egan, J. (1985) A developmental classification of feeding disorders associated with failure to thrive: diagnosis and treatments. In D. Drotar (ed.) *New Directions in Failure to Thrive: Implications for Research and Practice*. New York: Plenum Press.

Crane, S. (1987) Feeding the handicapped child, a review of intervention strategies. *Nutrition and Health*, 5, 109–118.

Crisp, A. H., Douglas, J. W. B., Ross, J. M. and Stonehile, E. (1970) Some developmental aspects of disorders of weight. *Journal of Psychosomatic Research*, 14(3), 313–320.

Crook, C. (1978) Taste perception in the newborn infant. *Infant Behaviour and Development*, 1, 52–69.

Cucchlara, S., Staianal A. and Boccieri, A. (1990) Effects of cisapride on parameters of oesophageal motility and on the prolonged intraoesophageal pH test in infants with gastro-oesophageal reflux disease. *Gut*, 31, 21–25.

Derivan, A. T. (1982) Disorders of bonding. In P. J. Accardo (ed.) *Failure to Thrive in Infancy and Early Childhood: A Multi-disciplinary Approach*. Baltimore: University Park Press.

Eppright, E. S., Fox, H. M., Fryer, B. S., Lamkin, G. H. and Vivian, V. M. (1969) Eating behaviour of pre-school children, *Journal of Nutrition Education*, 1, 16–19.

Geertsma, M. A., Hyams, J. S., Pelletier, J. M. and Reiters, S. (1985) Feeding resistance after parenteral hyperalimentation, *American Journal of Diseases in Childhood*, 139, 255–256.

Gisel, E. G. and Patrick, J. (1988) Identification of children with cerebral palsy unable to maintain a normal nutritional state. *Lancet*, i, 283–286.

Handen, B., Mandell, F. and Russo, D. (1986) Feeding induction in children who refuse to eat. *American Journal of Diseases in Children*, 140, 52–54.

Harnsberger, J. K., Corey, J. J., Johnson, D. G. and Herbst, J. J. (1983) Long-term follow-up of surgery for gastro-oesophageal reflux in infants and children. *Journal of Pediatrics*, 102, 505–508.

Harper, L. and Sanders, K. (1975) The effect of adults' eating on young children's acceptance of unfamiliar foods. *Journal of Experimental Child Psychology*, 20, 206–214.

Harris, G. (1988) Determinants of the introduction of solid food. *Journal of Reproductive and Infant Psychology*, 6, 241–249.

Harris, G. (1997) Development of taste perception and appetite regulation. In G. Bremner, A. Slater and G. Butterworth (eds) *Infant Development; Recent Advances*. Hove: Psychology Press.

Harris, G. (2000) Developmental, regulatory and cognitive aspects of feeding disorders. In A. Southall and A. Schwartz (eds) *Feeding Problems in Children: A Guide for Health Professionals*. Abingdon: Radcliffe Medical Press.

Harris, G. and Booth, D. A. (1987) Infants' preference for salt in food: its dependence upon recent dietary experience. *Journal of Reproductive and Infant Psychology*, 5, 97–104.

Harris, R. J., Armstrong, D., Ali, R. and Loynes, A. (1983) Nutritional survey of Bangladeshi children aged under 5 years in the London Borough of Tower Hamlets. *Archives of Disease in Childhood*, 58, 428–432.

Harris, G., Thomas, A. M. and Booth, D. A. (1990) Development of salt taste in infancy. *Developmental Psychology*, 268, 535–538.

Harris, G., Blissett, J. and Johnson, R. (2000) Food refusal associated with illness. *Child and Adolescent Mental Health*, 5, 4, 148–156.

Herbert, M. (1987) *Behavioural Treatment of Children with Problems: A Practice Manual*. London: Academic Press.

Illingworth, R. S. (1969) Sucking and swallowing difficulties in infancy: diagnostic problem of dysphagia. *Archives of Disease in Childhood*, 44, 655–665.

Illingworth, R. S. and Lister, J. (1964) The critical or sensitive period with specific reference to certain feeding problems in infants and children. *Journal of Pediatrics*, 65, 839–848.

Johnson, R. (1999) Development of taste preferences in infancy. Unpublished PhD thesis, University of Birmingham.

Jones, V. M. (1987) Current infant weaning practices within the Bangladeshi community in the London Borough of Tower Hamlets. *Human Nutrition: Applied Nutrition*, 41A, 349–352.

Krick, J. and Van Duyn, M. S. (1984) The relationship between oral-motor involvement and growth: a pilot study in a paediatric population with cerebral palsy. *Journal of the American Dietary Association*, 44, 555–569.

Lepper, M., Sagotsky, G., Dafoe, J. and Greene, D. (1982) Consequences of superfluous social constraints on young children's social inferences and subsequent intrinsic interest. *Journal of Personality and Social Psychology*, 2, 1, 51–65.

Lindberg, L., Bohlin, G., Hagekull, B. and Thunstrom, M. (1994) Early food refusal; infant and family characteristics. *Infant Mental Health Journal*, 15, 3, 262–277.

Linscheid, T. R. and Rasnake, L. K. (1986) Behavioural approaches to the treatment of failure to thrive. In D. Drotar (ed.) *New Directions in Failure to Thrive: Implications for Research and Practice*. New York: Plenum Press.

Linscheid, T. R., Tarnowski, K. J., Rasnake, L. K. and Brams, J. S. (1987) Behavioural treatment of food refusal in a child with short-gut syndrome, *Journal of Pediatric Psychology*, 12, 3, 451–459.

Mason, S., Harris, G. and Blissett, J. (2005) Tube feeding in infancy: implications for the development of normal eating and drinking skills. *Dysphagia*. 20, 1.

Milla, P. J. (1986) Intestinal motility and its disorders. ® *MDBR Clinical Gastroenterology*, 15(i), 121–136.

Moss, A. L. H., Jones, K. and Piggott, R. W. (1990) Submucous cleft palate in the differential diagnosis of feeding difficulties. *Archives of Disease in Childhood*, 65, 182–184.

Northstone, K., Emmett, P., Nethersole, F. and the ALSPAC Study Team (2001) The effect of age of introduction to lumpy solids on foods eaten and reported feeding difficulties at 6 and 15 months. *Journal of Human Nutrition and Dietetics*, 14, 43–54.

Ottenbacher, K., Scoggins, A. and Wayland, J. (1981) The effectiveness of oral sensory-motor therapy with the severely and profoundly developmentally disabled. *Occupational Therapy Journal of Research*, 147–160.

Palmer, S., Thompson, R. J. and Linscheid, T. R. (1975) Applied behaviour analysis in the treatment of childhood feeding problems. *Developmental Medicine and Child Neurology*, 17, 333–339.

Patrick, J., Boland, M. P., Stoski, J. and Murray, G. E. (1986) Rapid correction of wasting in children with cerebral palsy. *Developmental Medicine and Child Neurology*, 28, 724–739.

Pliner, P. and Loewen, E.R. (1997) Temperament and food neophobia in children and their mothers. *Appetite*, 28, 239–254.

Price, C. E., Rona, R. J. and Chinn, S. (1988) Height of primary school children and parents' perceptions of food intolerance. *British Medical Journal*, 196, 1696–1700.

Puntis, J. W. L., Ritson, D. G., Holden, C. E. and Buick, R. G. (1989) Growth and feeding problems after repair of oesophageal atresia. *Archives of Disease in Childhood*, 65, 84–88.

Robinson, P. H., Clarke, M. and Barrett, J. (1988) Determinants of delayed gastric emptying in anorexia and bulimia nervosa. *Gut*, 29, 458–464.

Rozin, P. (1986) One trial acquired likes and dislikes in humans; disgust as a US, food predominance and negative learning predominance. *Learning and Motivation*, 17, 180–189.

Skuse, D. (1990) Failure to thrive: clinical and developmental aspects. In H. Reinschmidt and M. Schmidt (eds) *Child and Youth Psychiatry: European Perspectives. Vol. II: Developmental Psychopathology*. Stuttgart: Hans Huben.

Smith, H. L., Newell, S. J., Puntis, J. W. L., Hollins, G. W. and Booth, I. W. (1989) Use of epigastric impedance recording to measure gastric emptying in two infants with dumping syndrome. *European Journal of Gastroenterology and Hepatology*, 1, 77–132.

Sondheimer, J. M. (1988) Gastrooesophageal reflux: update pathogenesis and diagnosis. *Pediatric Clinics of North America*, 35(i), 103–116.

Thomas, A., Chess, S. and Birch, H. G. (1968) *Temperament and Behaviour Disorders in Children*. London: University of London Press.

Williamson, D., Prether, R., Heffer, R. and Kelley, M. (1988) Eating disorder; psychological therapies. In J. L. Marston (ed.) *Handbook of Treatment and Approaches in Childhood Psychopathology*. New York: Plenum Press.

Chapter 4

Body dissatisfaction and dieting in children

Andrew J. Hill

In a review of the body image literature Grogan notes the ubiquity of discontent: 'It seems that some body dissatisfaction is the common experience of most people raised in Western culture' (Grogan, 1999). Gender shapes this experience as women are more dissatisfied with their bodies than men. Furthermore, these dissatisfactions drive behaviour and lead to attempts at change. Dieting is commonplace, indeed regarded as the normative eating behaviour of American women (Polivy and Herman, 1987). The commercial sector that supports dieting, exercise and cosmetic surgical alteration is proliferating. The underlying collective belief is that the body is infinitely malleable and that with dieting or exercise, or the two in the correct combination, every woman can reach her ideal.

It is against this cultural backdrop that children's regard of their own weight and shape must be examined. Children do not grow up in a social vacuum. They are sensitive to prevailing social mores, and anticipate adulthood, looking around for clues to the most important issues. And appearance is important. But at what age do shape and weight concerns emerge? Do they show the same patterns of dissatisfaction expressed by adults, the gender differences, the specific body areas? How are these concerns linked in with dieting and other weight control attempts? Above all, how are they acquired and maintained? And how might we limit them or prevent their escalation?

This chapter will seek answers from the current research literature. The focus will be on younger age groups, primarily 7–12 year olds, the so-called pre-adolescents. In knowledge terms, they are the poor relations of their adolescent siblings in whom we are accustomed to the jagged landscape of body discontent. Accordingly, these answers will be partial at best.

The emergence of shape and weight concerns

The question of when and how shape and weight concerns show themselves draws from research with adolescents. Those investigations that have stratified their sample by age report concerns even in the youngest groups. For example, Richards *et al.* found extreme weight and eating concerns in 15 per cent of their 11–13 year olds (in contrast with 32 per cent of those aged 14–15) (Richards and Casper, 1990). Similarly, Cooper and Goodyer found that 15 per cent of the 11–12 year old girls studied had significant shape and weight concerns, as measured by the Eating Disorders Examination (Cooper and Goodyer, 1997). As it is unlikely that such concerns arise on the first day of high school, some girls of junior school age must share these views.

One research method that has become increasingly popular has been to investigate children's body figure preferences. Taking their lead from Fallon and Rozin's studies of undergraduate preferences (Fallon and Rozin, 1985), researchers have used or developed their own pictorial body shape scales. Among the first to examine pre-adolescents was Collins (1991). She used a scale of seven female or male figures, ranging from thin to obese, to examine the current and ideal figure choices of over 1,000 children with a mean age of 8. The boys' ideal shape was very close to their choice of current shape. In contrast, the girls' ideal shape was much thinner than either their current self-perception or the boys' ideal. In other words, even at this early age girls were expressing a basic dissatisfaction with body shape that was not shared by boys.

Using a similar methodology of scaled drawings we compared the body shape preferences of 9 year old girls and boys (Hill *et al.*, 1994). Overall 41 per cent of the girls placed their preferred body shape at a thinner point than their current shape. Of the boys, 41 per cent placed their ideal at a point broader than their current perception, with only 28 per cent choosing a thinner ideal. Similar gender differences and levels of preference have been reported by same age children elsewhere in the UK (Parkinson *et al.*, 1998), in America (Thompson *et al.*, 1997) and in Australia (Rolland *et al.*, 1997).

Brodie *et al.* added a distorting mirror method of body image appraisal to the scales of body shape drawings described above (Brodie *et al.*, 1994). Girls aged 9 and 14 years old wearing black leotards used the distorting mirror to indicate their current and ideal body shape. They showed a very slight tendency to perceive themselves as fatter than they really were. But, and in line with results from the pictorial scales, their ideal shape was significantly thinner than their current perception. Importantly, there were no clear age differences in the setting of this ideal.

A very different approach to understanding the emergence of shape and weight concerns has been the development of a children's version of the Eating Attitudes Test (ChEAT). Maloney *et al.* gave the ChEAT to over 300 children aged 7–13 and found that 8.8 per cent of the girls scored at or above the cut-off used to indicate eating disorders in adults (Maloney *et al.*, 1989). Excluding the youngest group of boys, only one (less than 1 per cent) of the boys achieved such a score. Accompanying questions showed that 55 per cent of the girls and 34 per cent of the boys answered 'yes' to 'Have you ever wanted to be thinner?' Clear age trends were apparent with 40 per cent of the youngest girls and 79 per cent of the oldest girls agreeing with this statement.

Another study to have used ChEAT scores to define probable caseness is that by Rolland *et al.* (1997). Overall, 14 per cent of the 10 year old girls and 8 per cent of the boys had a score of 20 or above. Disconcertingly, caseness decreased with increasing age. The very high scores gained by the youngest children in this study and that of Maloney *et al.* therefore raise doubts over children's understanding of the questions asked and the concepts addressed (Maloney *et al.*, 1989).

One issue largely absent from the above literature is the degree to which body shape satisfaction relates to actual body weight. Shape and weight discontent may be legitimised if such feelings are expressed only by those girls who are overweight or obese. In a study of 15 year old girls Wadden *et al.* found that those who were overweight were indeed significantly more dissatisfied with their weight and figure than their leaner peers (Wadden *et al.*, 1989). These girls, however, did not have a monopoly on such dissatisfaction. Girls in all weight categories, with the exception of the very underweight, wished to lose some weight.

In an extension of this research, we examined 9 year olds' body shape preference in relation to their actual body weight (Hill *et al.*, 1994). Nearly 10 per cent of the underweight and 35 per cent of the average weight girls had a thinner ideal shape than perceived current shape, double the proportion of boys in these weight categories. This gender difference disappeared for the heaviest children of whom around 80 per cent of both girls and boys indicated a desire to be thinner.

Having a measure of their actual weight allowed the scaling of body shape satisfaction against group average weight (Figure 4.1). A critical feature of this scaling is the point at which there is congruence between current and preferred body shapes, the point of body shape satisfaction. The overweight children apart, boys tended to fall above the line and the majority of girls below the line. Knowing the mean body weight of each group makes it possible to estimate the weight that corresponds to the collective point of body shape satisfaction. For boys the point at which preferred shape was equal to current shape was 12 per cent above their mean weight. For girls, this was at 11 per cent below their mean weight. The discrepancy between preference and reality is in harmony with the impending development of boys, but in opposition to that of girls. And because of the timing of puberty, girls have to negotiate this conflict between preferred shape and physical change at an earlier age.

The emergence of dieting

In many studies the emergence of dieting has been considered alongside that of shape and weight concerns. Maloney *et al.*, for example, reported that 41 per cent of the 7–13 year old girls studied and 31 per cent of same age boys had already tried to lose weight, the most likely method being some form of

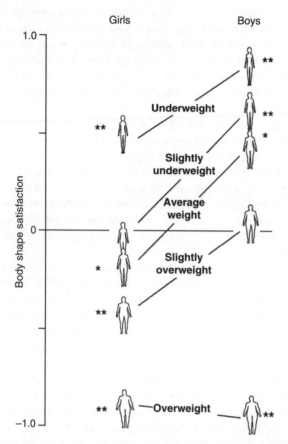

Figure 4.1 Body shape satisfaction (the difference between current and preferred body shapes) of 9 year old girls and boys in different weight categories. Significant difference between current and preferred shapes, * p<.05, ** p<.01.

Source: Hill *et al.*, 1994.

dieting (Maloney *et al.*, 1989). Unsurprisingly, these children scored higher on the ChEAT. Considering dieting concurrently with shape and weight concerns is a valuable strategy since it permits an analysis of consistency. Social desirability effects must be possible in such research given the widespread legitimacy of dieting and the social value of slimness. A key question must be whether early dieting reports co-exist with body shape or weight concerns.

One way of investigating such a relationship is to contrast the self-perception of girls who report that they are dieting with that of their peers who do not. Accordingly, Hill *et al.* examined the dieting reports of a group of 9 year old and 14 year old girls from the same school environment (Hill *et al.*, 1992). No significant difference was found in the mean levels of dietary restraint of the two age groups. Likewise, the distribution of scores was similar, indicating that there were girls who were highly restrained and reporting frequent dieting practices even among the 9 year olds. Identifying girls in the upper and lower quarters of the distribution of dietary restraint scores enabled an analysis of the effects of restraint and age on body perception. While the older girls expressed greater body discontent overall, several themes were shared by the restrained girls of both ages. The highly restrained girls were significantly more dissatisfied with their weight, their body build, and areas of their body such as their waist, hips and thighs. They also scored significantly lower on a global measure of body esteem. Looking at their body figure preferences, the unrestrained girls showed little discrepancy between their current and preferred body shape choices. In contrast, the highly restrained girls' preferred body shape was significantly slimmer than their current figure. Again, the pattern of discontent was a function of dietary restraint and unrelated to age.

Given the previous discussion of the loose coupling of shape and weight concerns with actual body weight, it is important to examine the relationship between weight and reported dieting. In the study by Hill *et al.*, the highly restrained girls were significantly heavier than the unrestrained girls, giving their dieting motivation and body discontent a flavour of legitimacy (Hill *et al.*, 1992). Indeed, over half of the restrained 14 year olds and nearly 40 per cent of the 9 year olds were more than 10 per cent above their age-standardised weight norm. But what is particularly revealing is the number of girls who were highly restrained but not overweight. Not only were the rest below this arbitrary (and low) weight threshold, but three girls (out of forty-two) could be considered underweight (<90 per cent of weight norm). For many of these girls, their motivation to diet was only loosely connected to their actual body weight. Rather, and as noted in the older girls from Wadden *et al.*'s study (1989), it was their self-perception of weight and/or shape that appeared to be the basis of their motivation to diet.

Other studies have followed this strategy of contrasting pre-adolescent 'dieters' with their non-dieting peers. Edlund *et al.*, for example, found that eleven of the fifty 7 year olds they interviewed reported already having tried to lose weight (Edlund *et al.*, 1996). This precocious group had a stronger desire to be thinner, had a significantly higher ChEAT score, perceived their current shape as larger, but were not heavier than their peers. Nor did they score higher on a simplified measure of dietary restraint. While it appears that dieting has some salience for 7 year olds, these inconsistencies in outcome and the small number of children interviewed limit the reliability of the findings and the capacity to generalise.

A more cautious approach was taken by Hill and Pallin (1998). We gave two forms of a shortened and simplified version of the DEBQ dietary restraint scale (Van Strien *et al.*, 1986) to 8 year old girls and boys. One form asked children about their own dieting behaviour. The second asked about whether a fictitious character, 'Mary-Jane', should engage in dieting behaviour. Children's responses showed that dieting was a familiar concept to them. Faced with a girl saying she was feeling fatter, and asked what she should do, both dieting and exercise were highly recommended. Again, this could be a socially desirable response to such feelings. More importantly perhaps, self-ratings of dieting practices were significantly related to children's own discontent with their appearance. Furthermore, self-rated dieting in girls was also related to elements of self-esteem such as low perceived behavioural conduct, social acceptance, and global self-worth, even when controlling for body weight. This was not the case for boys. Overall, these findings are consistent with the view that girls are drawn to weight control as a means of improving their self-worth (Hill, 1993), and that for some this starts before the age of 8.

Evidence of dieting behaviour

Two questions regularly asked of research into early dieting are, 'What proportion of these children are dieting?' and, 'How do you know they really are dieting?' Both can be hard to answer with certainty. Take the prevalence of early dieting. Although the use of dietary restraint scales is regarded as an appropriate method of measuring the regularity with which someone is attempting to diet in order to control or lose weight, it does not lend itself to simple categorisation. Frequencies do not convert easily to yes–no decisions. Therefore, while some of the research cited above focuses on the top quartile of restraint scores, it cannot be assumed that 25 per cent of these children are necessarily dieting.

A more straightforward way of estimating prevalence is to ask about current or past dieting attempts. In a cross-sectional study of American children, Thelen *et al.* found that 28 per cent, 33 per cent and 35 per cent of the 8, 10 and 12 year old girls respectively indicated they had already dieted (Thelen *et al.*, 1992). High levels of past dieting are also reported by British 12 year olds. We found that 40 per cent of 12 year old girls said they had previously dieted to lose weight, in comparison with only 15 per cent of same age boys (Edmunds and Hill, 1999). In addition, significantly more girls (20 per cent) than boys (8 per cent) were currently dieting, and there was a strong positive association between reports of current dieting and dietary restraint scores. Past and current dieting was also associated with attempts at fasting. Overall, 22 per cent of these girls reported previous episodes of fasting, although it should be recognised that a proportion of these girls were Muslim and their reports reflected observance of religious practice rather than rigorous weight control.

The association between dieting and extreme weight control methods has been observed in adolescent girls (French *et al.*, 1995a) but is more difficult to establish in younger girls. Part of the reason is the low frequency of these behaviours. In a large-scale survey of American children, Field *et al.* found that the use of laxatives or vomiting to control weight was very rare (<1 per cent) among 9–12 year old girls, despite over a quarter of this age group reporting trying to lose weight (Field *et al.*, 1999a). By the age of 14, however, 3 per cent of girls said they purged at least monthly.

But to what extent are reports of dieting behaviour accurate descriptions of alterations to eating behaviour? Experiments designed to describe and measure the eating behaviour of dietary restrained adults outside a laboratory environment have generally confirmed the picture of the restricting eater (Laessle *et al.*, 1989; Tuschl *et al.*, 1990). In addition, adolescents show a low but significant negative correlation between restraint and daily energy intake (Wardle *et al.*, 1992). But what of younger children? Do they have the ability, or the opportunity, to translate dieting motivation into dieting behaviour?

In another of our studies, a group of 9 year old girls kept a prospective record of everything they ate and drank over a seven-day period (Hill and Robinson, 1991). Parents were asked to help where possible and the diaries were checked every day to maintain quality of the recording. Analysis of the diaries revealed that restrained girls consumed 15 per cent less daily energy than their unrestrained peer group, and 11 per cent less than the dietary reference value for their age. Despite their lower energy intake, most of the indicators of nutritional quality (e.g. intake of protein, dietary fibre, calcium) showed their diets to be adequate. Only iron intake was below the reference value for this age group.

This study contrasts with three failures to associate dietary restraint or dieting with under-eating. First, Field *et al.* used a semi-quantitative food frequency questionnaire to assess daily diet over the previous year (Field *et al.*, 1993). The youngest group of girls (approx. 11 years old) showed a negative but non-significant correlation of 0.06 between self-reported frequency of dieting and estimated daily energy intake. Secondly, de Castro and Goldstein had children complete seven-day diet diaries, the instructions and all subject contact conducted by telephone and mail (de Castro and Goldstein, 1995). Although the youngest group (mean age 9.7) showed no association between restraint and daily intake, the authors acknowledged the absence of highly restrained girls in this sample. Thirdly, Braet and Van Strien found a non-significant correlation between dietary restraint and food intake recall (by children and parents) in 9–12 year old children (Braet and Van Strien, 1997). Measures of emotional eating and external eating were significantly and positively related to energy intake. However, it is important to note that the measures of dietary restraint (and other eating styles) were completed by the children's parents and not by the children themselves.

The studies described above cannot be used to dismiss the actuality of dieting behaviour in young children. First, there are several methodological features displayed in the above studies that militate against describing a simple relationship. These include the nature of food intake recording and its period, the representation of a full range of dietary restraint scores, and the opportunity for children rather than parents to describe their own dieting motivation.

Second, measures of diet quality or eating structure may be better expressions of dieting behaviour than summary energy intake. Hill and Robinson observed that restrained 9 year olds were more likely to miss meals, particularly breakfast (Hill and Robinson, 1991). These girls also had significantly higher levels of daily hunger than their unrestrained peers. Edmunds and Hill found that highly restrained 12 year old girls were less likely to eat all meals (excluding supper) and snacked less than their peers (Edmunds and Hill, 1999). Indeed, three times as many of the highly restrained girls 'never' ate breakfast. Gustafson-Larson and Terry noted a significant association between reported dieting behaviour and the frequency of adding a low calorie sweetener to food in a group of 10 year olds (Gustafson-Larson and Terry, 1992). The frequency of drinking diet soft drinks was positively associated with ten of the twelve weight-related concern statements. In addition, there was a positive correlation between the frequency of drinking diet soft drinks and body weight in girls but not in boys. Furthermore, Engell et al. have observed an association between fat content information labelling and preference for types of biscuits (cookies) in 10 year olds (Engell et al., 1998). Although the influence of restraint was not investigated in this study, it shows that children are aware of and sensitive to certain nutritional information, particularly that regarding fat.

Third, even in adults, real-life dieting is not synonymous with a rigorous and sustained restriction in food intake. The susceptibility to dieting failure is elegantly demonstrated by Herman and Polivy's research (Herman and Polivy, 1980). The experimental scenario is simple, but very powerful in its capacity to distinguish the behaviour of dieters and non-dieters. In this setting, dieting individuals can be led into a pattern of counter-regulatory eating (overeating) as compared with their usual eating or with that of non-dieters. It is a robust phenomenon with obvious face validity, and occurs in response to several disinhibiting stimuli including preloading, perceived dietary transgression, mood, alcohol and social facilitation. It is also a phenomenon that has been observed in girls aged 12 and 14 years (Hill et al., 1989). Girls at the start of adolescence who profess to diet are as liable to circumstances that lead to overeating as are older girls and women. Their pattern of eating may therefore be represented as attempts at restriction interspersed with episodes of unplanned or unwanted eating.

Transmission and acquisition

The increasing recognition of shape and weight concerns and dieting in younger age groups has prompted enquiry into the primary routes of acquisition. Just how do young children learn about the social value attached to weight and shape? From where do they learn about dieting and other methods of weight control?

Socio-cultural accounts of the development of eating disorders ask the same questions, albeit of an older age group (Stice, 1994). Generally, three channels are identified via which important cultural themes such as the thin ideal and the centrality of appearance to women are transmitted. They are the media, families, and peers. Each will be briefly reviewed according to what we do and don't know in regard to pre-adolescents.

The media

The role of the media in the development and prevention of eating disorders has been the subject of two excellent and authoritative reviews (Levine and Smolak, 1996, 1998). Many of the points discussed are pertinent to the present chapter. Take as an example our understanding of what the media comprises and the nature of its message. The slenderness of fashion models and their representation as icons of current female beauty in fashion magazines and on television is commonly seen as a primary route for media influence on young women. Outbursts of protest, however, have resulted in little change to the body shapes of chosen top models and a flat refusal to acknowledge any role in the development of eating disorders: 'Young women who tend towards anorexia do not get it from magazines, but from feelings of loss of self-worth that are instilled in them long before they are looking in Vogue' (Alexandra Shulman, editor of *Vogue*, *Guardian*, 31 May 1996).

In fact this argument is a gross over-simplification of how the media may influence eating disorders. First, as the term implies, the mass media is a vast and expanding conglomerate of communication encompassing television, radio, magazines, newspapers, books and other printed media, advertising, the internet, and more. It engages a heterogeneous, anonymous and enormous audience with a variety of purposes including selling, education and entertainment. So while parts of the mass media may be culpable, others consider themselves broadly innocent. Second, the diversity of the mass media is commensurate with the complexity of its message. Levine and Smolak have listed a variety of possible negative media effects in terms of the belief system that is expressed (Table 4.1; Levine and Smolak, 1996). Promoting thinness as the 'gold standard' for women's body shape is a small part of the media endorsed package. The confusion of image with reality and the marketing of impossible expectations are pernicious and widespread.

Third, little distinction is apparent in the audience that receives this belief system. This collection of values is broadcast in so many forms that there is little segregation in terms of women from men, or young from old. Even if they focus on the lives of young women, everyone is invited to endorse these values. This failure to protect the younger sections of society will be discussed further below, but the amount of access to visual media by children is now

Table 4.1 Media-endorsed beliefs relevant to eating disorders

Creation of slenderness as the 'gold standard' for a narrow range of ideal body shapes.

Promotion of slenderness as the path to social, sexual and occupational success for women.

Emphasis on the possibility and desirability of personal transformation through fashion and dieting.

Promotion of the importance (i.e. reality) of image as substance.

Establishment of gender roles based on impossible expectations.

Fatness as a sign of personal loss of control and failure.

Source: After Levine and Smolak, 1996.

quantifiable. Between the ages of 8 and 12 the amount of time spent watching TV programmes increases from 2.5 to 4 hours per day. During the 8.00 to 9.00 p.m. prime-time slot, more than half of all American children are watching television (Levine and Smolak, 1998). Children view up to 20,000 advertisements per year, over half of which are for food products of debatable nutritional quality (Dibb, 1996).

But what of the research evidence? Can this extent of exposure be shown to result in early weight and shape concerns, dieting, and more? The answer is a qualified 'no'. Levine and Smolak conclude that content analyses of relevant magazines and television programmes broadly show the expected glorification of thinness and weight loss (Levine and Smolak, 1996). However, the small number of experimental studies that have manipulated exposure to such content do not generally demonstrate increases in body dissatisfaction. Only in studies that establish participants' pre-existing weight and shape concerns is there evidence of media impact. For those young women who have such concerns, exposure to thin models and weight-loss information exacerbates their conflicts and problems, in the short term at least. Critically, however, there is virtually no research that identifies the media in the development of such a predisposition in children or adolescents.

Two studies published since Levine and Smolak's reviews demonstrate some of the problems in this area. Field *et al.* examined the perceived influence of fashion magazines on shape and weight contentment and weight control from survey data collected in 1991 (Field *et al.*, 1999b). Of the 500-plus girls aged 9–17, 85 per cent reported some exposure to fashion magazines, with 26 per cent reading such magazines at least twice a week. Two-thirds of the girls agreed with the statement, 'Do you think that pictures of women in magazines influence what you think is the perfect body shape?' Nearly half agreed with 'Do pictures of women in magazines make you want to lose weight?' Importantly there was an association between the perceived influence of the media and the frequency of reading women's fashion magazines. In particular, girls who were frequent readers were two to three times more likely than infrequent readers to report dieting or exercising because of a magazine article, and to agree that magazines influence what they believe is the ideal body shape. On the face of it this appears strong evidence of the impact of fashion magazines on the initiation of weight and shape concerns. However, causality is a major problem. It is just as likely that girls already dissatisfied with their body weight and shape are drawn to media that enforce their negative and possibly distorted weight and shape beliefs.

In an experimental investigation, Champion and Furnham showed pictures of thin models, overweight/obese women, or house interiors to girls aged 12, 14 and 16 (Champion and Furnham, 1999). This brief exposure had no effect on the girls' self-perception even when analysed according to their pre-existing levels of body shape satisfaction. In accounting for this absence of expected outcome the authors identify a problem inherent in otherwise tightly controlled experimental research: the weakness of a brief exposure to media images in comparison with a continuous, often unnoticed, bombardment.

A further problem with this literature is that it is descriptive rather than theory-driven. Levine and Smolak present alternative perspectives from the communications literature that have potential in this regard: cultivation theory, and uses and gratification theory (Levine and Smolak, 1998). Theories from social psychology may also prove useful (Waller and Shaw, 1994). Social comparison theory, for example, describes the need to use others as a source of information about social phenomena such as body shape ideals in order to evaluate one's own attitudes and self-perception. It follows that those with high social comparison needs should be more likely to use media images and be more sensitive to their portrayal in evaluating their own body image. Using this framework, Martin and Kennedy found that brief exposure to pictures of highly attractive models raised the comparison standards for physical attractiveness in adolescent girls but not in 10 year olds (Martin and Kennedy, 1993). In other words, the perceived attractiveness of a 'standard' model was dependent on the attractiveness of a preceding set of fashion images. This did not, however, generalise to the girls' own self-perception. We have also shown this change in comparison standard to occur in ratings of thinness made by 10 year old girls following exposure to pictures of thin versus more normal-weight young women (Atchison, 1999).

In short, what studies in this area must focus on is the characteristics of individuals that make them more or less susceptible to media images. The acceptance that media engagement is an active process is an essential step to take. Rather than asking what types of media have the most impact on children's shape and weight concerns we should be asking what types of children or what characteristics of children make them more vulnerable to body focus media. And all the time we should be reminding ourselves that for most of the time children's engagement with media is informative and pleasurable (Levine and Smolak, 1996).

Families

For the family as a route of transmission and acquisition it is more accurate to read 'parental', or indeed to change this to 'maternal'. The great majority of the research to be described has focused on mothers and their influence on their daughters. Mothers are still regarded as the gatekeepers of family nutrition. Moreover they are the most obvious role models of eating and weight issues for their growing daughters. A reasonable prediction, therefore, would be of a close correspondence between the weight and eating attitudes of mothers and daughters. Accordingly, Pike and Rodin looked at the mothers of 16 year old girls selected on the basis of their daughter's degree of disordered eating (Pike and Rodin, 1991). The mothers of girls who scored highly on such symptoms themselves scored significantly higher than mothers of girls with low scores on a compound of three subscales of the Eating Disorders Inventory (Garner et al., 1983): drive for thinness, bulimia, and body dissatisfaction.

If this association is apparent for extreme attitudes, can it also be shown for dieting behaviour at a much younger age? We examined the dietary restraint of a group of 10 year old girls and interviewed the mothers of high and low scoring girls (Hill et al., 1990). A strong correlational relationship was found ($r = 0.68$) between the degree of dietary restraint expressed by the girls and their mothers. In addition, the highly restrained girls shared with their mothers a perceived susceptibility in their eating control to the disinhibitory effects of negative mood states. Not only did the girls appear to be modelling their dieting behaviour on that of their mothers, but they learned and gave the same reasons for dieting failure. Further evidence comes from our study of 8 year olds. The perception of whether mum would diet if she felt fat was a strong predictor of children's dieting awareness (Hill and Pallin, 1998).

Central to accounts of this relationship is an explanation based on social learning mechanisms of transmission. However, the notion that girls are simply modelling mothers' current concerns is over-simplistic. Although some studies have reported significant correlations between the current dieting of mothers and daughters (Ruther and Richman, 1993), others have not. For example, Hill and Franklin found no difference in the dietary restraint of mothers of dieting and non-dieting 12 year old girls (Hill and Franklin, 1998). Nor was there a difference in the age these mothers first dieted, the maximum weight loss achieved, or their current weight. Part of the problem is that 70 per cent of all the mothers had previously dieted. However, on closer examination it was noted that the mothers of dieting girls had a greater lifetime weight range, and were more likely both to fast and to snack between meals. Against a background of commonplace weight control, therefore, these subtle differences may be markers of more intense past dieting behaviour or of current dieting failure.

Parents are not merely passive in modelling their weight concerns for their children. There is evidence of active involvement. Striegel-Moore and Kearney-Cooke reported that parents of 6–11 year olds, who themselves had been on a weight-loss diet in the past year, were more likely to have tried to help their child lose weight than parents who had not been on a diet (Striegel-Moore and Kearney-Cooke, 1994). Parental encouragement to control weight was also found to be positively associated with dieting in a study of 9 and 10 year old girls (Thelen and Cormier, 1995). In addition, mothers' comments have been observed to be especially influential (Keel et al., 1997).

In considering active parental involvement, two further issues arise from the literature. First, children's own self-reports implicate parental comments (Schreiber et al., 1996), as do studies that have directly asked parents themselves (Smolak et al., 1999). These two sources of information will not necessarily correspond as parents may be unaware of the hurt caused by their comments or children may differ in their resilience to parental comments. However, it is children's perception of parental involvement that is most important. Second, the comments made by fathers should not be overlooked. Two studies have specifically identified father's pressure for thinness (Shisslak et al., 1998a) and father's own weight dissatisfaction and comments on their daughter's weight (Keel et al., 1997) in contributing to their daughter's weight concerns.

If this intergenerational transmission implicates fathers as well as mothers, then siblings and other members of an extended family need to be considered. Again, this complexity is not reflected in the research literature, with virtually no research that includes other family members. A clue to the relevance of family environment comes from studies of girls from Asian families. Mumford et al. found a higher prevalence of eating disorders in 15 year old Asian girls living in the UK, compared with their Caucasian peers (Mumford et al., 1991). Importantly, abnormal eating attitudes and body shape dissatisfactions were unrelated to the degree of Westernisation of the family but were positively related to the family's traditional orientation. In other words, the most symptomatic Asian girls came from the most traditional Asian family environment.

We found a similar association between levels of dietary restraint and a measure of traditional orientation in British-born 9 year old Asian girls (Hill and Bhatti, 1995). Those girls who were most concerned with dieting and had greater body dissatisfaction came from a more traditional Asian family environment. One interpretation is that these girls are torn between competing cultural values operating outside and inside the home. For girls growing up within a traditional Asian family, conflict may arise over several issues, including arranged marriages, norms regarding dress, contact with the opposite sex, the role of women, mealtimes and cooking. Intercultural and intrafamilial conflicts add to the difficulties in achieving the developmental tasks of adolescence and in combination with the Western focus on body image and thinness make these girls especially vulnerable. This vulnerability is likely to increase during adolescence as the cultural contrast in social roles increases (McCourt and Waller, 1995).

A final perspective on family involvement in weight concern and dieting is that of perception of family functioning. Alongside shared high levels of weight concern, Pike and Rodin observed that both the mothers and their symptomatic daughters desired more family cohesion than they currently had (Pike and Rodin, 1991). Similarly Attie and Brooks-Gunn noted that mothers of adolescent girls with eating problems perceived their families as having less cohesion, organisation and expressiveness (Attie and Brooks-Gunn, 1989). In our study of 12 year old girls (Hill and Franklin, 1998), both the daughters who reported dieting and their mothers were less satisfied with current family cohesion, family organisation and moral-religious emphasis than the non-dieting comparison group. Dissatisfaction with characteristic areas of perceived family functioning is evident in families with a young dieter and in families with eating disordered adolescents. This suggests that the observed differences in family functioning are not merely consequences of coping with a dieting or eating disordered individual. Weight and shape dissatisfactions and the resultant alterations to eating behaviour do not occur in isolation from other domains of family existence. This is an important reminder of the dynamic nature of family functioning, with dissatisfactions in self-perception having the potential to influence dissatisfactions in other domains, and vice versa.

Peers

Early adolescence sees a change in the balance of children's social support from parents to peers. From the age of 12 and onwards parents become less important as support providers, although they rarely become unimportant (Berndt and Hestenes, 1996). The role of peers in the transmission and prioritisation of weight and shape issues should also increase and change with age. Unfortunately, this intragenerational transmission is largely unexamined in girls prior to adolescence. This is despite Maloney et al. observing that 45 per cent of their 7–13 year old girls had a friend who was dieting and 16 per cent agreed that their friends would like them more if they were thinner (Maloney et al., 1989).

The literature examining peer influences on adolescent dieting has been reviewed by Paxton (1996). She gives several examples of the ways in which talking about weight and dieting ('fat talk') could be functional in adolescent peer group interactions. One that is indicated by having high numbers of dieting friends is the giving and receiving of weight control information and advice. Although studies of adolescents find little evidence of direct encouragement to diet (Paxton *et al.*, 1991), some patients with eating disorders cite encouragement from a friend to lose weight as a trigger (and others, specific media images). But talking about dieting with friends also serves to highlight issues such as the importance of thinness, and shared negative perception of particular body areas. The sharing of these sentiments enhances the feeling that they are normative and may also serve to promote affiliation within a group.

The potential for body shape dissatisfaction and weight-loss behaviours to exert influence on adolescent friendship groupings has recently been examined by Paxton *et al.* (1999). Using social network analysis to identify girls' friendship clusters or cliques, these authors found higher within-group similarity for body image concern, dieting and extreme weight-loss behaviours than occurred between groups. In addition, groupings of 15 year old girls scoring high in body dissatisfaction and dieting showed high levels of peer engagement in weight and shape related issues.

Research with younger age groups has not asked similar sophisticated questions regarding peer influence. Rather, questions about numbers of friends dieting, and talking about weight and weight loss with friends, have been combined into single 'peer messages' factors for predictive analyses. In a study of 10–14 year old girls, Levine *et al.* found this peer messages factor to be correlated with both dieting and ChEAT scores (Levine *et al.*, 1994). Likewise, the perceived importance that peers put on weight and eating, strongly predicts weight concern in 9–12 year old girls (Barr Taylor *et al.*, 1998). So while there is evidence that peer opinion and behaviour are important before adolescence, we know far less about how they operate. Do the same mechanisms operate at age 9 as have been described at 15?

One possible exception is peer teasing about weight. If 'fat talk' is broadly a positive peer engagement, then 'fat teasing' is negative and excluding. Broadly assessed measures of peer teasing about weight have been shown to predict weight concern in 11–15 year old girls, but not in 9–12 year olds (Barr Taylor *et al.*, 1998). Similarly, Thompson *et al.* found past episodes of teasing related to later adolescent shape and weight concerns (Thompson *et al.*, 1995). Unfortunately, neither of these studies distinguished teasing about overweight from teasing about underweight. Nor did they evaluate how common such experiences are. In response, we have examined the levels of overweight-related victimisation in 12 year old girls and boys (Murphy and Hill, 1999). Of the 450 children studied, 12 per cent of the girls and 16 per cent of the boys described themselves as victimised for being overweight. As would be expected, these children were heavier than their non-victimised peers, although half were classified as normal weight for their age. Importantly, this victimisation was significantly associated with dietary restraint and was also associated with a range of weight-loss behaviours including fasting.

Peer behaviour is clearly relevant to early weight concern and dieting. The functional nature of 'fat talk' depends on the priority of appearance at different ages. It may be of less importance at an age when attractiveness to boys has lower social value. However, being attractive is relatively more important for girls than for boys at any age. Accordingly, there are gender differences in the direction of 'fat talk' and 'fat teasing'. For example, weight-related talk is more frequent between girls, but boys are more likely to tease girls about overweight than girls are to tease boys (Murphy and Hill, 1999). It is also worth noting that children teased about overweight are more likely to be teased for reasons unrelated to their overweight. The functions of peer behaviour in this regard are complex and demand far more research attention than they have so far received.

Views of overweight

It will be apparent from the above that children's body dissatisfactions and dieting are not simply expressions of a desire to fulfil the promise that a thin body holds. They are also a response to the social view of overweight and fatness. In their attitudes to obesity, children can be even more frank than adults. In one well-known study by Richardson *et al.* (1961), 10 and 11 year olds were asked to rank order six line drawings, one of which depicted a child who was physically normal, and the other five depicting children with physical disabilities, one of whom was obviously overweight. The drawing of the child with no physical handicap was consistently preferred. More surprisingly, the overweight child was ranked bottom – below the child in leg brace or on crutches, or in a wheelchair, or the hand amputee, or the child with facial disfigurement.

A review of the research that followed noted the consistency of this rank ordering with American children almost always placing the overweight child last or next to last (DeJong and Kleck, 1986). The following conclusions were drawn from the mass of subsequent replication and extensions. First, the least accepting attitudes to overweight peers are found in industrialised Western cultures. Second, girls are less accepting of overweight same-sex peers than are boys.

Complementing this body of research has been an exploration of the personality characteristics attributed to particular body shapes. As with adults, children more frequently assign negative characteristics to fat figures and positive personality qualities to thin figures (Staffieri, 1967). So, for example, a figure with a fat shape is more frequently described as lazy, stupid and ugly. In an addition to this literature we have extended the range of attributes studied in order to examine 9 year old children's perception of health and fitness (Hill and Silver, 1995). Their ratings of silhouette pictures depicting thin or overweight children confirmed expectations. Both fat boy and fat girl figures were rated as having far fewer friends than their thin counterparts, as less liked by their parents, very unhappy with their appearance, and as likely to perform less well at school. In addition, these overweight figures were seen as extremely unhealthy, very unfit, and very unlikely to eat healthy food.

Research by Wardle *et al.* has shown an effect of social class background on children's stereotyping (Wardle *et al.*, 1995). Overall, children from higher socio-economic status schools assigned fewer positive characteristics to fat figures than those from low socio-economic status schools. Looking at specific attributes, high socio-economic status school children evaluated the fat figures as less happy, less pretty/handsome, would like to play with least, and unhealthy. Furthermore, they were significantly more likely than low socio-economic status children to label the fat figures as, 'eats the most'.

Pre-adolescent girls and boys have safely received the contemporary messages concerning the association between overweight, social penalty, unhealthy nutrition, and poor health. Their push against overweight has a strong social and health mandate. The question of which is stronger, the appeal of thinness or the rejection of fatness, is largely immaterial. The consequence is that by 9, and possibly earlier, children know why they should lose weight and should not be fat.

Changing circumstances

Certain features of the socio-cultural support for dieting have remained constant during the last four decades. The high preference for thinness expressed by adolescent girls was apparent within the American affluence of the 1960s (Hill, 1993). Similarly, the negative views of obesity were detectable early that same decade. However, there have been changes in society that have further inflated the appeal of dieting. These changes are observable at various levels: at that of the individual, the family, and at a broader cultural level. Briefly, they are illustrated below.

The approach to health in the Britain of the new millenium has placed a great emphasis on lifestyle – individual lifestyle. Integral to this is a way of living that embraces healthy eating, exercise and healthy body weight. The onus has been on the individual to take responsibility for their own healthy eating. Because some elements of healthy eating overlap with strategies used in weight-loss dieting, this has led to confusion and has certainly endorsed the appropriateness of dieting in the public mind. The last twenty to thirty years have also seen major advances in food technology, and the accompanying commercial progress has resulted in an enormous variety of foodstuffs that are available for our purchase. It is not a coincidence that British and American studies have described an increase in average population weight and in the proportion of obese people (Prescott-Clarke and Primatesta, 1999; Flegal *et al.*, 1998). The biological system has shown efficiency in adapting to an 'obesogenic' environment that is rich in nutrition and discouraging of physical activity by storing some of the surplus (Egger and Swinburn, 1997).

This rise in weight has fuelled, and will continue to fuel, the acceptability of dieting.

The tension between the opposing forces of health and commerce is also relevant to the circumstances of children. Surveys have noted changes in children's lifestyle, such as an increase in the amount of time spent watching TV and a reduction in physical activity. Both have been linked to children's obesity (Gortmaker *et al.*, 1996). Children also have a greater freedom in food consumption as reflected in food product sales targeting, the variety of child-oriented food available, and their own purchasing power. Initiatives intended to promote healthy eating invite children to try to resolve these conflicting issues, something that adults continue to fail to do. For girls, one solution to achieving healthy eating in the face of delicious foods and a demand for thinness is self-imposed deprivation or dieting.

Looking at change from a broader perspective, the last thirty years have seen a change in family structure. An example of the way in which this social change has affected eating is the decline of the family meal (Ritzer, 1993). The evening meal is often now the only meal eaten by all the family sitting down together. Mealtimes are becoming less of a communal act as they are sacrificed to the competing demands of other time commitments, individual menus driven by personal likes and dislikes, and watching TV. This loss of structure not only encourages a grazing or snacking style of eating but diminishes parental monitoring of children's eating.

Probably the most profound change to have occurred over this period is at a broader cultural level, and it is the accessibility of information. In a provocative essay Postman has described ways in which this has changed the world of children (Postman, 1983). The advent of TV in particular has undermined any adult notion of tailoring the provision of information according to a child's age. Television demands passive attention to what is a full disclosure medium. It requires no instruction to understand it. Television makes no complex demands of the viewer, nor does it segregate its audience. What is there for adults is also there for children, and vice versa. And because it is visual, comprehension of its message is not reliant on verbal skills. It is easy to see how adult values concerning fatness, thinness and dieting strategies are available to children, even if they were never intended for this age group.

Possibilities for prevention

Recognising body dissatisfaction and dieting in children is in itself important. But it also requires us to consider how we should respond. Should we for example launch a full-scale primary prevention programme for eating disorders directed at 9–12 year olds? And would it be successful? The evidence available on primary prevention suggests the answers to be 'no' and so raises a further set of questions.

School-based primary prevention programmes dominate the eating disorders prevention literature. Most involve teaching sessions delivered to whole class groups and include a range of issues such as the health consequences of eating disorder symptoms, coping with pressures towards thinness, physical and psychological changes during puberty, and many others. Of those programmes that have been properly evaluated most have been unsuccessful. Take as an example the study by Killen *et al.* (1993), frequently cited as one of the most comprehensive of these studies. These researchers used their experience in the primary prevention of smoking and reducing cardiovascular risk factors to design a series of eighteen weekly fifty-minute classroom sessions. Nearly a thousand 11–13 year old Californian girls were randomised to treatment or control classes. Those in the treatment condition received teaching sessions that included slide-show presentations and workbooks with written assignments. The result was a significant increase in relevant knowledge but no effect on eating attitudes, dieting or extreme weight regulation practices.

This outcome typifies that of school-based primary prevention programmes. Generally, these programmes are effective in promoting knowledge, less so in terms of attitudes, and poor at changing behaviour. This conclusion is consistent with a good deal of research in social and health psychology. One response has been to question whether these programmes are targeting the right age groups. Most published interventions have been directed at adolescents. Given the evidence presented above, a strong case could be made for primary school prevention programmes. Accordingly, Smolak *et al.* designed 'Eating smart, eating for me', a ten-lesson school programme that was delivered to 147 9 year old girls and boys (Smolak *et al.*, 1998). Compared with the non-intervention children these 9 year olds showed an increase in some areas of knowledge and a decrease in their negative perception of fat people. However, the programme resulted in no change to children's body esteem, exercise behaviour, eating, dieting or 'fat teasing'. Programmes directed at pre-adolescents therefore fare no better than adolescent interventions.

A further problem with these programmes lies in the choice of criteria used to assess their effectiveness. True efficacy is difficult to assess because of the very low rates of eating disorder onset. A similar argument has been applied to the primary prevention of adolescent suicide (Hazel and King, 1996). The result is the selection of 'softer' outcomes representing aspects of knowledge, attitudes and behaviour, of which dieting is the most common. In fact dieting is viewed as a key behaviour and has become almost analogous with a full eating disorder in the appraisal of success. This is unacceptable. Whatever the position of dieting in the etiological scheme for eating disorders, the demonisation of dieting is unsustainable in a circumstance of escalating adult and pediatric obesity. Moreover, just because extreme dieting can be shown to be a major risk factor for adolescent onset eating disorders (Patton *et al.*, 1990,

1999) it does not follow that the same association between dieting and eating disorder onset applies to much younger groups. This is a leap of faith that urgently requires research evidence. In fact it is much more likely, given the very low rates of early eating disorder onset, that early expressions of dieting concern represent a vulnerability to adolescent eating disorders when in conjunction with specific developmental tasks or life events (Levine and Smolak, 1992). Dieting cannot be outlawed and any attempt to do so is doomed to failure. Instead we should be considering more sophisticated and complex combinations of outcome measures in studies with large samples, rather than targeting dieting because of its convenience.

Of prime importance is the absence of strong connections between programme design and research-supported theory. Education-led prevention programmes are unlikely to be successful if they do not involve the conduits of influence that inform and support children in their experience of body dissatisfaction. The involvement of parents (Smolak and Levine, 1994; Graber and Brooks-Gunn, 1996), the appreciation of media influence via media literacy skills, and peer-led or -assisted interventions (Martz et al., 1997) all have strong claims for inclusion in primary prevention programmes.

Prevention programmes should also acknowledge that the development of eating disorders involves more than just risk factors for body dissatisfaction. Connors has proposed a two-component model that distinguishes vulnerability to develop body dissatisfactions with subsequent dieting and eating disturbance, from factors that predispose to interpersonal and self-regulatory difficulties (Figure 4.2). Connors argues that both lines of development are necessary (Connors, 1996) for a diagnosable eating disorder. Body dissatisfaction in the absence of emotional disturbance results in normal dieting. An at-risk group for eating disorders may consist of those with relatively high dissatisfaction and some vulnerability for affective dysregulation under stress.

In line with this conceptualisation is the argument that there should be a shift away from a disease prevention approach to a health promotion model in the formulation of prevention programmes (Huon et al., 1998). Implicit in this is a focus on general protective factors rather than the targeting of specific risk factors. Observations that adolescent girls who most frequently report dieting or purging are also those most likely to use alcohol and tobacco (French et al., 1995b) support this call for generic health promotion programmes. Central to any such approach would be work on broad personal issues such as self-esteem. Not only are there several suggested routes for enhancing self-esteem (Shisslak et al., 1998b), but there is preliminary evidence of the effectiveness of a self-esteem focused intervention on the body image and eating attitudes of 11–14 year olds (O'Dea and Abraham, 1999). Key to the success of this approach is the reinforcement of school-conveyed messages by teachers and parents.

This overview of the presence of body dissatisfactions and dieting in children, the process of their acquisition, and how we should respond, must end

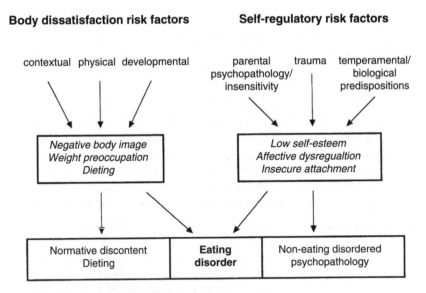

Figure 4.2 Two-component model of eating disorders.

Source: Connors, 1996.

by reiterating the importance of the adult world. Too often primary prevention requires that children take on attitudes and behaviours that are in conflict with their experience outside school and those expressed by adults around them. Why are we trying to instil in our children values and expectations that we do not hold ourselves? It is this disparity that presents the greatest challenge to effecting change. Children's open access to the adult world demands that the responsibility is ours. If the prioritisation of thinness and rejection of fat are important, if we judge our self-esteem by our physical appearance, then it is our collective attitudes that must change. We cannot abrogate our responsibility and then wail because our children fall into similar relationships with their appearance and their bodies.

References

Andersen, R.E., Crespo, C., Bartlett, S.J. and Pratt, S.J. (1998) Relationship of physical activity and television watching with body weight and level of fatness among children. *Journal of the American Medical Association*, 280, 1231–1232.

Atchison, L. (1999) Media effects on body shape perception in children. Unpublished DClinPsychol thesis, University of Leeds.

Attie, I. and Brooks-Gunn, J. (1989) Development of eating problems in adolescent girls: a longitudinal study. *Developmental Psychology*, 25, 70–79.

Barr Taylor, C., Sharp, T., Shisslak, C., Bryson, S., Estes, L.S., Gray, N., McKnight, K.M., Crago, M., Kraemer, H.C. and Killen, J.D. (1998) Factors associated with weight concerns in adolescent girls. *International Journal of Eating Disorders*, 24, 31–42.

Berndt, T.J. and Hestenes, S.L. (1996) The developmental course of social support: family and peers. In *The Developmental Psychopathology of Eating Disorders*, Smolak, L., Levine, M.P. and Striegel-Moore, R. (eds). Lawrence Erlbaum Associates, Mahwah, NJ, pp. 77–106.

Braet, C. and Van Strien, T. (1997) Assessment of emotional, externally induced and restrained eating behaviour in nine to twelve-year-old obese and non-obese children. *Behaviour Research and Therapy*, 35, 863–873.

Brodie, D.A., Bagley, K. and Slade, P.D. (1994) Body-image perception in pre- and post-adolescent females. *Perceptual and Motor Skills*, 78, 147–154.

Champion, H. and Furnham, A. (1999) The effect of the media on body satisfaction in adolescent girls. *European Eating Disorders Review*, 7, 213–228.

Collins, M.E. (1991) Body figure perceptions and preferences among preadolescent children. *International Journal of Eating Disorders*, 10, 199–208.

Connors, M.E. (1996) Developmental vulnerabilities for eating disorders. In *The Developmental Psychopathology of Eating Disorders*, Smolak, L., Levine, M.P. and Striegel-Moore, R. (eds). Lawrence Erlbaum Associates, Mahwah, NJ.

Cooper, P.J. and Goodyer, I. (1997) Prevalence and significance of weight and shape concerns in girls aged 11–16 years. *British Journal of Psychiatry*, 171, 542–544.

de Castro, J.M. and Goldstein, S.J. (1995) Eating attitudes and behaviours of pre- and post-pubertal females: clues to the etiology of eating disorders. *Physiology and Behaviour*, 58, 15–23.

DeJong, W. and Kleck, R.E. (1986) The social psychological effects of overweight. In *Physical Appearance, Stigma, and Social Behaviour: The Ontario Symposium*, Herman, C.P., Zanna, M.P. and Higgins, E.T. (eds). Lawrence Erlbaum, Hillsdale, NJ, pp. 65–87.

Dibb, S. (1996) *A Spoonful of Sugar. Television Food Advertising Aimed at Children: An International Comparative Survey*. Consumers International, London.

Edlund, B., Halvarsson, K. and Sjödén, P. (1996) Eating behaviours, and attitudes to eating, dieting, and body image in 7-year-old Swedish girls. *European Eating Disorders Review*, 4, 40–53.

Edmunds, H. and Hill, A.J. (1999) Dieting and the family context of eating in young adolescent children. *International Journal of Eating Disorders*, 25, 435–440.

Egger, G. and Swinburn, B. (1997) An 'ecological' approach to the obesity pandemic. *British Medical Journal*, 315, 477–480.

Engell, D., Bordi, P., Borja, M., Lambert, C. and Rolls, B. (1998) Effects of information about fat content on food preferences in pre-adolescent children. *Appetite*, 30, 269–282.

Fallon, A. and Rozin, P. (1985) Sex differences in the perceptions of desirable body shape. *Journal of Abnormal Psychology*, 94, 102–105.

Field, A.E., Wolf, A.E., Herzog, D.B., Cheung, L. and Colditz, G.A. (1993) The relationship of caloric intake to frequency of dieting among preadolescent and adolescent girls. *Journal of the American Academy of Child and Adolescent Psychiatry*, 32, 1246–1252.

Field, A.E., Camargo, C.A., Barr Taylor, C., Berkey, C.S., Frasier, A.L., Gillman, M.W. and Colditz, G.A. (1999a) Overweight, weight concerns, and bulimic behaviours among girls and boys. *Journal of the American Academy of Child and Adolescent Psychiatry*, 38, 754–760.

Field, A.E., Cheung, L., Wolf, A.M., Herzog, D.B., Gortmaker, S.L. and Colditz, G.A. (1999b) Exposure to the mass media and weight concerns among girls. *Pediatrics*, 103, E36.

Flegal, K.M., Carroll, M.D., Kuczmarski, R.J. and Johnson, C.L. (1998) Overweight and obesity in the United States: prevalence and trends, 1960–1994. *International Journal of Obesity*, 22, 39–47.

French, S.A., Perry, C.L., Leon, G.R. and Fulkerson, J.A. (1995a) Dieting behaviours and weight change history in female adolescents. *Health Psychology*, 14, 548–555.

French, S.A., Story, M., Downes, B., Resnick, M.D. and Blum, R.W. (1995b) Frequent dieting among adolescents: psychosocial and health behaviour correlates. *American Journal of Public Health*, 85, 695–701.

Garner, D.M., Olmstead, M.P. and Polivy, J. (1983) Development and validation of a multidimensional Eating Disorder Inventory for anorexia-nervosa and bulimia. *International Journal of Eating Disorders*, 2, 15–34.

Gortmaker, S.L., Must, A., Sobol, A.M., Peterson, K., Colditz, G.A. and Dietz, W.H. (1996) Television viewing as a cause of increasing obesity among children in the United States, 1986–1990. *Archives of Pediatric and Adolescent Medicine*, 150, 356–362.

Graber, J.A. and Brooks-Gunn, J. (1996) Prevention of eating problems and disorders: including parents. *Eating Disorders: The Journal of Treatment and Prevention*, 4, 348–363.

Grogan, S. (1999) *Body Image. Understanding Body Dissatisfaction in Men, Women and Children*. Routledge, London.

Gustafson-Larson, A.M. and Terry, R.D. (1992) Weight-related behaviours and concerns of fourth-grade children. *Journal of American Dietetic Association*, 92, 818–822.

Hazel, P. and King, R. (1996) Arguments for and against teaching suicide prevention in schools. *Australian and New Zealand Journal of Psychiatry*, 30, 633–642.

Herman, C.P. and Polivy, J. (1980) Restrained eating. In *Obesity*, Stunkard, A.J. (ed.). Saunders, Philadelphia, pp. 208–235.

Hill, A.J. (1993) Pre-adolescent dieting: implications for eating disorders. *International Review of Psychiatry*, 5, 87–100.

Hill, A.J. and Bhatti, R. (1995) Body shape perception and dieting in pre-adolescent British Asian girls: links with eating disorders. *International Journal of Eating Disorders*, 17, 175–183.

Hill, A.J. and Franklin, J.A. (1998) Mothers, pre-adolescent daughters, and dieting: investigating the transmission of weight control. *British Journal of Clinical Psychology*, 37, 3–13.

Hill, A.J. and Pallin, V. (1998) Dieting awareness and low self-worth: related issues in 8-year old girls. *International Journal of Eating Disorders*, 24, 405–413.

Hill, A.J. and Robinson, A. (1991) Dieting concerns have a functional effect on the behaviour of 9-year old girls. *British Journal of Clinical Psychology*, 30, 265–267.

Hill, A.J. and Silver, E. (1995) Fat, friendless and unhealthy: 9-year old children's perception of body shape stereotypes. *International Journal of Obesity*, 19, 423–430.

Hill, A.J., Rogers, P.J. and Blundell, J.E. (1989) Dietary restraint in young adolescent girls: a functional analysis. *British Journal of Clinical Psychology*, 28, 165–176.

Hill, A.J., Weaver, C. and Blundell, J.E. (1990) Dieting concerns of 10-year old girls and their mothers. *British Journal of Clinical Psychology*, 29, 346–348.

Hill, A.J., Oliver, S. and Rogers, P.J. (1992) Eating in the adult world: the rise of dieting in childhood and adolescence. *British Journal of Clinical Psychology*, 31, 95–105.

Hill, A.J., Draper, E. and Stack, J. (1994) A weight on children's minds: body shape dissatisfactions at 9-years old. *International Journal of Obesity*, 18, 383–389.

Huon, G.F., Braganza, C., Brown, L.B., Ritchie, J.E. and Roncolato, W.G. (1998) Reflections on prevention in dieting-induced disorders. *International Journal of Eating Disorders*, 23, 455–458.

Keel, P.K., Heatherton, T.F., Harnden, J.L. and Hornig, C.D. (1997) Mothers, fathers, and daughters: dieting and disordered eating. *Eating Disorders: The Journal of Treatment and Prevention*, 5, 216–228.

Killen, J.D., Barr Taylor, C., Hammer, L.D., Litt, I., Wilson, D.M., Rich, T., Hayward, C., Simmonds, B., Kraemer, H. and Varady, A. (1993) An attempt to modify unhealthful eating attitudes and weight regulation practices of young adolescent girls. *International Journal of Eating Disorders*, 13, 369–384.

Laessle, R.G., Tuschl, R.J., Kotthaus, B.C. and Pirke, K.M. (1989) Behavioural and biological correlates of dietary restraint in normal life. *Appetite*, 12, 83–94.

Levine, M.P. and Smolak, L. (1992) Toward a model of the developmental psychopathology of eating disorders: the example of early adolescence. In T*he Etiology of Bulimia Nervosa: The Individual and Familial Context*, Crowther, J.H, Tennenbaum, D.L., Hobfoll, S.E. and Stephens, M.A.P. (eds). Hemisphere Publishing, Kent State University, pp. 59–80.

Levine, M.P. and Smolak, L. (1996) Media as a context for the development of disordered eating. In *The Developmental Psychopathology of Eating Disorders*, Smolak, L., Levine, M.P. and Striegel-Moore, R (eds). Lawrence Erlbaum Associates, Mahwah, NJ, pp. 235–257.

Levine, M.P. and Smolak, L. (1998) The mass media and disordered eating: implications for primary prevention. In *The Prevention of Eating Disorders*, Vandereycken, W. and Noordenbos, G. (eds). Athlone Press, London.

Levine, M.P., Smolak, L., Moodey, A.F., Shuman, M.D. and Hessen, L.D. (1994) Normative developmental challenges and dieting and eating disturbances in middle school girls. *International Journal of Eating Disorders*, 15, 11–20.

Lewis, M.K. and Hill, A.J. (1998) Food advertising on British children's television: a content analysis and experimental study with 9-year olds. *International Journal of Obesity*, 22, 206–214.

McCourt, J. and Waller, G. (1995) Developmental role of perceived parental control in the eating psychopathology of Asian and Caucasian schoolgirls. *International Journal of Eating Disorders*, 17, 277–282.

Maloney, M.J., McGuire, J, Daniels, S.R. and Specker, B. (1989) Dieting behaviour and eating attitudes in children. *Pediatrics*, 84, 482–489.

Martin, M.C. and Kennedy, P.F. (1993) Advertising and social comparison: consequences for female preadolescents and adolescents. *Psychology and Marketing*, 10, 513–530.

Martz, D.M., Graves, K.D. and Sturgis, E.T. (1997) A pilot peer-leader eating disorders prevention program for sororities. *Eating Disorders: The Journal of Treatment and Prevention*, 5, 294–308.

Mumford, D.B., Whitehouse, A.M. and Platts, M. (1991) Sociocultural correlates of eating disorders among Asian schoolgirls in Bradford. *British Journal of Psychiatry*, 158, 222–228.

Murphy, J. and Hill, A.J. (1999) Fat-teasing in young adolescent children: links with dieting? Paper presented at the 4th International Conference on Eating Disorders, London.

O'Dea, J.A. and Abraham, S. (1999) Improving the body image, eating attitudes and behaviours of young male and female adolescents: a new educational approach which focuses on self-esteem. *International Journal of Eating Disorders*, 28, 43–57.

Parkinson, K.N., Tovée, M.J. and Cohen-Tovée, E.M. (1998) Body shape perceptions of preadolescent and young adolescent children. *European Eating Disorders Review*, 6, 126–135.

Patton, G.C., Johnson-Sabine, E., Wood, K., Mann, A. and Wakeling, A. (1990) Abnormal eating attitudes in London schoolgirls – a prospective epidemiological study: outcome at twelve months. *Psychological Medicine*, 20, 382–394.

Patton, G.C., Selzer, R., Coffey, J.B., Carlin, J.B. and Wolfe, R. (1999) Onset of adolescent eating disorders: population based cohort study over 3 years. *British Medical Journal*, 318, 765–768.

Paxton, S.J. (1996) Prevention implications of peer influences on body image dissatisfaction and disturbed eating in adolescent girls. *Eating Disorders: The Journal of Treatment and Prevention*, 4, 334–347.

Paxton, S.J., Wertheim, E.H., Gibbons, K., Szmukler, G.I. and Petrovich, J.C. (1991) Body image satisfaction, dieting beliefs and weight loss behaviour in adolescent girls and boys. *Journal of Youth and Adolescence*, 20, 361–379.

Paxton, S.J., Schutz, H.K., Wertheim, E.H. and Muir, S.L. (1999) Friendship clique and peer influences on body image concerns, dietary restraint, extreme weight-loss behaviours, and binge eating in adolescent girls. *Journal of Abnormal Psychology*, 108, 255–266.

Pike, K.M. and Rodin, J. (1991) Mothers, daughters, and disordered eating. *Journal of Abnormal Psychology*, 100, 198–204.

Polivy, J. and Herman, C.P. (1987) Diagnosis and treatment of normal eating. *Journal of Consulting and Clinical Psychology*, 55, 635–644.

Postman, N. (1983) *The Disappearance of Childhood*. Allen, London.

Prescott-Clarke, P. and Primatesta, P. (1999) *Health Survey for England 1997*. HMSO, London.

Richards, M.H. and Casper, R.C. (1990) Weight and eating concerns among pre- and young adolescent boys and girls. *Journal of Adolescent Health Care*, 11, 203–209.

Richardson, S.A., Hastorf, A.H., Goodman, N. and Dornbusch, S.M. (1961) Cultural uniformity in reaction to physical disabilities. *American Sociological Review*, 26, 241–247.

Ritzer, G. (1993) *The McDonaldisation of Society*. Pine Forge Press, Thousand Oaks, Calif.

Rolland, K., Farnill, D. and Griffiths, R.A. (1997) Body figure perceptions and eating attitudes among Australian schoolchildren aged 8 to 12 years. *International Journal of Eating Disorders*, 21, 273–278.

Ruther, N.M. and Richman, C.L. (1993) The relationship between mothers' eating restraint and their children's attitudes and behaviours. *Bulletin of the Psychonomic Society*, 31, 217–220.

Schreiber, G.B., Robins, M., Striegel-Moore, R., Obarzanek, E. and Wright, D.J. (1996) Weight modification efforts reported by black and white preadolescent girls: National Heart, Lung and Blood Institute Growth and Health Study. *Pediatrics*, 98, 63–70.

Shisslak, C.M., Crago, M., McKnight, K.M., Estes, L.S., Gray, N. and Parnaby, O.G. (1998a) Potential risk factors associated with weight control behaviours in elementary and middle school girls. *Journal of Psychosomatic Research*, 44, 301–313.

Shisslak, C.M., Crago, M., Renger, R. and Clark-Wagner, A. (1998b) Self-esteem and the prevention of eating disorders. *Eating Disorders: The Journal of Treatment and Prevention*, 6, 105–118.

Smolak, L. and Levine, M.P. (1994) Toward an empirical basis for primary prevention of eating problems with elementary school children. *Eating Disorders: The Journal of Treatment and Prevention*, 2, 293–307.

Smolak, L., Levine, M.P. and Schermer, F. (1998) A controlled evaluation of an elementary school primary prevention program for eating problems. *Journal of Psychosomatic Research*, 44, 339–353.

Smolak, L., Levine, M.P. and Schermer, F. (1999) Parental input and weight concerns among elementary school children. *International Journal of Eating Disorders*, 25, 263–271.

Staffieri, J.R. (1967) A study of social stereotype of body image in children. *Journal of Personality and Social Psychology*, 7, 101–104.

Stice, E. (1994) Review of the evidence for a sociocultural model of bulimia nervosa and an exploration of the mechanisms of action. *Clinical Psychology Review*, 14, 633–661.

Striegel-Moore, R.H. and Kearney-Cooke, A. (1994) Exploring parents' attitudes and behaviours about their children's physical appearance. *International Journal of Eating Disorders*, 15, 377–385.

Thelen, M.H. and Cormier, J.F. (1995) Desire to be thinner and weight control among children and their parents. *Behaviour Therapy*, 26, 85–99.

Thelen, M.H., Powell, A.L., Lawrence, C. and Kuhnert, M.E. (1992) Eating and body image concerns among children. *Journal of Clinical Child Psychology*, 21, 41–46.

Thompson, J.K., Coovert, M.D., Richards, K.J., Johnson, S. and Cattarin, J. (1995) Development of body image, eating disturbance, and general psychological functioning in female adolescents: covariance structure modeling and longitudinal investigations. *International Journal of Eating Disorders*, 18, 221–236.

Thompson, S.H., Corwin, S.J. and Sargent, R.G. (1997) Ideal body size beliefs and weight concerns of fourth-grade children. *International Journal of Eating Disorders*, 21, 279–284.

Tuschl, R.J., Platte, P., Laessle, R.G., Stichler, W. and Pirke, K.M. (1990) Energy expenditure and everyday eating behaviour in healthy young women. *American Journal of Clinical Nutrition*, 52, 81–86.

Van Strien, T., Frijters, J.E.R., Bergers, G.P.A. and Defares, P.B. (1986) Dutch Eating Behaviour Questionnaire for the assessment of restrained, emotional, and external eating behaviour. *International Journal of Eating Disorders*, 5, 295–315.

Wadden, T.A., Foster, G.D., Stunkard, A.J. and Linowitz, J.R. (1989) Dissatisfaction with weight and figure in obese girls: discontent but not depression. *International Journal of Obesity*, 13, 89–97.

Waller, G. and Shaw, J. (1994) The media influence on eating problems. In *Why Women? Gender Issues and Eating Disorders*, Dolan, B. and Gitzinger, I. (eds). Athlone Press, London, pp. 44–54.

Wardle, J., Marsland, L., Sheikh, Y., Quinn, M., Federoff, I. and Ogden, J. (1992) Dietary restraint and eating behaviour in adolescents. *Appetite*, 18, 167–183.

Wardle, J., Volz, C. and Golding, C. (1995) Social variation in attitudes to obesity in children. *International Journal of Obesity*, 19, 562–569.

Chapter 5

The influence of maternal eating disorder on children

Alan Stein, Helen Woolley and Heather Williams

Introduction

Eating disorders occur commonly amongst women of childbearing age
(Szmukler, 1985; Fairburn and Beglin, 1990) and the prevalence seems to be
on the increase (Treasure *et al.*, 1996). Estimates indicate that at least 2 per cent
of women aged 16–40 suffer from bulimia nervosa or anorexia nervosa, and
this figure rises to 4 per cent when other eating disorders are considered
(Fairburn and Beglin, 1990; Hoek, 1993). It is now well established that
children of parents who have psychiatric disorders are at risk of developing
disturbances themselves (Rutter, 1989; Garmezy and Masten, 1994) and these
may persist after remission of the parental disorder (Murray and Cooper,
1996; Barnes and Stein, 2000). It is therefore surprising that the potential
implications for children of mothers with eating disorders have received little
attention until recently. Knowledge of whether these children are at risk and
the mechanisms underlying any transmission of disturbance is important so
that appropriate treatment can be instituted and preventative strategies put in
place.

Eating disorders have the potential to interfere with parenting in a number
of ways. First, the core symptoms of eating disorders are extremely pervasive
and potentially disruptive of daily activities and sensitive parenting. Particularly debilitating are the preoccupations with body shape, weight and food,
which may draw parental attention away from the needs of their child. The
behaviours which characterise eating disorders and which may disrupt har-
monious parent–child interaction include episodes of binge eating, and the
extreme behaviours adopted to compensate for over-eating, such as vomiting,
the use of purgatives and excessive exercise. Second, a number of studies (e.g.
Humphrey, 1989) have shown that people with eating disorders have difficulties in their interpersonal relationships. These difficulties may extend to their
relationships with their children.

Developmental risk

Particular stages of development may render children especially susceptible to the influence of parental eating disorders. Infancy may be a vulnerable time given that feeding and mealtimes take up a significant part of the day during the first months and years of life, and are one of the most important times for close communication between parents and children. Feeding, particularly after weaning has begun, provides a context in which infants can experiment with some of their new developmental capacities, such as self-gratification and autonomy. At these times they require particularly sensitive and facilitative parenting to promote their exploratory behaviour. However, the attitudes, preoccupations and behaviours parents with eating disorders manifest may interfere with their ability to prepare meals, to sit patiently feeding their infants, and to respond appropriately to hunger and satiety cues. Whilst eating disorder symptomatology may diminish during pregnancy, recent research has shown that the disturbance rises in the postpartum period to above pre-pregnancy levels, with mothers trying to regain their pre-pregnancy body shape and weight in the context of the significant disruption of their own mealtimes and sleep routines whilst feeding and caring for their baby (Fairburn et al., 1993; Stein et al., 1996).

Adolescents may also be more vulnerable in relation to parental eating disorders. Teenagers become increasingly aware of societal pressures while also developing an interest in body shape and attractiveness. Weight control was found to be the single most important concern in an epidemiological study of health concerns amongst a large sample of Californian teenagers (Evans et al., 1995). Parents' attitudes towards their own body shape and weight, and their own behaviour with respect to eating, may affect their adolescent children in two ways. First, the children may model themselves on their parents; and second, the parents may influence them directly through their attitudes towards their children's weight, shape and eating habits.

Most of the papers on the development of children of parents with eating disorders have consisted of clinical case reports and case series in which concerns are raised about the risk of adverse sequelae for the children. Given the nature of these reports it is not easy to evaluate their significance. Papers have concentrated on mothers with eating disorders with little reference to fathers. Two of these reports found evidence that the mother's disorder impinged directly on the child. Lacey and Smith (1987) found that some women with bulimia nervosa were concerned that their babies were overweight and had tried to slim them down, while Stein and Fairburn (1989) found that some mothers with bulimia nervosa were excessively worried about their children's shape and size and also had significant difficulties with feeding their children. Others have also found that the mothers' eating disorders interfered with parenting more generally (Fahy and Treasure, 1989; Woodside and Shekter-Wolfson, 1990; Timimi and Robinson, 1996). Fahy and Treasure (1989) described the conflicting demands of child rearing for parents coping with severe bulimic episodes while having to feed their young children, when the very presence of food may stimulate a binge. Hodes and colleagues (Hodes *et al.*, 1997) studied twenty-six children (age range 9 months to 25 years) of thirteen mothers with eating disorders, and found that 50 per cent had psychiatric disorders, including severe conditions such as anorexia nervosa and obsessive compulsive disorder.

There is also evidence that the physical growth of children of mothers with eating disorders might be adversely affected. Brinch *et al.* (1988) followed up a group of women with a history of anorexia nervosa, who had subsequently had children, and reported that 17 per cent of these children had failed to thrive in their first year. However, these findings were based largely on retrospective maternal reports of child development and on a broad definition of failure to thrive and should be regarded with caution. Van Wezel-Meijler and Wit (1989) reported that seven children from three eating disordered mothers presented with features of growth retardation, which the authors believed was due to under-nutrition of the child. Furthermore, Hodes *et al.* (1997) found that one-third of the children in their case series were significantly lighter or smaller than expected for their age.

In one controlled study that employed direct observation of 1-year-old children of mothers with eating disorders of a bulimic type, mothers and infants were observed during both mealtimes and play in the home (Stein *et al.*, 1994). The main findings were that, compared with controls, the index mothers were more intrusive with their infants during both mealtimes and play, and expressed more negative emotion (critical and derogatory remarks) during mealtimes but not during play. The most common precipitant of such expressed negative emotion was the mothers' concern that their infants were making a 'mess'. There were, however, no differences between the groups in the extent of their positive expressed emotion towards their infants. There was considerably more conflict between index infants and their mothers during mealtimes, with the index mothers showing much more reluctance to allow their infants to attempt self-feeding. Mess avoidance and the need to keep control of food intake seemed particularly important to these mothers. Furthermore, the index infants weighed less than the control infants, and infant weight was found to be independently and inversely related to the amount of conflict during mealtimes. While a significant proportion of these mothers and infants were having problems, this was not invariable. Some mothers were coping well with their babies, who were growing and developing healthily (Stein *et al.*, 1994). Interestingly, a smaller more recent study of older toddlers (aged 1–4 years, mean = 30 months) which also employed direct mealtime observation found that case mothers made significantly fewer positive eating comments than control mothers and tended to avoid eating with their children (Waugh and Bulik, 1999).

In order to establish whether growth faltering amongst children of mothers with eating disorders was specific, Stein and his colleagues extended the study reported above. The infants of mothers with eating disorders were compared with infants of mothers with postnatal depression and a large normal comparison group (Stein *et al.*, 1996). It was found that infants of mothers with eating disorders were smaller, both in terms of weight and length for age, than either the normal comparison group or the infants of mothers with postnatal depression; and the latter two groups did not differ from each other. This indicated that the growth faltering was specific to the infants of mothers with eating disorders. The same sample was also used to determine whether higher levels of mother–infant conflict during mealtimes were the result of general or specific psychopathology. Mothers with eating disorders, mothers with postnatal depression, and mothers in a healthy comparison group and their infants were observed during play and mealtimes (Stein *et al.*, 2001). Eating disordered mothers used more verbal control, especially strong control, but there were no differences between the groups in their use of gentle verbal control or physical contact. Maternal dietary restraint was the one feature of eating disorder psychopathology which was associated with the use of verbal control. This suggests that aspects of maternal control are not a result of general psychopathology or negative affect, but specific to maternal eating disorder psychopathology.

The same three groups were used to examine whether or not there were more direct influences than conflict on growth disturbance. Two features of maternal psychopathology might lead the mothers to limit their children's food intake and potentially bring about growth disturbance in the children. First, people with eating disorders tend to misjudge their own body shapes, by perceiving themselves to be fatter than they actually are. Second, they have a strong desire to be thin. If these mothers' misjudgements about their own body shape extended to their evaluation of their infants' body shape, and they desired their infants to be thin, this might well lead them to limit their children's food intake. However, empirical examination revealed that, compared with the depressed mothers and the comparison group, the eating disordered mothers did not prefer thinner babies or misperceive their children's size. On the contrary, they were highly sensitive to their children's shape and, compared to the other two groups, were significantly more accurate at judging their children's size (Stein *et al.*, 1996).

The strength and specificity of the association between maternal eating disorder psychopathology and child feeding disturbance was confirmed by a study using a different strategy, namely one which used the child's disturbance as a starting point (Stein *et al.*, 1995). In this study the mothers of a consecutive series of young children referred to child psychiatric clinics with ICD-10 feeding disorders were compared to a matched group of children with behavioural disorders and a large unselected control group. ICD-10 criteria require that a feeding disorder in infancy or childhood 'generally involves refusal of food and extreme faddiness' (World Health Organisation,

1992). Only the children with feeding disorders had mothers with significantly disturbed eating habits and attitudes. These findings received support from a study of 4-year-old children, conducted by Whelan and Cooper (2000). They studied three groups of children: children with feeding problems, children with non-feeding disturbance (shyness, fearfulness or behavioural disturbance) and a group with no disturbance. They then compared their mothers' mental state and found that the mothers of the children with feeding problems had a raised rate of current and past eating disorder, but not affective disorder, compared to the other two groups. The finding that children's feeding disorders were specifically linked to the mothers' eating habits and attitudes suggests that maternal eating psychopathology may play a significant role in the development of children's feeding disorders (Stein et al., 1995).

This issue has been further investigated by Stice and his colleagues in a prospective study of parents and children from birth to 5 years (Stice et al., 1999). The emergence of childhood eating disturbances, such as inhibited or secretive eating, over-eating and vomiting, was related to both parental and child factors. Maternal body dissatisfaction, internalisation of the thin ideal, dieting and bulimic symptoms, maternal and paternal body mass, and infant body mass and feeding behaviour during the first month of life were found to predict the emergence of eating disturbances in the child. A subgroup of these children, whose mothers had a past or present eating disorder, was examined in more detail (Agras et al., 1999). The daughters of eating disordered mothers showed a higher suckling rate and later weaning from bottle-feeding compared with children of non-eating disordered mothers. Furthermore, children of eating disordered mothers demonstrated greater negative affect at 5 years old, with no differences between boys and girls.

A few studies have looked at the potential relationship between eating disorders in older children and those of their mothers, the aim being to consider whether mothers' attitudes and behaviours regarding food are a factor in determining whether or not their daughters would have disordered eating. A follow-up of the sample originally studied by Stice and colleagues examined the influence of maternal eating habits on children's eating habits and attitudes when the children were 8 years old (Jacobi et al., 2001). They found that higher maternal restraint and higher maternal disinhibition scores, measured when the infant was between 2 and 4 weeks of age, predicted worries about being too fat and weight control behaviours in daughters but not sons. Furthermore, by 8 years of age, daughters of mothers with eating psychopathology were more likely to demonstrate disturbed eating behaviours and attitudes. However, there were no differences between girls and boys in the frequencies of the children's self-reported eating disturbances.

A US study by Pike and Rodin (1991) used self-report measures in groups of middle-class mothers and adolescent daughters to compare mothers of daughters with disordered eating with controls. They found that mothers whose daughters' eating was disordered had more eating problems themselves. Mothers of girls with disordered eating also thought that their daughters should lose more weight than did the mothers of girls who were not eating disordered, and saw their daughters as less attractive than the girls judged themselves. However, a study by Attie and Brooks-Gunn (1989) did not support these findings. Thus, these issues remain largely unresolved and research has yet to be carried out to establish any clear causal link between disordered eating behaviours in mothers and their children.

Summary of mechanisms of transmission

From the relatively limited number of studies conducted to date, it is possible to describe five broad mechanisms by which parents with eating disorders may influence child rearing and their children's development. First, parents' extreme attitudes to eating, body shape and weight may have direct effects on the child. For example, parents' fear of fatness may cause them to underfeed their children, and their over-concern with shape, weight and food intake may lead to mealtime conflict with their younger children and to their becoming critical of their adolescent children's eating habits, body shape, and appearance. Second, eating disorders may interfere with general parenting functioning. For example, these parents' preoccupations with food, body shape, and weight may impair their concentration in such a way as to interfere with their sensitivity and responsiveness to their children's needs. Third, parents' disturbed eating behaviours may act as a poor role model for their children. Fourth, parents' eating disorders may be associated with discordant marital and family relationships which have been shown to have their own adverse effects on child development (Rutter and Quinton, 1984). Fifth, while relatively little has been done to illuminate how parental eating disorders may influence the children's development through genetic factors, there is now evidence that there is a genetic component to eating disorders (Holland et al., 1984; Kendler et al., 1991; Lilenfeld et al., 1998; Strober et al., 2000).

Clinical implications

From the research evidence available it is clear that the children of some mothers with eating disorders are themselves at risk. Those working with families with young children – for example, general practitioners and health visitors – and those working with parents with eating disorders are well-placed to identify any difficulties which occur in parent–child interaction or in child development (Berg and Hodes, 1997), and either to deal with these themselves or refer on when appropriate. It is essential that the parental eating disorder itself is treated. In addition, attention to the developing parent–child interaction may help to prevent the intergenerational transmission of disorder and support optimal child development.

Given the relative paucity of research to date, only tentative guidelines can be proposed. However, on the basis of our research work and clinical experience, we have developed a clinical approach to families with young children where a parent has an eating disorder. Most of our comments are confined to helping families with young children although a number of the issues are relevant to older children as well.

At the outset it is important that the quality of the interactions between parents with eating disorders and their children be carefully assessed, as should the children's growth and nutritional status. As part of the assessment of parent–child interaction it is helpful to observe mealtimes sensitively and unintrusively in the home. When making such assessments, it is important to remember that much communication between parents and infants occurs around mealtimes, and many issues and potential conflicts may arise. It is part of everyday experience for parents and infants to resolve the common disputes and mismatches that occur during feeding. Indeed, the working out of the struggles for autonomy through attempts to self-feed, and the explanations and negotiation that lead to resolution, signal to the child that such disputes are normal events and model means of solution. Some parents, however, overburdened by their own eating difficulties, get locked into disputes with their infants, and extensive conflictual interaction becomes the norm, causing great distress to all concerned.

A parent's ability to recognise, acknowledge, and respond sensitively to the infant's signals and to understand about an infant's age-appropriate needs is crucial. If, however, a parent cannot recognise, acknowledge, and own their own concerns, they may persist in seeing the child's actions exclusively through adult eyes and fail to understand the child's eye view of the world. Parental concerns then cut across the infant's developmental needs. A sympathetic non-judgemental approach to these parents' difficulties is crucial. They may need help to recognise and set aside their own concerns and so recognise their infants as separate with their own needs and motivations.

Particular help may be needed in recognising an infant's hunger and satiety cues. Infants may have difficulty learning about their own somatic and emotional cues if parents constantly misread them and reflect back those misperceptions (Chatoor et al., 1988). Help in learning to pace food offers is also important, that is, in recognizing when an infant is ready for more food. If feeding has become intensely unhappy, parents may be encouraged to widen the mealtime focus of attention upon food, by, for instance, talking about pleasurable family activities or events. Above all, helping parents to remain available (physically and emotionally) to their infants, to sit back at times and allow the infant to experiment a little without intruding or cutting across the infant's efforts, is important.

Some small practical steps may help parents who are particularly concerned about mess. Help them to recognise that some mess is inevitable as an infant learns to self-feed; and suggest using a waterproof tablecloth under the high chair, using two spoons (one for parent, one for the infant) and possibly two feeding dishes so that the infant can experiment with a smaller amount of food. They may also need help in setting realistic and age-appropriate rules, in particular with setting limits without being angry. Recognition of how the parent feels when rules are broken, and how to contain and manage those feelings, may be crucial in avoiding the escalation of dispute into full conflict. It is important to help parents to identify their own flashpoints and to work out some simple ways of dealing with their own feelings and concerns. For some parents even a minor breaching of a rule represents a threatening loss of control. Simple low-key ploys may help them to keep a sense of control without heavy-handed intrusion.

If older children are involved, help might take the form of working with parents to lessen the attention and criticism directed at their children's body weight and shape. Again, the parents may be helped to widen the focus of their interaction with their children during mealtimes, encouraging discussion of the day's events, trying to focus on areas of mutual enjoyment.

Struggling to feed an infant can be a very lonely experience, especially if parent and infant have got into intractable conflict. It is especially in these cases that the health professional can usefully involve the partner or relative in supporting, sharing the feeding, or even taking over the feeding at some mealtimes. This needs to be done in a sensitive way, so as not to undermine the parent. The presence of another adult can help to diffuse the intense conflict and the partners can work together and learn to identify the child's feeding patterns, cues and needs.

Finally, it should be emphasised that the children of parents with eating disorders are not invariably adversely affected. Some parents manage well and their children develop without apparent problems. Thus, the importance of assessing each family carefully cannot be overemphasised.

References

Agras, S., Hammer, L. and McNicholas, F. (1999) A prospective study of the influence of eating-disordered mothers on their children. *International Journal of Eating Disorders*, 25, 253–262.

Attie, I. and Brooks-Gunn, J. (1989) Development of eating problems in adolescent girls: a longitudinal study. *Developmental Psychology*, 25, 70–79.

Barnes, J. and Stein, A. (2000) The effects of parental psychiatric and physical illness on child development. In M.G. Gelder, J.J. Lopez-Ibor and N.C. Andreasen (eds), *New Oxford Textbook of Psychiatry*. Oxford: Oxford University Press, 759–775.

Berg, B. and Hodes, M. (1997) Adult psychiatrists' knowledge of children whose mothers have eating disorders. *European Eating Disorders Review*, 5, 25–32.

Brinch, M., Isager, T. and Tolstrup, K. (1988) Anorexia nervosa and motherhood: reproduction pattern and mothering behaviour of 50 women. *Acta Psychiatrica Scandinavica*, 77, 611–617.

Chatoor, I., Egan, J., Getson, P., Menvielle, E. and O'Donnell, R. (1988) Mother–infant interactions in infantile anorexia nervosa. *Journal of the American Academy of Child and Adolescent Psychiatry*, 27, 535–540.

Evans, N., Gilpin, E., Farkas, A.J., Shenassa, E. and Pierce, J.P. (1995) Adolescents' perceptions of their peers' health norms. *American Journal of Public Health*, 85, 1064–1069.

Fahy, T. and Treasure, T. (1989) Children of mothers with bulimia nervosa. *British Medical Journal*, 299, 1031 (letter).

Fairburn, C.G. and Beglin, S. (1990) Studies of the epidemiology of bulimia nervosa. *American Journal of Psychiatry*, 147, 401–408.

Fairburn, C.G., Jones, R. and Stein, A. (1993) Eating habits and attitudes during pregnancy. *Psychosomatic Medicine*, 54, 665–672.

Garmezy, N. and Masten, A. (1994) Chronic adversities. In M. Rutter and L. Hersov (eds), *Child and Adolescent Psychiatry*. Oxford: Blackwell, 191–208.

Hodes, M., Timimi, S. and Robinson, P. (1997) Children of mothers with eating disorders: a preliminary study. *European Eating Disorders Review*, 5, 11–24.

Hoek, H.W. (1993) Review of the epidemiological studies of eating disorders. *International Review of Psychiatry*, 15, 346–348.

Holland, A.J., Hall, A., Murray, R., Russell, G.F.M. and Crisp, A.H. (1984) Anorexia nervosa: a study of 34 twin pairs and one set of triplets. *British Journal of Psychiatry*, 145, 414–419.

Humphrey, L.L. (1989) Observed family interactions among subtypes of eating disorders using structural analysis of social behaviour. *Journal of Consulting and Clinical Psychology*, 57, 206–214.

Jacobi, C., Agras, W.S. and Hammer, L. (2001) Predicting children's reported eating disturbances at 8 years of age. *Journal of the American Academy of Child and Adolescent Psychiatry*, 40, 364–372.

Kendler, K.S., MacLean, C., Neale, M., Kessler, R., Heath, A. and Eaves, L. (1991) The genetic epidemiology of bulimia nervosa. *American Journal of Psychiatry*, 148, 1627–1637.

Lacey, J.H. and Smith, G. (1987) Bulimia nervosa: the impact of pregnancy on mother and baby. *British Journal of Psychiatry*, 150, 777–781.

Lilenfeld, L.R., Kaye, W.H., Greeno, C.G., Merikangas, K.R., Plotnicov, K., Pollice, C., Rao, R., Strober, M., Bulik, C.M. and Nagy, L. (1998) A controlled family study of anorexia nervosa and bulimia nervosa: psychiatric disorders in first-degree relatives and effects of proband comorbidity. *Archives of General Psychiatry*, 55, 603–610.

Murray, L. and Cooper, P. (1996) The impact of postpartum depression on child development. *International Review of Psychiatry*, 8, 55–63.

Pike, K.M. and Rodin, J. (1991) Mothers, daughters, and disordered eating. *Journal of Abnormal Psychology*, 100, 198–204.

Rutter, M. (1989) Psychiatric disorder in parents as a risk factor for children. In D. Schaffer, I. Phillips and N.B. Enger (eds), *Prevention of Mental Disorder, Alcohol and Other Drug Use in Children and Adolescents*. Rockville, Md.: Office for Substance Abuse, USDHHS, 157–189.

Rutter, M. and Quinton, D. (1984) Parental psychiatric disorder: effects on children. *Psychological Medicine*, 14, 853–880.

Stein, A. and Fairburn, C.G. (1989) Children of mothers with bulimia nervosa. *British Medical Journal*, 299, 777–778.

Stein, A., Woolley, H., Cooper, S.D. and Fairburn, C.G. (1994) An observational study of mothers with eating disorders and their infants. *Journal of Child Psychology and Psychiatry*, 35, 733–748.

Stein, A., Stein, J., Walters, E.A. and Fairburn, C.G. (1995) Eating habits and attitudes among mothers of children with feeding disorders. *British Medical Journal*, 310, 228.

Stein, A., Murray, L., Cooper, P. and Fairburn, C.G. (1996) Infant growth in the context of maternal eating disorders and maternal depression: a comparative study. *Psychological Medicine*, 26, 569–574.

Stein, A., Woolley, H., Murray, L., Cooper, P., Cooper, S., Noble, F., Affonso, N. and Fairburn, C.G. (2001) Influence of psychiatric disorder on the controlling behaviour of mothers with 1-year-old infants: a study of women with maternal eating disorder, postnatal depression and a healthy comparison group. *British Journal of Psychiatry*, 179, 157–162.

Stice, E., Stewart Agras, W. and Hammer, L.D. (1999) Risk factors for the emergence of childhood eating disturbances: a five-year prospective study. *International Journal of Eating Disorders*, 25, 375–387.

Strober, M., Freeman, R., Lampert, C., Diamond, J. and Kaye, W. (2000) Controlled family study of anorexia nervosa and bulimia nervosa: evidence of shared liability and transmission of partial syndromes. *American Journal of Psychiatry*, 157, 393–401.

Szmukler, G. (1985) The epidemiology of anorexia nervosa and bulimia nervosa. *Journal of Psychiatric Research*, 19, 143–153.

Timimi, S. and Robinson, P. (1996) Disturbances in children of patients with eating disorders. *European Eating Disorder Review*, 4, 183–188.

Treasure, J.L., Troop, N.A. and Ward, A. (1996) An approach to planning services for bulimia nervosa. *British Journal of Psychiatry*, 169, 551–554.

Van Wezel-Meijler, G. and Wit, J.M. (1989) The offspring of mothers with anorexia nervosa: a high risk group for under-nutrition and stunting? *European Journal of Paediatrics*, 149, 130–135.

Waugh, E. and Bulik, C.M. (1999) Offspring of women with eating disorders. *International Journal of Eating Disorders*, 25, 123–133.

Whelan, E. and Cooper, P.J. (2000) The association between childhood feeding problems and maternal eating disorder: a community study. *Psychological Medicine*, 30, 69–77.

Woodside, D. and Shekter-Wolfson, L. (1990) Parenting by patients with anorexia nervosa and bulimia nervosa. *International Journal of Eating Disorders*, 9, 303–309.

World Health Organisation (1992) The ICD-10 classification of mental and behavioural disorders; clinical descriptions and diagnostic guidelines. Geneva: WHO.

Chapter 6

Anorexia nervosa of early onset and its impact on puberty

Gerald F. M. Russell

Anorexia nervosa in childhood and early adolescence is less common than in later adolescence, but its occurrence at an early age gains in importance because of its impact on puberty. The first accounts of anorexia nervosa of early onset were more concerned with arbitrary age limits such as onset from 8 to 16 years (Lesser *et al.*, 1960; Blitzer *et al.*, 1961; Tolstrup, 1965). One of the first accounts to time the onset of anorexia nervosa in relation to puberty was that of Warren (1968) who distinguished between 'pre-pubertal', pubertal and post-pubertal onset. Puberty, however, is a complex developmental process spanning two to three years (Tanner, 1962), and varying in its timing from child to child. For the purpose of the present account, the onset of anorexia nervosa will be timed in relation to the pubertal process rather than the patient's age.

1   **True pre-pubertal anorexia nervosa:** in these children anorexia nervosa commences before the very first signs of puberty. Thus, in girls the illness precedes the appearance of pubic hair and breast growth; and in boys it precedes the first signs of genital growth.
2   **Intra-pubertal anorexia nervosa:** this is the commoner early manifestation of anorexia nervosa. The first signs of puberty will have appeared (breast growth in girls and genital enlargement in boys), but puberty will still be incomplete. In girls the illness precedes the first menstrual period so that this early form of anorexia nervosa has been called pre-menarchal (Russell, 1985a).

These two forms of anorexia nervosa in many ways resemble classical anorexia nervosa which commences after the completion of puberty. But they carry additional importance which will be stressed throughout this chapter and can now be summarised as follows:

First, the physical and psychological immaturity of the patient may modify considerably the clinical presentation of the illness. Accordingly, the diagnostic criteria of pre-pubertal and pre-menarchal anorexia nervosa will require modified definitions. Secondly, such an early onset of anorexia nervosa is likely to delay or arrest the developmental process of puberty itself. There may be temporary or more permanent effects on growth and repro- ductive development. This carries implications for the assessment of the long- term outcome of the illness, which should include measures of physical growth, and sexual and reproductive maturity. Finally, the pre-pubertal occurrence of anorexia nervosa may carry a theoretical significance for our understanding of the illness. In particular, it has been suggested by Crisp (1965, 1980) that anorexia nervosa represents a profound psychobiological regression consequent on the maturational challenges of puberty. If anorexia nervosa can occur before even the first stages of pubertal development, this theory may no longer be tenable without some modification which would allow for this exception.

Incidence and prevalence

There have been several population-based studies aimed at estimating the incidence of anorexia nervosa from diagnostic data recorded on psychiatric case registers (Kendell *et al.*, 1973; Jones *et al.*, 1980; Willi and Grossmann, 1983; Hoek and Brook, 1985; Szmukler *et al.*, 1986). The incidence has been found to range from 1 to 5 cases per 100,000 population per year. Moreover, these investigators have generally reported an increasing incidence of ano- rexia nervosa over recent decades. Another approach has been to survey specific and vulnerable populations such as schoolgirls in the private school sector. These surveys have yielded prevalence rates as high as 1.1 per cent (Crisp *et al.*, 1976; Szmukler, 1983).

Among the studies of vulnerable populations, that by Råstam *et al.* (1989) is particularly relevant because it was aimed at the youngest population so far surveyed epidemiologically, children aged 15 and under. The total population of 15-year-old schoolchildren in Göteborg, Sweden, was screened in 1985 for anorexia nervosa, using questionnaires, growth charts and individual school nurse reports. This population consisted of 4,291 children in all. After full clinical assessments and interviews with the mothers, twenty-three were found to have an eating disorder. Among these, seventeen had a full anorexia nervosa syndrome, three had a partial anorexia nervosa syndrome and three had bulimia nervosa. The accumulated prevalence for anorexia nervosa among the girls (those who had or had had the disorder) was 0.84 per cent. Among the twenty cases of anorexia nervosa only nine had been referred to a psychiatric or pediatric clinic. Yet all the children, including the three with a partial syndrome, had severe and conspicuous symptoms. Eighty-five per cent of the cases satisfied DSM-III-R criteria for anorexia nervosa. An additional search of Göteborg psychiatric and pediatric clinics did not reveal any new cases that might have escaped detection during the population screening.

Of interest in this survey of young schoolchildren is the finding that six girls had an onset of anorexia nervosa at age 13 years, eight girls and two boys at age 14 years, and four girls at age 15 years. The onset of the anorexia coincided with early puberty in two of the girls and in the two boys but the remaining girls presented with secondary amenorrhoea. The authors also conclude that the peak age of onset was 14 years and they take issue with other investigators who have reported a peak age of onset at 18 years (Crisp and Stonehill, 1971; Szmukler et al., 1986). On the other hand, it must be questioned whether this conclusion is justified in view of the fact that Råstam and her colleagues concentrated their survey on the youngest population so far surveyed. They could not therefore ascertain patients whose illness commenced at a later age. Nevertheless their study is of great value and they reached the arresting conclusion that anorexia nervosa is even commoner in the general schoolgirl population than had been thought by previous investigators.

The incidence rate for anorexia nervosa in the Swedish study exceeds that reported by earlier investigators who tended to concentrate on smaller selected populations of schoolgirls. The most comparable study, that of Crisp et al. (1976) conducted in London private girls' schools, yielded a prevalence of only 0.2 per cent in girls aged 15 years and under. Another London study, again conducted in private schools, estimated a prevalence rate of 0.8 per cent in girls aged 14 to 18 years, and 1.1 per cent in girls aged 16 to 18 years (Szmukler, 1983). The failure of another London study to detect any cases of anorexia nervosa may have been due to the lower social class of the schoolgirls surveyed as they were attending state schools (Mann et al., 1983).

In conclusion, in view of the excellent methodology employed, including the scrutiny of the girl's growth chart and the internal validation which showed that no cases had been missed, the high prevalence rate in 15-year old schoolgirls in Sweden is likely to be the most accurate measure to date.

Sex ratio

Most studies of anorexia nervosa consistently show that 90 to 95 per cent of the patients are female (Garfinkel and Garner, 1982). There have, however, been exceptions among clinical series of children with anorexia nervosa. Thus six out of twenty pre-pubertal children reported by Jacobs and Isaacs (1986) were male, as were thirteen out of forty-eight early onset patients reported by Fosson et al. (1987), and four out of twenty-one children in Hawley's (1985) series. It may be surmised that the preponderance of females will be less marked when illness precedes puberty, before the accentuation of gender differences which follows puberty. This hypothesis is not supported, however, by looking at the sex ratio of the largest series of young patients reported in the literature so far. In his review of seven series of early onset anorexia nervosa, Swift (1982) provides data in support of a sex ratio of girls to boys of 9.5 to 1, a ratio not very different from that commonly reported in classical anorexia nervosa.

Causation of anorexia nervosa in the young

This discussion of causation will concentrate on those factors most pertinent to an illness of early onset, in order to avoid repeating material from the chapter on anorexia nervosa in adolescence (Chapter 7). Nevertheless, it is necessary to outline current thinking on the aetiology of anorexia nervosa generally. It should be recalled that the main clinical landmarks were reached over one hundred and thirty years ago when Gull (1874) and Lasègue (1873) came to recognise that anorexia nervosa was primarily a psychological disorder. They were both extremely cautious about the precise nature of the psychological disorder: Gull merely referred to a morbid mental state, whereas Lasègue thought the illness was hysterical *faute de mieux*. Since these two early classical contributions we have advanced extremely slowly. At this stage, it will suffice to mention the multidimensional perspective adopted by Garfinkel and Garner (1982), which is of heuristic value in promoting research on a broad front.

The multidimensional causation of anorexia nervosa

A multidimensional view of causation permits one to accept that a range of causal factors may interact in a cumulative or specific manner so as to cause anorexia nervosa. The causes may vary according to the different forms of the illness: for example pre-pubertal anorexia nervosa may have origins which differ wholly or partly from those of classical anorexia nervosa. A multi-dimensional view of causation goes further and allows for anorexia nervosa to occur only when a given constellation of causal factors interact with an individual patient's constitutional make-up. Thus the patient's constitution may result in a predisposing vulnerability for the illness. This vulnerability may remain concealed as a genetic predisposition, or it may reveal itself through the expression of a disturbed personality. The assessment of possible predisposing and precipitating causes (as well as perpetuating factors) in the individual patient is crucial if the responsible clinician is to understand her illness and devise an optimum plan of treatment. In keeping with the multidimensional approach, biological and psychosocial causes of anorexia nervosa will now be considered.

Biological causes

Genetic factors

There is increasing evidence that genetic factors contribute to the causation of anorexia nervosa. It has been known for some time that there is an increased familial incidence of the illness – 6.6 per cent among the sisters of patients (Theander, 1970). But the strongest evidence for a genetic basis comes from twin studies. The first decisive twin study, with at least one twin suffering from anorexia nervosa, was that by Holland *et al.* (1984). Among thirty female twin pairs, 55 per cent of the monozygotic and only 7 per cent of the dizygotic twins were concordant for anorexia nervosa. The authors of this twin study thought it likely that their findings could best be explained by a genetic predisposition to anorexia nervosa, which would express itself openly following adverse conditions such as excessive dieting.

In an extension of this first study, enlarging the series to forty-five twin pairs, Holland *et al.* (1988) found that there was again a significant difference between the concordance rates in the monozygotic pairs (56 per cent) and in the dizygotic pairs (5 per cent). They elaborated further the multidimensional model for the causation of anorexia nervosa: they suggested that the propensity for the illness is genetically determined and consists of a weakness of the homeostatic mechanisms which normally ensure restoration of weight after a period of weight loss. This model predicts that in a society where dieting and weight loss are common, individuals who are genetically vulnerable would be most at risk of developing anorexia nervosa.

The hypothalamic disorder

In the classical post-pubertal forms of anorexia nervosa it has been firmly established that the illness is associated with a hypothalamic disorder, manifest by an endocrine disturbance involving the hypothalamic-anterior pituitary-gonadal axis (Mortimer *et al.*, 1973; Boyar *et al.*, 1974; Mecklenberg *et al.*, 1974; Russell, 1977; Treasure *et al.*, 1988). The hypothalamic disorder in pre-menarchal anorexia nervosa is probably even more important as it is associated with an arrest of growth and pubertal development (Russell, 1983, 1985a). These younger patients have not yet been systematically investigated with modern methods of endocrine research. We know even less about the form of anorexia nervosa which has a true pre-pubertal onset.

The endocrine disorder is, to a large extent, due to weight loss and malnutrition, entirely so according to Ploog and Pirke (1987). Another view is that the endocrine disorder is not wholly due to weight loss but depends on additional factors such as the psychological disturbance which is always present in anorexia nervosa (Russell, 1965, 1977; Halmi and Falk, 1983; Wakeling and De Souza, 1983). The impact of weight loss in pre-pubertal anorexia nervosa is also crucial, and again controversial.

The dependence of puberty on an adequate nutritional state was expressed, perhaps in an extreme form, by Frisch and her colleagues who suggested that the onset of menarche depended on attaining a critical weight, or at least a critical body composition (17 per cent as stored fat) (Frisch and Revelle, 1971; Frisch and McArthur, 1974; Frisch, 1976). The notion of a specific weight threshold being necessary for the initiation and completion of puberty has been severely criticised (Tanner *et al.*, 1966; Billewicz *et al.*,

1981). Nevertheless, it is certain that in the presence of malnutrition due to anorexia nervosa puberty may be delayed or even arrested.

The effects of weight loss on endocrine function can be surmised by following the stages of endocrine recovery as effective treatment leads to a progressive increase in weight. Blood levels of gonadotrophins (LH and FSH) and oestrogen gradually rise. Early on, the action of gonadotrophin-releasing hormone (LHRH) is restored to normal, indicating a return of the functional capacity of the anterior pituitary. Most significant is the return of hypothalamic responsiveness to administered oestrogen which influences the release of LH. The negative-feedback effects are restored first, but the return of the positive-feedback effects may be considerably delayed (Wakeling et al., 1977). Endocrine recovery is also reflected in three stages of ovarian growth and differentiation demonstrated by the use of pelvic ultrasonography. To date, this sequence of events has been established in those patients with classical post-pubertal anorexia nervosa who are responding favourably to treatment as shown by a progressive gain in weight eventually followed by a return of menstruation (Treasure et al., 1985, 1988). During the first stage, severe undernutrition is associated with small amorphous ovaries. In the second stage, following partial weight gain, the ovaries are somewhat larger and contain follicles. This second stage is associated with a rise in blood levels of FSH, and LH to a lesser extent. During the third stage of ovarian differen-tiation one of the follicles grows to become a dominant follicle. This is associ-ated with the main rise of blood LH and oestrogens, the latter leading to an enlargement of the uterus.

Pelvic ultrasound examination of the ovaries and uterus is also a useful method of ascertaining regression or recovery in children with anorexia nervosa (Lai et al., 1994). A series of young patients were first tested when the children were of low weight and their menstruation had not yet been established. Their ovarian and uterine volumes were found to be reduced when compared with normal pubertal girls. On retesting eighteen months after the first scan, the patients who had achieved menstruation showed significantly higher ovarian and uterine volumes than the patients in whom amenorrhoea persisted. A comparison of the weight in these two groups led the authors to conclude that the advent of ovarian and uterine maturity required the young patients to achieve a mean weight of 48 kg and a mean weight/height of 96.5 per cent. This is a higher target weight than that usually set.

Cerebral lesions and disturbances

There were early clinical reports of patients diagnosed with anorexia nervosa who were later found to have one of a variety of cerebral lesions, for example, a tumour of the hypothalamus (Bauer, 1954; Diamond and Averick, 1966). There has been renewed interest in this subject from a report on occult intracranial tumours masquerading as anorexia nervosa in young children (De Vile *et al.*, 1995).

Functional neuroimaging techniques have also been applied in anorexia nervosa. Fifteen children were investigated with single photon emission computerised tomography (SPECT) (Gordon *et al.*, 1997). The method provides a measure of regional cerebral blood flow (RCBF). In most of the children there was a significant difference of over 10 per cent in the RCBF between the temporal lobes. Hypoperfusion was found on the left side in eight children and on the right in five. Unfortunately the method involves the intravenous injection of a radioactive ligand, which has made it impossible to have a control series of normal children. However, the authors retested three children in whom treatment had resulted in a normal weight. The reduced RCBF in the temporal lobe persisted on the same side as in the initial scan. It was tentatively concluded that the asymmetry in RCBF indicated an underlying neurological imbalance of the limbic system which in turn led to a hypothalamic-pituitary disturbance contributing to the onset of anorexia nervosa in these children. Clearly this work requires to be replicated.

Psychosocial causes

This section will again review causal factors contributing to anorexia nervosa in general, as well as causes more specific to the illness of early onset.

Sociocultural factors are clearly of crucial importance in causing anorexia nervosa which occurs predominantly within Westernised cultures. Brumberg (1988) has observed that certain social and cultural systems encourage women to control their food intake, but for different reasons and purposes which may vary over historical periods. In particular, the modern anorectic is said to strive for perfection in terms of society's ideal of physical beauty. In modern Western societies this ideal has increasingly valued thinness. This has led to dieting behaviour becoming popularised and highly prevalent even among young schoolgirls in whom it is probably harmful (Nylander, 1971; Patton, 1988). Increased vulnerability to anorexia nervosa has also been found in certain subcultures where professional demands and competitiveness lead to thinness being valued. Thus a high prevalence of anorexia nervosa has been identified among ballet students and models (Garner and Garfinkel, 1980; Szmukler *et al.*, 1985). On the other hand, some social groups within Western societies appear protected from anorexia nervosa, possibly because thinness is less valued among them. Thus this illness has been documented infrequently among non-whites. Among black American patients with anorexia nervosa, other causal factors are dominant, such as family bereavements or associated psychiatric illness (Robinson and Andersen, 1985).

Anorexia nervosa is relatively uncommon in parts of the world remote from Western influences including third world countries. Not surprisingly, there are few epidemiological studies from these countries, but one exception is a survey of a school in the islands of Sâo Miguel, a Portuguese territory of the Azores (de Azevedo and Ferreira, 1992). No case of frank anorexia nervosa was found although partial syndromes were identified in 0.7 per cent of the girls and 0.3 per cent of the boys interviewed. A prevalence of 0.3 per cent for DSM-III bulimia was found among the girls. These low prevalence rates for frank eating disorders were attributed by the author to an absence of sociocultural pressures to control eating and weight. Cultural determinants of eating disorders can affect young students whose nationality previously protected them. For example, Greek girls in Munich have a higher rate of anorexia nervosa than Greek girls in Greece (Fichter *et al.*, 1983), and Arab female students in London have a higher incidence of bulimia nervosa than students in Cairo (Nasser, 1986).

The family culture has been the subject of interesting theoretical ideas regarding its possible role in causing anorexia nervosa. Thus Bruch (1974) thought that a failure by the parents to encourage self-expression underlies the anorexic patient's 'paralysing sense of ineffectiveness'. Minuchin and his colleagues identified faulty patterns of interaction between members of the anorexic patient's family and concluded that the illness was a dysfunctional method used in an attempt to resolve the family's problems (Liebman *et al.*, 1974; Minuchin *et al.*, 1975). As well as identifying abnormal patterns of communication within these families, Palazzoli (1978) described abnormal relationships between the family members. It is assumed that anorexia nervosa is a logical adjustment to an illogical interpersonal system. Although these abnormal interactions can be identified in the families of anorexic patients, it remains uncertain whether they are to blame for the illness, or develop as a secondary adaptation by the parents faced with a starving child or adolescent.

More direct evidence of adverse familial influences is available from studies of mothers who themselves suffered from eating disorders and caused weight loss and sometimes anorexic attitudes in their children. Thus in a series of eight mothers with anorexia nervosa it was found that nine out of thirteen children had their food intake reduced by their mothers, who might prolong breast feeding and delay weaning, dilute the bottle feeds, reduce the amount of food available in their home, confine eating to mealtimes, and forbid the consumption of sweets (Russell *et al.*, 1998). In addition, in a minority of the children, anorexic attitudes were induced so that they would refuse food offered to them, for example at school, possibly out of misguided loyalty to their mothers. The resulting food deprivation led to a low weight and reduced growth in stature. The problems were remediable by a whole family approach. Catch-up growth was correlated with the degree of engagement in treatment of both mother and child. Similar findings have been reported by Van Wezel-Meijler and Wit (1989) and Hodes *et al.* (1997).

Adverse psychological factors can often be identified as precipitants shortly before the onset of anorexia nervosa. A major life event is thought to precede the illness more often with a pre-pubertal than a post-pubertal onset (Jacobs and Isaacs, 1986). These life events include bereavements, family disruptions and losses, physical illnesses causing weight loss, and scholastic pressures. The patient often experiences a high expectation of scholastic achievement. This is often self-imposed with the parents firmly denying that these expectations originate from them, but at the same time they express pride in their daughter's success at school. The onset of the illness may coincide with the stresses of preparing for school examinations, such as the ordinary or advanced certificates in Britain (Mills, 1973). In recent years interest in these somewhat banal causes has been displaced by a frenetic concern with the harmful effects of sexual abuse in childhood. It has been reported that about one-third of a series of eating disordered patients reported sexual experiences in childhood with persons who were significantly older (Palmer et al., 1990; McClelland et al., 1991). These rates indeed exceed substantially those found in non-psychiatric populations according to the evidence based on a community study in New Zealand (Mullen et al., 1988). The question has been examined whether childhood sexual abuse is a specific risk factor in patients who develop eating disorders, but it has been concluded that this is not the case as the rates for childhood sexual abuse in these patients are similar to those in various other psychiatric comparison groups (Wonderlich et al., 1997). It remains uncertain at present whether sexual abuse plays a significant part in causing anorexia nervosa, but whenever it is uncovered it assumes great importance in the treatment of the anorexic patient.

Interaction of biological and psychosocial causes at puberty

It is now time to turn to the interesting question of the possible role of puberty in the genesis of anorexia nervosa. The peak age of onset of the disorder is 17 to 18 years, some three to four years after the completion of puberty. Crisp (1980) has stated that anorexia nervosa arises out of puberty and is specifically related to the meaning that body shape and weight have for the patient. He therefore tries to bridge the psychological and biological determinants of anorexia nervosa. He views the illness as a regression into an existence which is simpler for the patient, removed from the conflicts of growth, sexuality and personal independence. The patient achieves this by losing weight through the systematic avoidance of carbohydrate-containing foods. Consequently the weight loss interrupts the central nervous mechanisms controlling sex hormone activity. This regression brings relief so that food avoidance becomes reinforced.

That anorexia nervosa occasionally represents an adverse reaction to the physical changes of puberty in vulnerable patients has received empirical support from the observations of Brown (1989). She ascertained systematically the reaction to menarche and puberty in a series of forty-seven patients with eating disorders. About one-third of them reported very negative experiences such as revulsion, disgust and fear of the first menstrual bleeding or embarrassment when breasts began to develop. The majority of the patients, however, were rated as having no problems or only minor difficulties in adjusting to their puberty. The minority of patients with a negative response tended to be lighter in weight and more depressed than those with a positive response to puberty. Brown concluded that, at least for a minority of patients with eating disorders, the developmental conflict of puberty may play a role in the causation of the illness.

As long ago as 1968 Warren questioned whether Crisp's hypothesis was tenable in the patients he described as afflicted with 'pre-pubertal' (meaning pre-menarchal) anorexia nervosa. Crisp (1980) argued correctly that puberty is a prolonged process with menarche a late feature, so that when the patient's illness commences before the menarche it may still be in response to the emotional upheavals occurring during the earliest phases of the pubertal process. An argument against Crisp's hypothesis of a regression from pubertal conflicts was provided by Jacobs and Isaacs (1986) in their retrospective study of a series of true pre-pubertal patients with anorexia nervosa. They compared them with a series of post-pubertal patients and found both series to experience very similar illnesses. In particular there were no differences in the high levels of 'sexual anxiety' consisting of fears of growing up, sexual maturity, menstruation, motherhood or fatherhood. In their appraisal of Crisp's hypothesis, the authors endorsed a multidimensional approach to causation. They surmised that instead of pubertal conflicts pre-pubertal patients would reveal other predisposing causes. Their study confirmed the more frequent occurrence of major life events before the onset of the illness, higher levels of family preoccupations with feeding, and early feeding difficulties in the patients themselves. The patients also showed more behavioural difficulties in childhood. These authors concluded that in pre-pubertal anorexia nervosa there occurs an interaction between a high premorbid level of emotional disturbance and external pressures or precipitating life events. On the other hand, post-pubertal patients would appear to have had a lower level of stress until they experience what for them are the major conflicts of puberty and adolescence. If this interpretation is sustained by further research, it would support a multidimensional approach to anorexia nervosa, with the conflicts of puberty amounting to powerful contributory causes.

Clinical features

Anorexia nervosa occurs much more frequently in girls than in boys. Accordingly the illness will first be described in girls, and the few points of difference will be left to a later short section.

Subclassification and terminology

The sequence of events when a girl passes through her puberty has been described by Tanner (1962). Early signs are the growth of breast buds and the appearance of pubic hair. The menarche is usually a late event, but varies in its occurrence between the ages of 10 and 16 years. Puberty is accompanied by accelerated growth and weight gain. Anorexia nervosa may be classified according to its onset in relation to the timing of puberty.

Pre-pubertal anorexia nervosa

This has its onset before any of the signs of puberty have even begun to appear. It evidently coincides with the earliest ages of onset, 9 to 11 years.

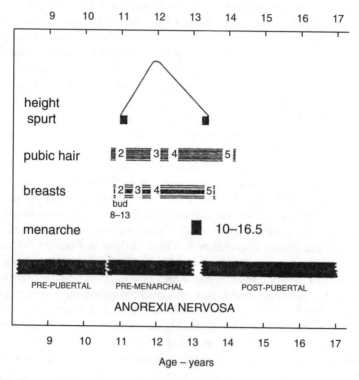

Figure 6.1 The normal sequence of pubertal events in girls. From above downwards: (i) changes in the rate of linear growth; (ii) the growth of pubic hair and breast development, each shown on a five-point scale. The appearance of breast buds ranges from 8 to 13 years; (iii) the menarche occurs late during the pubertal sequence, but varies from 10 to 16.5 years. The three solid black lines depict the time of onset of anorexia nervosa in relation to pubertal events: pre-pubertal, pre-menarchal and post-pubertal.

Source: Modified from Tanner, 1962.

Pre-menarchal anorexia nervosa

This occurs some time during the pubertal process itself. Early breast growth and scanty pubic hair will be evident on examination. Growth in stature will usually have become arrested. The age of onset of pre-menarchal anorexia nervosa varies from 10 to 14 years.

Post-pubertal anorexia nervosa

This is the commonest form of the illness, and occurs some time after the completion of puberty and the establishment of menstruation. The age of onset usually extends from 13 years upwards.

The value of this subclassification is that it alerts the clinician to the risk of pre-pubertal anorexia nervosa delaying the onset of puberty. In the case of a pre-menarchal onset, pubertal development will already have commenced, only to become arrested. In either case the completion of puberty is likely to be delayed, so that even in patients who recover fully the menarche is usually late. Until recovery occurs, primary amenorrhoea is a feature of the illness, but not recognised as significant until the girl becomes older, for example after the age of 16 years. This, of course, is in contrast to the secondary amenorrhoea of post-pubertal anorexia nervosa, a symptom which is of diagnostic significance in this classical form of the illness.

The time of onset of anorexia nervosa in relation to the pubertal process is also of significance in terms of weight changes in the patient. With a post-pubertal onset there occurs a weight loss, below the optimum level previously achieved by the healthy adolescent. This optimum level has been defined as the 'healthy weight' (Russell, 1979, 1985b) or 'premorbid weight' (Treasure *et al.*, 1988). In the case of pre-pubertal or pre-menarchal onset, however, the patient has not yet achieved her mature weight: had she not become ill she would still have been gaining weight. The early phase of the illness is associated with an arrest of this normal weight gain. Thereafter, there often occurs an actual loss of weight. These observations are relevant to the diagnostic criteria for cases of early onset, which will be formulated later. They also bear on the prediction of what weight should be gained in order to induce an endocrine recovery. Whereas in post-pubertal anorexia nervosa menstruation is resumed on returning to the premorbid weight, in pre-menarchal anorexia nervosa a completion of puberty cannot readily be predicted from the girl's weight history.

The estimation of the patient's optimum weight is further complicated by her probable failure to have reached an optimum stature. She will have missed the growth spurt associated with a normal puberty. This removes an important guide to a patient's optimum weight, because it should not be based on a sub-optimal height. Yet it is essential to assess the weight necessary for an early resumption of puberty. In order to do this, standardised weight charts for children and adolescents are consulted so as to ascertain the 50th percentile weight to be expected at the patient's age, irrespective of her stature. A more reliable figure can be reached if a serial record of weights well before the onset of the illness is available, as this will provide a better impression of the percentile weight achieved by the individual child while she was still growing normally. Extrapolation on the same percentile weight chart will provide a 'healthy' weight to be aimed at in the course of treatment so as to ensure a normal completion of puberty.

Clinical presentation of anorexia nervosa of early onset

Precipitating events may or may not have been evident. It has been previously indicated that they may range from a family bereavement to a physical illness associated with a loss of weight, the stress of school examinations or apparently trivial teasing by other children.

The presentation of the illness is highly variable and the onset is liable to be insidious (Fosson et al., 1987). The child appears fretful, withdraws from her friends and may refuse to go to school. On the other hand, she may voice no complaint, and the omission of school meals may remain undetected. Thus the parents notice nothing amiss until they become aware that she has become thinner. The key feature is a failure to gain weight followed by actual weight loss. Because the child may not yet have reached her optimum weight, the superadded weight loss may result in a very low weight indeed, as low as 25 kg or even lower.

When the weight loss is eventually detected the child is likely to complain of insomnia, constipation, cold extremities, and even tiredness. This last symptom may be displaced, however, when the patient exercises to excess – jogging, walking or cycling long distances. When parents attempt to reduce this excessive activity she may continue to practise press-ups or other exercises in solitude in her bedroom. Repeated rubbing of the skin on pressure points may result in abrasions or sores, evidence of the repetitiveness of a particular exercise.

Closer observation by the parents reveals that their child is avoiding food. Even young children may become preoccupied with the caloric values of foods. They may resort to deviousness and secrecy. The marked resistance to eating becomes manifest when attempts are made to reverse the loss of weight. Although typical bulimia nervosa is rare in young children, these patients may experience episodes of overeating in secret, and then induce vomiting or take laxatives (Lask and Bryant-Waugh, 1986).

Symptoms of depression and tension are common (Fosson et al., 1987) and may be more frequent than in illnesses of later onset. Indeed, severe depression was found in 69 per cent of youngsters in the Göteborg community-based study (Råstam *et al.*, 1989). Crying may be frequent, as may be the expression of guilt, particularly when asked to eat food she feels she does not deserve. When depression is severe, self-injuries including lacerations with sharp objects or actual suicidal attempts may occur. Obsessional features are also frequently encountered. In the Göteborg study one-third of the patients had an obsessive compulsive personality disorder, and 8 per cent developed hand washing and other compulsions (Råstam *et al.*, 1989). Thus the majority of anorexic patients displayed personality traits of conscientiousness and orderliness. Frank obsessional rituals including the counting of calories are also frequently evident.

Mental state

When the child is asked why she avoids food, she is most likely to disclose that it is through a fear of fatness. This is in keeping with the principal psychological disturbance in anorexia nervosa – an over-valued idea that to be fat is not only unattractive, but also unlovable. A sizeable minority of patients express their difficulties in terms of a physical symptom such as abdominal pain, nausea, feelings of fullness or loss of appetite (Fosson *et al.*, 1987). A small group of patients will disclose fears that may be viewed as a reluctance to grow up or develop into sexual maturity. These may include fears of puberty and especially menstruation. On the other hand, girls with a prolonged illness who have failed to develop breasts become sensitive about this obvious lack of femininity. Some of these patients specifically request treatment to induce breast growth and their motivation may improve when it is explained that a general management which includes weight gain is the best approach.

A reluctance to grow up may be expressed in social terms, the patient feeling much uncertainty about a future which includes greater personal responsibility and the prospect of leaving home. She may also display 'manipulative' behaviour. Whereas most patients will express regret about upsetting their parents, some may frankly revel in their discovery of newly gained power over the family.

Physical examination

Very low weights may be recorded in these patients, who will also show general wasting, hollow cheeks, stick-like limbs, and a flat belly and buttocks. The extremities are blue and cold. The skin is dry with downy hair (lanugo) over the cheeks, back of the neck and limbs. The heart rate is slow and the blood pressure low (e.g. 90/60 mm Hg).

Delay or arrest of puberty

In addition to these general signs of malnutrition, the impact of the illness on pubertal development may also be evident, according to the time of onset. If the onset was pre-pubertal, the absence of any sign of pubertal development and the failure of growth will become increasingly conspicuous as the child becomes older and with continued duration of the illness. A pre-menarchal onset will cause arrest of pubertal development which will be most severe if the weight loss occurs during the early stages of puberty. Thus, the young girl may only have reached a height corresponding to less than the second percentile (usually 1.47 m to 1.50 m). Pubic hair will be scanty. The breasts may show early growth only (Tanner, 1962: Stages 1 or 2). Menarche will be delayed beyond the normal age. The impact of anorexia nervosa on puberty is variable. Fortunately most patients with a pre-pubertal or pre-menarchal onset eventually recover, with a mere delay of their menarche, as in the first clinical illustration.

Patient I

This girl's illness began when she was 12 years of age: her weight was static at first but then diminished until she weighed only 30 kg at 14 years. She was then very thin and short in stature (1.525 m), with tiny breasts (Tanner Stage 1) and scanty pubic hair. She responded well to in-patient treatment and subsequent out-patient family therapy. At the age of 16 years 11 months when she had recovered she weighed 53 kg and her height had increased to 1.56 m. Menstruation had begun at 15 years 8 months. She had made a full psychological recovery.

A very different course was shown by the next patient to be described.

Patient 2

This girl's parents blamed themselves for having taken her to a pediatrician at the age of 10 in order to reduce her slight plumpness. One year later she was admitted to hospital weighing only 25 kg. This admission and nine subsequent re-admissions failed to bring about a stable weight gain. She was reassessed at 18 years when she weighed only 24 kg. Her height was only 1.505 m and her breasts had hardly developed (Tanner Stage 1). Intensive in-patient treatment resulted in a weight of 46 kg which was maintained for three months, but there was no gain in stature, no significant breast development and primary amenorrhoea persisted. After discharge from hospital she again lost weight, and six years later had not gone through her puberty.

This patient illustrates the adverse effects which early anorexia nervosa may have on growth, breast development and menstrual function. These will now be discussed in turn.

Growth failure

Examples of failures of linear growth were provided in a study of twenty patients in whom the onset had been identified as pre-menarchal; only two of them had reached the 50th percentile in height (Russell, 1985a). In the case of seven of these patients, catch-up growth of 2 to 5 cm was achieved as a result of treatment resulting in weight gain. This favourable response only occurred, however, in patients aged 17 years or less.

Breast development

In the same series (Russell, 1985a) only six patients had normal breasts, four had small breasts and the remaining ten patients had only infantile breasts. After weight gain, sustained for at least three months, eight of the fourteen patients with underdeveloped breasts showed a considerable response. Because of individual variations it is difficult to determine whether an optimum breast growth has been achieved. There is some evidence that even in these patients the response was less than optimum. For example, one patient required the additional administration of ethinyl estradiol and norethisterone to enable her breasts to develop fully to Tanner Stage 5 (Russell, 1983). Further evidence of a permanent arrest of breast growth was provided by a case of monozygotic twins who both suffered from 'pre-menarchal anorexia nervosa' from the age of 13 (Russell, 1983). Twin A had experienced a less severe illness and had developed normal breasts. Twin B, however, had suffered an unremitting illness and her breasts were infantile. Hospital admission caused both patients to gain weight to 44 kg in six weeks. Twin B responded with growth of her breasts which she welcomed. However, they remained smaller than her sister's. As these twins possessed identical genetic material it is unlikely that the failure of full breast growth was due to end-organ insensitivity to hormonal control. Instead, it is probable that there occurred a more permanent failure of breast development as a result of severe prolonged malnutrition interfering with puberty.

Menstrual function

Pre-pubertal and pre-menarchal anorexia nervosa will also cause a delay in the onset of menstruation. Amenorrhoea will persist until after weight gain and recovery, and even then there might be a prolonged delay. In the same series of twenty pre-menarchal patients (Russell, 1985a), only four had menstruated by the age of 16 years. A further three patients menstruated between 16 and 18 years. Among the remaining thirteen patients, four had begun to menstruate at ages ranging from 18 to 25. The remaining nine patients had prolonged amenorrhoea well beyond the age of 18.

It is perhaps curious that the arrest of puberty resulting from anorexia nervosa has only recently been studied systematically (Russell, 1983, 1985a). Earlier writers have, on the whole, been unconcerned about the risk of physical sequelae. In one study it was noted that normal menstruation would become established in late adolescence after recovery (Warren, 1968). In another study most of the young girls reported on progressed well physically, and any sequelae were more likely to be in the psychological sphere (Silverman, 1974). Such optimism may indeed be justified for the majority of patients. Arrest of puberty may occur uncommonly when a severe and chronic form of anorexia nervosa coincides with a critical pubertal stage. This explains why attempts to study the effects of the illness on linear growth during adolescence have, on the whole, provided inconclusive or reassuring results (Crisp, 1969; Lacey et al., 1979; Pfeiffer et al., 1986). In none of these studies was a distinction made between post-pubertal and earlier onset, though all of them concentrated on young patients (e.g. an onset before 18 years in the study by Lacey et al.). The study by Pfeiffer and colleagues would have included patients with a pre-menarchal onset as the average age at diagnosis was 13.8 years. These authors concluded that most patients with anorexia nervosa continue to grow at the expected rate and to reach their expected height despite considerable earlier weight losses. They agree, however, that exceptions do occur. It is probable that these exceptions are the patients who fail to recover at a sufficiently early age to allow growth to be resumed. They may have been missed in previous studies and, while relatively few in number, these patients obviously present the clinician with an important therapeutic challenge.

Special investigations

Plasma levels of follicular stimulating hormone (FSH), luteinizing hormone (LH) and oestrogens are certain to be low in these patients and may remain reduced for months after weight gain, until the pubertal process is set in train. With these investigations there are often delays before the results become available. They are thus less likely to be clinically useful than serial pelvic ultrasound scans, which yield immediate observations. In the post-pubertal patient who is severely malnourished the ovaries will be seen to be small and amorphous in structure. If she is less severely undernourished the ovaries will appear somewhat larger with multiple small follicles (3 to 9 mm in diameter). With approaching recovery, in about 50 per cent of patients, one of the follicles overtakes the others in size, reaching 10 mm or more, a sign that a return of menstruation is imminent (Treasure et al., 1988). In the pre-menarchal patient the ovaries will be small (e.g. 1.5 cubic cm), as will the uterus (e.g. 6.7 cubic cm). The precise pattern of ovarian recovery on ultrasound, following weight gain, has yet to be determined. It is likely that multifollicular ovaries eventually develop as this is a normal morphological appearance in pre-pubertal girls (Treasure and Thompson, 1988).

Bone age, estimated from X-rays of the wrist, will be delayed by up to three years. Although the initial haemoglobin is often normal, it may show a moderate to severe fall after weight gain. Other abnormalities due to malnutrition may also be found, such as leucopenia, thrombocytopenia, raised blood urea, hypercarotenemia and electrocardiographic changes (Mester, 1981; Silverman, 1983).

Anorexia nervosa in boys

Anorexia nervosa is still far less common in young boys than in young girls. The clinical manifestations in young boys require clarification as only a few of them have been described in detail. It is clear, however, that, as with girls, in boys the illness can occur before the completion of puberty (Beumont et al., 1972). The precipitants include premorbid obesity or oversensitivity to teasing about their weight and appearance by other children. A few boys may express anxiety about their developing sexuality.

The clinical features of anorexia nervosa in boys are remarkably similar or equivalent to those in girls. This similarity renders the sex difference in the incidence of the illness all the more puzzling. The young boy becomes preoccupied with fatness and avoids food in order to lose weight. Again the food avoidance may be rationalised on the grounds of abdominal pain, constipation or other bodily complaints. The endocrine disorder in the male also consists of a disturbance of the hypothalamic-pituitary-gonadal axis, whose clinical consequences are equivalent to those in the female. With a prepubertal onset, and to a lesser degree with an intra-pubertal onset, the penis and scrotum remain infantile, there is only a scanty growth of pubic and facial hair, and the voice may not break.

Assessment of the family

Although caution has been recommended before concluding that pathological family processes underlie anorexia nervosa (Russell et al., 1987), it is desirable to make a thorough appraisal of family organisation to complement the assessment of the child. Fosson et al. (1987) have described parental overinvolvement in a high proportion of families, with a lack of privacy for individual members of the family. In addition they frequently observed communication problems such as individual members speaking for or interrupting others, and the issuing of mixed messages. Whereas overprotective or inconsistent parenting occurs in most families with an anorexic child, deficient parenting may occur in a minority of them. Marital conflict is also common and 'triangulation' may be a feature, when a third person (the patient) is drawn into the transactions occurring between two people (the parents) (Minuchin et al., 1978).

Diagnostic criteria of pre-pubertal and pre-menarchal anorexia nervosa

It follows from the preceding account that three sets of criteria can be formulated for the diagnosis of pre-pubertal and intra-pubertal anorexia nervosa:

1   There is a failure to gain weight at the time of the expected growth spurt (10–14 years), or an actual loss of weight may occur. This nutritional failure is the result of food avoidance often accompanied by excessive exercise.
2   The basic psychopathology of anorexia nervosa is similar to that in older patients, with evidence of an exaggerated dread of fatness.
3   There is an endocrine disorder that manifests itself as a retardation of normal pubertal development. In girls, growth in stature is reduced, breast development is incomplete and the menarche is delayed. In boys, in addition to the delay in growth, the penis and scrotum remain infantile, and there is only a scanty growth of pubic and facial hair.

The criteria for the diagnosis of pre-menarchal anorexia nervosa were put forward in 1985 (Russell, 1985a) and are incorporated in ICD-10 (1992).

The outcome of anorexia nervosa with an onset before or during puberty

Unfortunately there are few or no follow-up studies on the outcome of anorexia nervosa with a pre-pubertal or pre-menarchal onset, in comparison with the numerous studies on the post-pubertal form of the illness. The studies that are available were carried out on young patients in whom the onset was not defined with respect to the stages of pubertal development. There is another reason for dissatisfaction with the adequacy of outcome studies in pre-pubertal and pre-menarchal anorexia nervosa. Swift (1982), in reviewing follow-up studies, provided a long list of requirements: diagnostic criteria, specified patient selection, information about treatment, follow-up methodology and indicators of outcome; but he failed to include the measures of arrested puberty described above, except for the criterion of a return of menstruation. This omission is also a feature of most other studies, and it is to be hoped that future outcome research will include follow-up data on stature, secondary sexual characteristics, reproductive function and psychosexual development.

One of the principal aims of following up a series of patients is to determine the proportions who recover, remain chronically ill or die. It has to be conceded, however, that these proportions vary a great deal from one study to another. These variations almost certainly reflect differences in the severity of the patients' illnesses, rather than the efficacy of the treatment delivered in different centres. This can be illustrated with the findings from the follow-up studies on patients with the classical post-pubertal onset. A high recovery rate (58 per cent) was reported among patients treated mainly as out-patients (Morgan *et al.*, 1983), in comparison with recovery rates of 39 per cent (Morgan and Russell, 1975) and 48 per cent (Hsu *et al.*, 1979) among those treated mainly as in-patients. Higher recovery rates were also reported among first admissions to hospital rather than subsequent admissions, again under-lining the importance of selection factors in modifying apparent outcome. This, unfortunately, means that it is not possible to compare the efficacy of treatment in different centres on the basis of different patterns of outcome.

While bearing in mind the limitations of follow-up studies, comparisons are still worthwhile as they provide a general guide to the frequency of recoveries. Swift (1982) reviewed seven series, each of which included a high proportion of younger patients. Among them, the report by Minuchin *et al.* (1978) gave the highest recovery rate (78 per cent). In contrast, the study by Sturzenberger *et al.* (1977) yielded a 59 per cent rate for recoveries based on patients' menstrual function, and that by Warren (1968) provided a 56 per cent recovery rate.

Hawley (1985) followed up twenty-one children who were aged 13 years or less at the onset of anorexia nervosa and found a good nutritional outcome among 67 per cent of them. Bryant-Waugh *et al.* (1988) obtained a good outcome in 60 per cent of thirty-four children with a mean age of onset of 11.7 years. A lower rate of recovery could have been expected in this series of children treated at Great Ormond Street, London, as a high proportion of them would previously have been treated in other centres. Råstam *et al.* (2003) have more recently reported the outcome of anorexia nervosa in a community-based sample with a mean age of onset of 14.3 years. The 10-year outcome was relatively favourable with half of the 51 cases free from eating disorder and other axis I disorder. There were no deaths.

It is sad to observe that among the patients with the severest illnesses there is a definite risk of death. Swift (1982) estimated the mortality rate as 3.2 per cent among the 186 patients included in the seven studies he reviewed. This must be considered an imperfect estimate as he does not express it in terms of the average duration of the follow-ups. Among individual series, the more informative mortality rates are 6 per cent among 151 patients over the course of 12.5 years (Tolstrup *et al.*, 1985), 7 per cent over 7.2 years (Bryant-Waugh *et al.*, 1988) and, in the smallest series (Warren, 1968), 10 per cent over 8 years. The first of these is the largest study but included patients with a later age of onset: its mortality rate (0.5 per cent per year) should be com-pared with that found by Theander (1985) in adult patients (18 per cent over 33 years). It appears, therefore, that the risk of death in children and young adolescents is somewhat similar to that in adults. The causes of death in order of frequency were suicide, malnutrition and oesophageal rupture from vomiting.

A variable minority of patients fail to recover and remain chronically ill, sometimes into adulthood. Among them a small number of patients fail to complete their puberty, as described above. Consequently there is a persistence of primary amenorrhoea, some reduction in stature and a failure of breast development. Even if they eventually increase their weight, they may not commence menstruation and become fertile (Russell, 1985a). It remains uncertain whether every anorectic with persistent primary amenorrhoea remains capable of reproductive recovery after weight gain. The consequences for the patient's psychosexual development in the event of a delayed puberty have not been determined as the appropriate research has yet to be carried out.

Among the patients who fail to recover, the majority show persistent features of anorexia nervosa. In a minority, however, the anorexic features are gradually displaced by other psychological disturbances, especially depressive or obsessive-compulsive symptoms. One study stands apart, in that about 60 per cent of the patients manifested a range of depressive features on long-term follow-up. This is the study by Cantwell and his colleagues (1977) on patients with a mean age of onset of 13.47 years. Because of this finding the authors proposed that in at least some cases anorexia nervosa is a variant of an affective disorder. However, theirs was rather a small series with a successful follow-up of twenty-six patients. Moreover, at least three of them would now probably be diagnosed as bulimia nervosa, a disorder whose description only appeared two years later (Russell, 1979). Their findings stand in marked contrast to the larger series of Tolstrup and his colleagues (1985) in which persistent anorexia nervosa was the commonest psychiatric diagnosis among the patients who failed to recover. In conclusion, there may well be an overlap between some cases of anorexia nervosa and depressive illness, but this is no argument for minimising the diagnostic status of anorexia nervosa which generally runs its own course, and calls for a different therapeutic approach.

It is as well to concede that the course and outcome of anorexia nervosa in an individual patient are well nigh unpredictable. Prognosis remains a difficult task, and follow-up studies have yielded relatively few prognostic predictors to help the clinician. However, the long-term follow-up study by Bryant-Waugh and her colleagues (1988) is the most informative on this subject. Depressive features during the initial illness tended to be associated with a poorer future outcome. There was also a tendency for a less favourable outcome to be associated with an abnormal family structure – for example, one-parent families or families in which one or both parents had previously been married. Surprisingly, outcome did not appear to be related to the duration of the illness at referral, nor was it influenced by the patient's gender.

Age of onset of anorexia nervosa is one variable which has interested several investigators as a possible prognostic predictor. Age of onset has been shown to have a predictive value in post-pubertal patients, in that the older the age at onset, the worse the outcome (Morgan and Russell, 1975; Hsu *et al.*, 1979). The equivalent equation in pre-menarchal and pre-pubertal patients remains ambiguous. There are in fact two parts to the question:

1   Is a pre-menarchal or a younger age of onset (e.g. 15 years or less) associated with a better outcome?
2   Within this younger group of patients, is there a correlation between age of onset and eventual outcome?

Swift (1982) addressed himself to the first question and concluded that there was insufficient evidence to support the view that an early age of onset is associated with a good outcome. This view is also supported by Hawley (1985). As regards the second question, the clearest statement is by Bryant-Waugh *et al.* (1988) who found that a young age at referral was associated with a poorer outcome. This finding raises the possibility of a u-shaped relationship, with a worse outcome to be expected at both the very young and the older ends of the age spectrum.

In conclusion, the relationship between age of onset and outcome in pre-menarchal patients is still uncertain and requires further research for its clarification.

Conclusion

This chapter consists of a review of current knowledge on anorexia nervosa when its onset occurs in childhood or early adolescence, thus threatening normal pubertal development. Treatment is not considered as it is dealt with later in this volume (Chapter 9).

It is essential to subclassify the illness in terms of its onset in relation to the pubertal process, that is, pre-pubertal, intra-pubertal (or pre-menarchal) and post-pubertal (or classical) anorexia nervosa. A high prevalence of the illness (0.84 per cent) has been detected in a population of young schoolgirls in Göteborg in Sweden.

As in more mature patients, the aetiology of anorexia nervosa is best viewed from a multidimensional perspective. This explains why the illness occurs only when a constellation of factors interact with each other: for example, a constitutional vulnerability together with certain precipitating factors, or a specific mix of biological and psychosocial causes. An attractive multidimensional model is one of a genetically determined propensity for the illness which is brought to light only after weight loss is induced through fashionable dieting. This model applies equally to the later and the earlier onsets of anorexia nervosa. On the other hand, it may be argued that the psychobiological impact of puberty, which has been adduced as an important determinant of post-pubertal anorexia nervosa, cannot be considered as a likely cause of pre-pubertal anorexia nervosa. In the latter patients, a more important role is attributed to previous emotional disturbances, external pressures and adverse life events.

The clinical manifestations of pre- and intra-pubertal anorexia nervosa differ from those of the classical illness in important respects. First, pubertal development is likely to be delayed until after recovery, or may be arrested in severe and chronic cases. Thus there may be a failure of linear growth, the breasts may fail to develop and the menarche may be long delayed. Second, recovery must include as a criterion the resumption of endocrine function leading to a full pubertal development. Serial pelvic ultrasound examinations may be useful in determining hypothalamic-pituitary-ovarian recovery.

The lack of fully satisfactory follow-up studies of patients with early onset anorexia nervosa limits meaningful comparisons with those of later onset, although most reports suggest that the outcome is more favourable than in the classical later form of the illness. Prognostication is difficult with the individual patient. It remains uncertain whether age of onset is as useful a prognostic indicator as in classical anorexia nervosa.

References

Bauer, H. G. (1954) Endocrine and other clinical manifestations of hypothalamic disease. A survey of sixty cases with autopsies. *Journal of Clinical Endocrinology*, 14, 13.

Beumont, P. J. V., Beardwood, C. J. and Russell, G. F. M. (1972) The occurrence of the syndrome of anorexia nervosa in male subjects. *Psychological Medicine*, 2, 216–231.

Billewicz, W. Z., Fellowes, H. M. and Thomson, A. M. (1981) Pubertal changes in boys and girls in Newcastle upon Tyne. *Annals of Human Biology*, 8, 3, 211–219.

Blitzer, J. R., Rollins, N. and Blackwell, A. (1961) Children who starve themselves: anorexia nervosa. *Psychosomatic Medicine*, 23, 369–383.

Boyar, R. M., Katz, J., Finkelstein, J. W., Kapen, S., Weiner, H., Weitzman, E. D. and Hellman, L. (1974) Anorexia nervosa; immaturity of the 24-hour luteinizing hormone secretary pattern. *New England Journal of Medicine*, 291, 861–865.

Brown, R. M. A. (1989) Psychosexual development, adjustment and behaviour in women with anorexia nervosa, bulimia nervosa and neurotic (phobic) disorder. MPhil diss., University of London.

Bruch, H. (1974) *Eating Disorders: Obesity, Anorexia Nervosa and the Person Within*. London: Routledge and Kegan Paul.

Brumberg, J. J. (1988) *Fasting Girls: The Emergence of Anorexia Nervosa as a Modern Disease*. Cambridge, Mass.: Harvard University Press.

Bryant-Waugh, R., Knibbs, J., Fosson, A., Kaminski, Z. and Lask, B. (1988) Long term follow-up of patients with early onset anorexia nervosa. *Archives of Disease in Childhood*, 63, 5–9.

Cantwell, D. P., Sturzenberger, S., Burroughs, J., Salkin, B. and Green, J. K. (1977) Anorexia nervosa. An affective disorder? *Archives of General Psychiatry*, 34, 1087–1093.

Crisp, A. H. (1965) Some aspects of the evolution, presentation and follow-up of anorexia nervosa. *Proceedings of the Royal Society of Medicine*, 58, 814–820.

Crisp, A. H. (1969) Some skeletal measurements in patients with primary anorexia nervosa. *Journal of Psychosomatic Research*, 13, 125–142.

Crisp, A. H. (1980) *Let Me Be*. London: Academic Press.

Crisp, A. H. and Harding, B. (1979) Outcome of anorexia nervosa. *The Lancet*, 1, 61–65.

Crisp, A. H. and Stonehill, E. (1971) Relationship between aspects of nutritional disturbance and menstrual activity in primary anorexia nervosa. *British Medical Journal*, iii, 149–151.

Crisp, A. H., Palmer, R. L. and Kalucy, R. S. (1976) How common is anorexia nervosa? A prevalence study. *British Journal of Psychiatry*, 128, 549–554.

de Azevedo, M. H. and Ferreira, C. P. (1992) Anorexia nervosa and bulimia: a prevalence study. *Acta Psychiatrica Scandinavica*, 86, 6, 432–436.

De Vile, C. H., Sufraz, R., Lask, B. D. and Stanhope, R. (1995) Occult intracranial tumours masquerading as early onset anorexia nervosa. *British Medical Journal*, 311, 1359–1360.

Diamond, E. F. and Averick, N. (1966) Marasmus and the Diencephalic Syndrome. *Archives of Neurology*, 14, 270.

Fichter, M. M., Weyerer, S., Sourdi, L. and Sourdi, Z. (1983) In *Anorexia Nervosa. Recent Developments in Research* (ed. P. L. Darby, P. E. Garfinkel, D. M. Garner and D. V. Coscina). New York: Alan R. Liss.

Fosson, A., Knibbs, J., Bryant-Waugh, R. and Lask, B. (1987) Early onset anorexia nervosa. *Archives of Disease in Childhood*, 62, 114–118.

Frisch, R. E. (1976) In *The Physiological Basis of Reproductive Efficiency. In Meat Animals* (ed. D. Lister, D. J. Rhodes, V. R. Fowler and M. F. Fuller). New York: Plenum Publishing.

Frisch, R. E. and McArthur, J. W. (1974) Menstrual cycles: fatness as a determinant of minimum weight for height necessary for their maintenance or onset. *Science*, 185, 949–951.

Frisch, R. E. and Revelle, R. (1971) Height and weight at menarche and a hypothesis of menarche. *Archives of Disease in Childhood*, 46, 695–701.

Garfinkel, P. E. and Garner, D. M. (1982) *Anorexia Nervosa: A Multi-dimensional Perspective*. New York: Brunner-Mazel.

Garner, D. M. and Garfinkel, P. E. (1980) Sociocultural factors in the development of anorexia nervosa. *Psychological Medicine*, 10, 647–656.

Gordon, I., Lask, B., Bryant-Waugh, R., Christie, D. and Timimi, S. (1997) Childhood onset anorexia nervosa: towards identifying a biological substrate. *International Journal of Eating Disorders*, 22, 2, 159–165.

Gull, W. W. (1874) Anorexia nervosa (apepsia hysterica, anorexia hysterica). *Transactions of the Clinical Society of London*, 7, 180–185.

Halmi, K. A. and Falk, J. R. (1983) Behavioral and dietary discriminators of menstrual function in anorexia nervosa. In *Anorexia Nervosa: Recent Developments in Research* (ed. P. L. Darby, P. E. Garfinkel, D. M. Garner and D. V. Coscina). New York: Alan R. Liss.

Hawley, R. M. (1985) The outcome of anorexia nervosa in younger subjects. *British Journal of Psychiatry*, 146, 657–660.

Hodes, M., Timimi, S. and Robinson, P. (1997) Children of mothers with eating disorders: a preliminary study. *European Eating Disorders Review*, 5, 1, 11–24.

Hoek, H. W. and Brook, F. G. (1985) Patterns of care in anorexia nervosa. *Journal of Psychiatric Research*, 19, 155–160.

Holland, A. J., Hall, A., Murray, R. M., Russell, G. F. M. and Crisp, A. H. (1984) Anorexia nervosa: a study of 34 twin pairs and 1 set of triplets. *British Journal of Psychiatry*, 145, 414–419.

Holland, A. J., Sicotte, N. and Treasure, J. L. (1988) Anorexia nervosa: evidence for a genetic basis. *Journal of Psychosomatic Research*, 32, 561–571.

Hsu, L. K. G., Crisp, A. H. and Harding, B. (1979) Outcome of anorexia nervosa. *The Lancet*, i, 61–65.

ICD-10 Classification of Mental and Behavioural Disorders – Clinical Description and Diagnostic Guidelines (1992). Geneva: World Health Organization, 176–177.

Jacobs, B. W. and Isaacs, S. (1986) Pre-pubertal anorexia nervosa: a retrospective controlled study. *Journal of Child Psychology and Psychiatry*, 27, 237–250.

Jones, D. J., Fox, M. M., Babigian, H. M. and Hutton, H. E. (1980) Epidemiology of anorexia nervosa in Monroe County, New York: 1960–76. *Psychosomatic Medicine*, 42, 551–558.

Kendell, R. E., Hall, D. J., Hailey, A. *et al.* (1973) The epidemiology of anorexia nervosa. *Psychological Medicine*, 3, 200–203.

Lacey, J. H., Crisp, A. H., Kart, F. and Kirkwood, B. A. (1979) Weight and skeletal maturation-study of radiological and chronological age in an anorexia nervosa population. *Postgraduate Medical Journal*, 55, 381–385.

Lai, K., de Bruyn, R., Lask, B., Bryant-Waugh, R. and Hankins, M. (1994) Use of pelvic ultrasound to monitor ovarian and uterine maturity in childhood onset anorexia nervosa. *Archives of Disease in Childhood*, 71, 228–231.

Lasègue, C. (1873) De l'anorexie hystérique. *Archives Générales de Médecine*, 1, 385–403.

Lask, B. and Bryant-Waugh, R. (1986) Childhood onset anorexia nervosa. In *Recent Advances in Paediatrics* (ed. Roy Meadow). Vol. 8. Edinburgh: Churchill Livingstone, 21–31.

Lesser, L. I., Ashenden, B. J., Debuskey, M. and Eisenberg, L. (1960) Anorexia nervosa in children. *American Journal of Orthopsychiatry*, 30, 572–580.

Liebman, R., Minuchin, S. and Baker, L. (1974) An integrated treatment program for anorexia nervosa. *American Journal of Psychiatry*, 131, 432–436.

McClelland, L., Mynors-Wallis, L., Fahy, T. A. and Treasure, J. (1991) Sexual abuse, disordered personality and eating disorders. In *Women and Mental Health*. Supplement to the *British Journal of Psychiatry*, 158 (Suppl. 10), 63–68.

Mann, A. H., Wakeling, A., Wood, K., *et al.* (1983) Screening for abnormal eating attitudes and psychiatric morbidity in an unselected population of 15-year-old schoolgirls. *Psychological Medicine*, 13, 573–580.

Mecklenburg, R. S., Loriaux, D. L., Thompson, R. H., Anderson, A. E. and Lipsett, M. B. (1974) Hypothalamic dysfunction in patients with anorexia nervosa. *Medicine*, 53, 147–159.

Mester, H. (1981) *Die Anorexia Nervosa*. Monographien aus dem Gesamtgebiete der Psychiatrie, 26. Berlin: Springer-Verlag.

Mills, I. H. (1973) Endocrine and social factors in self-starvation amenorrhoea. In *Anorexia Nervosa and Obesity* (ed. R. F. Robertson and A. T. Proudfoot). Edinburgh: Royal College of Physicians.

Minuchin, S., Baker, L., Rosman, B. L., Liebman, R., Milman, L. and Todd, T. C.

(1975) A conceptual model of psychosomatic illness in children. *Archives of General Psychiatry*, 32, 1031–1038.

Minuchin, S., Rosman, B. L. and Baker, L. (1978) In *Psychosomatic Families. Anorexia Nervosa in Context*. Cambridge, Mass.: Harvard University Press.

Morgan, H. G. and Russell, G. F. M. (1975) Value of family background and clinical features as predictors of long-term outcome in anorexia nervosa: four-year follow-up study of 41 patients. *Psychological Medicine*, 5, 355–371.

Morgan, H. G., Purgold, J. and Wellbourne, J. (1983) Management and outcome in anorexia nervosa: a standardized prognostic study. *British Journal of Psychiatry*, 143, 282–287.

Mortimer, C. H., Besser, G. M., McNelly, A. S., Marshall, J. S., Harsoulis, P., Tunbridge, W. M. S., Gomez-Pan, A. and Hall, R. (1973) Luteinizing hormone and follicle stimulating hormone releasing test in patients with hypothalamic-pituitary-gonadal dysfunction. *British Medical Journal*, 4, 73–77.

Mullen, P. E., Romans-Clarkson, S. E., Walton, V. A. and Herbison, G. P. (1988) Impact of sexual and physical abuse on women's mental health. *The Lancet*, 1, 841–845.

Nasser, M. (1986) Comparative study of the prevalence of abnormal eating attitudes among Arab female students of both London and Cairo Universities. *Psychological Medicine*, 16, 621–625.

Nylander, I. (1971) The feeling of being fat and dieting in a school population; epidemiologic interview investigation. *Acta Sociomedica Scandinavica*, 3, 17–26.

Palazzoli, M. S. (1978) In *Self-starvation: From Individual to Family Therapy in the Treatment of Anorexia Nervosa*. New York: Jason Aronson.

Palmer, R. L., Oppenheimer, R., Dignon, A., Chaloner, D. and Howells, K. (1990) Childhood sexual experiences with adults reported by women with clinical eating disorders; an extended series. *British Journal of Psychiatry*, 156, 699–703.

Patton, G. C. (1988) The spectrum of eating disorder in adolescence. *Journal of Psychosomatic Research*, 32, 6, 579–584.

Pfeiffer, R. J., Lucas, A. R. and Ilstrup, D. M. (1986) Effect of anorexia nervosa on linear growth. *Clinical Pediatrics*, 24, 1, 7–12.

Ploog, D. W. and Pirke, K. M. (1987) Psychobiology of anorexia nervosa. *Psychological Medicine*, 17, 843–859.

Råstam, M., Gillberg, C. and Garton, M. (1989) Anorexia nervosa in a Swedish urban region. A population-based study. *British Journal of Psychiatry*, 155, 642–646.

Råstam, M., Gillberg, C. and Wentz, E. (2003) Outcome of teenage-onset anorexia nervosa in a Swedish community-based sample. *European Child and Adolescent Psychiatry*, 12 suppl. 1, 178–190.

Robinson, P. H. and Andersen, A. (1985) Anorexia nervosa in American blacks. *Journal of Psychiatric Research*, 19, 2/3, 183–188.

Russell, G. F. M. (1965) Metabolic aspects of anorexia nervosa. *Proceedings of the Royal Society of Medicine*, 58, 811–814.

Russell, G. F. M. (1977) Editorial: the present status of anorexia nervosa. *Psychological Medicine*, 7, 363–367.

Russell, G. F. M. (1979) Bulimia nervosa: an ominous variant of anorexia nervosa. *Psychological Medicine*, 9, 429–448.

Russell, G. F. M. (1983) Delayed puberty due to anorexia nervosa of early onset.

In *Anorexia Nervosa: Recent Developments in Research* (ed. P. L. Darby, P. E. Garfinkel, D. M. Garner and D. V. Coscina). New York: Alan R. Liss.

Russell, G. F. M. (1985a) Premenarchal anorexia nervosa and its sequelae. *Journal of Psychiatric Research*, 19, 2/3, 363–369.

Russell, G. F. M. (1985b) Bulimia revisited. *International Journal of Eating Disorders*, 4, 4, 681–692.

Russell, G. F. M., Szmukler, G. I., Dare, C. and Eisler, I. (1987) An evaluation of family therapy in anorexia nervosa and bulimia nervosa. *Archives of General Psychiatry*, 44, 1047–1056.

Russell, G. F. M., Treasure, J. and Eisler, I. (1998) Mothers with anorexia nervosa who underfeed their children: their recognition and management. *Psychological Medicine*, 28, 93–108.

Silverman, J. A. (1974) Anorexia nervosa: clinical observations in a successful treatment plan. *Journal of Pediatrics*, 84, 68–73.

Silverman, J. A. (1983) Medical consequences of starvation; the malnutrition of anorexia nervosa: caveat medicus. In *Anorexia Nervosa: Recent Developments in Research* (ed. P. L. Darby, P. E. Garfinkel, D. M. Garner and D. V. Coscina). New York: Alan R. Liss.

Sturzenberger, S., Cantwell, D. P., Burroughs, J., Salkin, B. and Green, J. K. (1977) A follow-up study of adolescent psychiatric in-patients with anorexia nervosa. The assessment of outcome. *Journal of the American Academy of Child Psychiatry*, 16, 703–715.

Swift, W. J. (1982) The long-term outcome of early onset anorexia nervosa. A critical review. *Journal of the American Academy of Psychiatry*, 21, 38–46.

Szmukler, G. I. (1983) Weight and food preoccupation in a population of English schoolgirls. In *Understanding Bulimia and Anorexia Nervosa*. Report on the fourth Ross Conference on Medical Research (ed. G. J. Bargman). Columbus, Ohio: Ross Laboratories.

Szmukler, G. I., Eisler, I., Gillies, C. and Hayward, M. E. (1985) The implications of anorexia nervosa in a ballet school. *Journal of Psychiatric Research*, 19, 2/3, 177–181.

Szmukler, G. I., McCance, C., McCrone, L., *et al.* (1986) Anorexia nervosa: a psychiatric case register study from Aberdeen. *Psychological Medicine*, 16, 49–58.

Tanner, J. M. (1962) *Growth at Adolescence*. Oxford: Blackwell Scientific Publications.

Tanner, J. M., Whitehouse, R. M. and Takaishi, M. (1966) Standards from birth to maturity for height, weight, height velocity and weight velocity: British children 1965. *Archives of Disease in Childhood*, 41, 454–471.

Theander, S. (1970) Anorexia nervosa: a psychiatric investigation of 94 female patients. *Acta Psychiatrica Scandinavica Supplement*, 214, 1–194.

Theander, S. (1985) Outcome and prognosis in anorexia nervosa and bulimia: some results of previous investigations, compared with those of a Swedish long-term study. *Journal of Psychiatric Research*, 19, 2/3, 493–508.

Tolstrup, K. (1965) Die Charakteristika der jüngeren Fälle von Anorexia Nervosa. In *Symposium, Göttingen* (ed. J. E. Meyer and H. Feldmann) Stuttgart: Georg-Thieme Verlag.

Tolstrup, K., Brinch, M., Isager, T., Nielsen, S., Bystrup, J., Severin, B. and Olesen, N. S. (1985) Long-term outcome of 151 cases of anorexia nervosa. *Acta Psychiatrica Scandinavica*, 71, 380–387.

Treasure, J. L. and Thompson, P. (1988) Anorexia nervosa in childhood. *British Journal of Hospital Medicine*, 40, 362–369.

Treasure, J. L., Gordon, P. A. L., King, E. A., Wheeler, M. J. and Russell, G. F. M. (1985) Cystic ovaries: a phase of anorexia nervosa. *The Lancet*, 2, 1379–1382.

Treasure, J. L., Wheeler, M., King, E. A., Gordon, P. A. L. and Russell, G. F M. (1988) Weight gain and reproductive function: ultrasonographic and endocrine features in anorexia nervosa. *Clinical Endocrinology*, 29, 607–616.

Van Wezel-Meijler, G. and Wit, J. M. (1989) The offspring of mothers with anorexia nervosa: a high-risk group for undernutrition and stunting? *European Journal of Pediatrics*, 49, 130–135.

Wakeling, A. and De Souza, V. F. A. (1983) Differential endocrine and menstrual response to weight change in anorexia nervosa. In *Anorexia Nervosa: Recent Developments in Research* (ed. P. L. Darby, P. E. Garfinkel, D. M. Garner and D. V. Coscina). New York: Alan R. Liss.

Wakeling, A., De Souza, V. F. A. and Beardwood, C. J. (1977) Assessment of the negative and positive feedback effects of administered oestrogen on gonadotrophin release in patients with anorexia nervosa. *Psychological Medicine*, 7, 397–405.

Warren, W. (1968) A study of anorexia nervosa in young girls. *Journal of Child Psychology and Psychiatry*, 9, 27–40.

Willi, J. and Grossmann, S. (1983) Epidemiology of anorexia nervosa in a defined region of Switzerland. *American Journal of Psychiatry*, 140, 564–567.

Wonderlich, S. A., Brewerton, T. D., Jocic, Z., Dansky, B. S. and Abbott, D. W. (1997) Relationship of childhood sexual abuse and eating disorders. *Journal of American Academy of Child and Adolescent Psychiatry*, 368, 1107–1115.

Chapter 7

The nature of adolescent anorexia nervosa and bulimia nervosa

David B. Herzog, Safia C. Jackson and Debra L. Franko

Introduction

Two psychiatric syndromes comprise the major eating disorders in adolescence: anorexia nervosa and bulimia nervosa. Both disorders feature disturbed eating patterns that reflect underlying fears of weight gain. Adolescence is the period of development most closely associated with the onset of both eating disorders, although they can develop in pre-pubescents (see Chapter 6) and adults. Anorexia nervosa typically develops in early (ages 13–14) or late (ages 17–18) adolescence, while bulimia nervosa commonly originates in the later teenage years or early adulthood. There has been an increase in interest in eating disorders that do not fulfill criteria for anorexia nervosa or bulimia and these are known either as 'eating disorders not otherwise specified' (EDNOS) or as 'atypical eating disorders'. It appears that they may be more common than anorexia nervosa or bulimia (Fairburn and Harrison, 2003; Rodriguez *et al.*, 2001) but they have not been well researched in this age-group and thus this chapter will concentrate exclusively on anorexia and bulimia. A host of biological, psychological, familial and sociological factors have been implicated in the etiology and maintenance of the disorders. In this chapter we will examine the epidemiology, clinical picture, and medical complications of anorexia nervosa and bulimia nervosa, and discuss risk profiles for the development of these eating disorders in adolescence.

Anorexia nervosa

Epidemiology

The syndrome of anorexia nervosa has been recognized for centuries, but until the last four decades it was a rarely diagnosed phenomenon. Several studies have documented substantial increases in incidence rate from the 1950s (Willi and Grossmann, 1983) and 1960s (Jones *et al.*, 1980) to the 1970s, although one study found no change in prevalence rate across four decades (Lucas *et al.*, 1988). In a review by Hoek and van Hoeken (2003), the average lifetime prevalence rate for anorexia nervosa was 0.3 percent for young females (15–19 years old). The authors also found that the incidence of anorexia nervosa has increased over the past century but has stabilized since the 1970s. An epidemiological sample of Swiss adolescent girls (14–17 years) found lifetime prevalence rates of anorexia nervosa to be 0.7 percent (Steinhausen *et al.*, 1997). Similarly, in a Scandinavian study of adolescent girls aged 14–15 years, Kjelsas and colleagues (2004) found the lifetime prevalence of anorexia nervosa to be 0.7 percent. In select groups, prevalence appears to be higher: approximately 1 percent of girls in British private secondary schools (Crisp *et al.*, 1976; Szmukler, 1985) manifest anorexia nervosa; and, among teenage girls in ballet schools in Canada and England, rates of the disorder have been estimated at 6.5 percent and 7 percent (Garner and Garfinkel, 1980; Szmukler *et al.*, 1985).

Anorexia nervosa occurs across races and cultures (Hoek *et al.*, 1998; Keel and Klump, 2003). Studies of adolescents in non-Western countries have reported significant rates of eating disorders among non-Western groups. In a large-scale study of eating disorder symptomatology in the People's Republic of China, 0.7 percent of 1,246 adolescent girls interviewed met criteria for partial diagnosis of anorexia nervosa (Huon *et al.*, 2002). In a study of eating disorders in 3,100 Iranian schoolgirls, Nobakht and Dezhkam (2000) found a prevalence rate of 0.9 percent for anorexia nervosa. In a recent review Makino and colleagues concluded that while the prevalence of eating disorders in non-Western countries is lower than that of Western countries, it is increasing in non-Western groups.

Relatively few males exhibit anorexia nervosa. Most studies suggest that 5–10 percent of individuals presenting with anorexia nervosa are male (Hoek and van Hoeken, 2003); however, there are increasing reports of body dissatisfaction in teenage males (Olivardia *et al.*, 1995; Pope *et al.*, 1993). Kjelsas and colleagues (2004) reported a prevalence rate of 0.2 percent in male adolescents aged 14–15 years old. When the clinical syndrome does arise in males it appears to be similar to that in females (Eliot and Baker, 2001; Olivardia *et al.*, 1995). Since the majority of adolescents who have anorexia nervosa are female, we will use the feminine pronoun unless discussing features particular to males.

Clinical features

Severe, deliberate weight loss, distorted body image and a profound fear of becoming fat are the cardinal symptoms of anorexia nervosa. Patients with anorexia nervosa present as substantially underweight – 15 percent or less of their normal body weight (American Psychiatric Association, 1994) – with many of the features associated with malnutrition and starvation. Despite their skeletal appearance, these patients insist that they are still fat. Another central aspect of anorexia nervosa is the patient's extreme fear of gaining weight. This feature has been characterized as a 'weight phobia' and 'a morbid fear of fatness'. However, younger patients may deny a fear of gaining weight, despite engaging in behaviors that strongly suggest an intense fear of fatness. Children as young as 7–12 may present with symptoms including nausea, abdominal pain, a feeling of fullness, and inability to swallow. In a recent study, Cooper *et al.* (2002) found that the clinical features associated with childhood onset anorexia nervosa (AN) are very similar to those seen in adolescent onset AN. The authors also found that some children may experience 'food avoidance emotional disorder' (FAED), a syndrome distinct from childhood AN in which food avoidance and weight loss are due to psychological reasons. Children with this disorder acknowledge their low weight and express desire to gain weight.

The onset of anorexia nervosa is often gradual. Healthy teenagers of normal or slightly heavy weight will begin to shed pounds in a sanctioned fashion, through dieting. Frequently behavior aimed at weight loss starts after being teased or criticized about weight by family or friends or a coach. Other precipitating factors include breaking-up with a boyfriend or developmental transition, such as leaving home. At some point, however, the diet becomes excessive, as the adolescent eliminates more and more food groups and increases restriction of the amount of food she allows herself to eat. Ever-increasing thinness becomes the *raison d'être* of the teenager's life, motivating all activities. Despite a severely restricted diet, individuals with AN will typically engage in frequent, vigorous exercise that consumes several hours of the day. Excessive physical activity may also predate frank anorexia nervosa and be a cue to a developing disorder. Adolescents with AN often develop rituals around food and mealtimes. They may cut food into tiny morsels, nibble off pieces of food or spend hours chewing a few bites. Food may be hidden, hoarded, fondled or crumbled. They may cook elaborate meals to serve to their families, goading relatives to eat more while they consume little or nothing. Some patients with AN secretly binge-eat and then try to rid themselves of what they have just eaten by vomiting or use of laxatives. These patients report having constant thoughts about food.

In addition to being preoccupied with food, individuals with AN tend toward 'black/white' thinking and personal rigidity. They are perfectionistic and engage in numerous activities at which they attempt to excel (Halmi *et al.*, 2000; Shafran *et al.*, 2002). Castro and colleagues (2004) recently found that adolescents with anorexia nervosa scored higher than healthy adolescents on the Multidimensional Perfectionism Scale; 40 percent of adolescents with anorexia nervosa showed high scores on dimensions of the scale relating to self-perfectionism. An adolescent with anorexia nervosa may apply herself rigorously to her studies in order to maintain good grades, while keeping a schedule crammed with extracurricular activities, often sleeping only a few hours a night. In addition to burning off calories, this frantic activity may serve the function of helping the adolescent manage overwhelming or intolerable feelings. Despite her many activities and often impressive accomplishments, the young woman with anorexia nervosa typically feels personally ineffective and unworthy of love. Other personality characteristics distinctive of anorexia nervosa include being overtly compliant, emotionally constricted, competitive, envious and obsessive. Patients with anorexia nervosa who regularly binge and purge show impulsivity and extroversion more characteristic of individuals with bulimia nervosa. Adolescents with anorexia nervosa can present as either passive and withdrawn or cheerful and perky, and frequently behave in a controlling manner. Concomitant depression is common, and over half of patients with anorexia nervosa have lifetime histories of major depressive disorder (Herzog et al., 1996).

At a stage in life when most teenagers begin to experience sexual urges and experiment with dating relationships, those with anorexia nervosa rarely date and report low levels or absence of romantic interest (Wiederman et al., 1996). Whether the lack of sexual appetite is a cause or a result of anorexia nervosa is difficult to determine. The effects of malnutrition and constant activity certainly reduce sexual drive, and attitudes of disgust and anxiety towards sexuality are common in these patients. These adolescents tend not to pursue friends or romantic relationships. Some studies indicate that homosexuality is a specific risk factor for disordered eating in men (Herzog et al., 1984; Russell and Keel, 2002; Yager et al., 1988). However, other studies have found little or no association between eating disorders and homosexual orientation in men (Mangweth et al., 1997; Olivardia et al., 1995). Some patients with anorexia nervosa have a history of sexual abuse (Hall et al., 1989; Sloan and Leichner, 1986), which may contribute to feelings of conflict with regard to sexuality. However, the incidence of sexual abuse in patients with anorexia nervosa does not exceed that of other psychiatric populations.

In keeping with her stoic stance, the adolescent with anorexia nervosa usually denies that she has a problem. Many claim that they have never felt better and cannot understand their family's concern. Indeed, one of the most difficult aspects of treatment with these patients is their perception that their extreme lifestyle is the route to happiness. Despite an almost continual state of hunger and exhaustion, they report feeling more in control of their lives than they have ever been. In some cases it is only after the adolescent accepts that she may die from her illness that she begins to change her behavior. In other cases, the patient may decide that she is bored with her illness or that for some other reason it is time to stop being anorexic (Beresin et al., 1989).

Course and outcome

Although the onset of AN can occur throughout the life span (Beck et al., 1996; Inagaki et al., 2002), the period of highest risk is around puberty (Halmi et al., 1979; Lucas et al., 1988, 1991). It is often difficult to ascertain when an adolescent first manifests anorexia nervosa, since it generally begins with normal dieting. Parents and friends may praise the teenager for her initial weight loss and tell her she has made herself more attractive. Gradually, however, the praise turns into complaints that she is 'too thin'. Usually, by this time, however, she is entrenched in a self-perpetuating anorexic behavior pattern that she is unwilling or unable to give up. Puberty may be a particularly precarious time during which girls may be more vulnerable to social pressures to be thin in the context of their changing bodies (Gowers and Shore, 2001). Hormonal changes associated with puberty may also trigger other relevant biological processes (Munoz and Argente, 2002). Additionally, high achieving, more anxious, post-menarchal females have been found to be at an increased risk for eating disorders (O'Dea and Abraham, 1999).

The course of the disorder appears to be varied. Some adolescents go through a single episode of relatively short duration. More commonly the disorder lasts for several years or becomes chronic. Approximately 50 to 70 percent of adolescents with AN recover, 20 percent are improved but continue to have residual symptoms, and 10 to 20 percent have chronic AN (Steinhausen, 2002). In follow-up studies of at least ten years, approximately 70 percent of patients recover from AN. Adolescents with AN continue to recover over time; Strober et al. (1997) reported that a 1 percent probability of reaching full recovery at three years increased to 72 percent at ten years. Those patients who improve or recover often persist in extreme attentiveness to weight and appearance and strange habits surrounding food and eating long after the syndrome subsides. In addition to symptoms related to the eating disorder, other psychiatric conditions may continue after recovery. One study found that more than one-third of a sample of these patients experienced repeated episodes of some kind of mood disorder, such as depression (Cantwell et al., 1977). Other studies indicate that recovered patients tend to retain feelings of social anxiety and of dependency on and hostility toward the family (Beresin et al., 1989; Hsu et al., 1979; Morgan and Russell, 1975). Personality traits associated with AN, including obsessionality, perfectionism and neuroticism, persist after recovery (Bulik et al., 2000; Kaye et al., 1993). Patients who experience persistent eating disorder symptoms display abnormalities with weight, eating behaviors, menstrual function, comorbid psychopathology, and difficulties with psychosocial functioning (Herpertz-Dahlmann et al., 2001; Steinhausen et al., 1997; Strober et al., 1997; Wentz et al., 2001). In addition, over half develop bulimic symptomatology during the course of AN (Eddy et al., 2002), and 10 to 15 percent go on to develop bulimia nervosa (Fichter and Quadflieg, 1999; Herpertz-Dahlmann et al., 1996, 2001). Relapse is common in weight-recovered hospitalized patients, with up to one-third of adolescent AN patients relapsing soon after discharge (Strober et al., 1997).

AN has one of the highest mortality rates among psychiatric disorders. Reported mortality rates range from 0 percent to 22 percent across different studies (Herzog *et al.*, 1988). Approximately 5.6 percent of patients diagnosed with AN die per decade of illness (Sullivan, 1995). A naturalistic follow-up study found that AN patients are twelve times more likely to die than women of a similar age in the general population (Keel *et al.*, 2003). The most common causes of death are suicide and the effects of starvation. The suicide rate among women with AN is up to fifty-seven times higher than for women of a similar age in the general population (Keel *et al.*, 2003).

Predictors of poor outcome for anorexia nervosa have included a longer duration of illness, presence of an underlying personality disorder, vomiting and disturbed family relationships (Herzog *et al.*, 1988). Some studies have also found that patients hospitalized at lower weights fare worse than those at higher weights (Patton, 1988). In general, however, results have been inconclusive.

Medical complications

The physical complications of anorexia nervosa are many and varied, affecting most major systems of the body: cardiovascular, hematologic, gastrointestinal, renal, endocrinologic and skeletal (Becker *et al.*, 1999; Misra *et al.*, 2004; Palla and Litt, 1988). Most of the complications are due to starvation. Patients who binge and purge have additional problems, which will be discussed in a later section on bulimia nervosa.

Despite her malnourished state, the patient with anorexia nervosa is typically full of energy. Patients who exhibit lethargy may be experiencing depression, or this symptom may indicate cardiovascular compromise. Characteristically, the adolescent with anorexia nervosa looks younger than her age, displaying cachexia and breast atrophy. The skin is often dry and, as a result of carotenemia, may be tinged yellow. Cyanosis of the extremities, especially when exposed to cold, is common, as are lanugo and hair thinning. Cardiovascular complications are typical, the most worrisome of which is bradycardia. Bradycardia can be difficult to assess in athletic patients because they maintain a low pulse rate. Those with a pulse rate of less than 50 beats per minute merit vigilance; if the rate dips below 40 per minute, the patient should be hospitalized. Hypotension and hypothermia are also frequently associated features that may require hospitalization.

Common electrocardiographic abnormalities in anorexia nervosa include low voltage bradycardia, T-wave inversions and ST segment depression. The gravest findings are arrhythmias, including supra-ventricular premature beats and ventricular tachycardia, with and without exercise, and following emetine use. Prolonged QT intervals are rare, but may predispose to life-threatening arrhythmias and explain cases of sudden death. All these changes return to normal with weight gain. Although cardiovascular complications are common, it is not possible to predict which patients will ultimately develop life-threatening symptoms.

Hematologic changes are common and include anemia, leukopenia, and thrombocytopenia. Although neutrophil counts are lowered in many patients, it does not appear to make these patients more susceptible to infection. Generally, the hematologic sequelae of anorexia nervosa do not result in clinical consequences.

Gastrointestinal abnormalities include retarded intestinal motility and delayed gastric emptying, which may result in complaints of constipation and abdominal bloating. Metacipromide has been successfully used in some cases to increase gastric motility and decrease dyspeptic flatulence. Frequent, small feeding can also help to reduce abdominal discomfort.

Dehydration is often associated with anorexia nervosa and can produce renal complications. The most common of these is increased blood urea nitrogen. Partial diabetes insipidus may also develop as a result of reduction in renal concentrating capacity and abnormalities in vasopressin secretion. This may explain the common complaint of polyuria. Renal calculi have been noted in cases of chronic dehydration. Hydration and weight gain reverse these changes.

The major endocrine abnormality in females with anorexia nervosa is amenorrhea secondary to a low estrogen state. The relationship between weight loss and amenorrhea, however, is not a simple one. Chronically underweight women can menstruate regularly, and in about 20 percent of cases amenorrhea predates noticeable weight loss in anorexia nervosa. Moreover, the return of menses often lags behind the return to normal body weight. Although thyroid function is disturbed in anorexia nervosa there is no evidence for primary hypothyroidism. T4 and TSH levels are usually in the low-normal to normal range. Males have decreased plasma testosterone levels, with concomitant loss of early morning erections.

Skeletal abnormalities are generating increasing concern in those who treat patients with anorexia nervosa. Fractures of the vertebrae, sternum and long bones have all been seen in patients presenting at the Massachusetts General Hospital. Recent studies have demonstrated that more than 90 percent of adolescents and young adults with AN have reduced bone mass at one or more skeletal sites (Golden, 2003; Grinspoon et al., 2000). Osteopenia that occurs in adolescence may not be completely reversible (Rigotti et al., 1991; Soyka et al., 2002). Rigotti et al. (1984) found that women with anorexia nervosa with a history of amenorrhea of at least one year were at increased risk for osteoporosis, with significantly decreased bone density as compared to normal controls. Physical exercise appeared to mitigate this effect, such that those who exercised moderately had bone density levels more similar to those of controls. The degree of osteopenia in AN is more severe than seen in women with osteopenia resulting from hypothalamic amenorrhea, suggesting that nutritional factors play an important role in bone density (Grinspoon et al., 1999). Adolescence is a critical period for building bone mass; about 60 percent of peak bone mass is accrued during the adolescent years. Biller *et al.* (1989) found that those at the greatest risk for osteoporosis were women whose amenorrhea had started in adolescence (prior to peak bone formation) and had persisted into adulthood. Moreover, malnutrition in prepubertal girls and pubertal males may also result in growth failure (see Chapter 6).

Bulimia nervosa

Epidemiology

Due to the use of different diagnostic criteria and the fact that behaviors associated with bulimia nervosa (such as binge-eating or vomiting after meals) are not uncommon in some adolescent populations (Killen *et al.*, 1986), prevalence rates of the clinical syndrome have been difficult to ascertain. Studies investigating the prevalence of this disorder have employed strict diagnostic criteria; as a result, prevalence rates may be misleading since adolescents who evidence the core features of bulimia nervosa (BN) may not have developed the requisite severity or duration of symptoms (Golden, 2003). For female adolescents and adults, low prevalence rates (0.5 percent or less) were reported in several European countries (Italy: Rathner and Messner, 1993; Switzerland: Steinhausen *et al.*, 1997; Hungary: Szabo and Tury, 1991; Netherlands: Verhulst *et al.*, 1997; Poland: WlodarczykBisaga and Dolan, 1996). In a more recent study, Kjelsas and colleagues (2004) found the lifetime prevalence rate of BN among adolescent girls (14–15 years) to be 1.2 percent. Studies have consistently found that this disorder is very rare among adolescent boys. Garfinkel and Garner (1982) suggest that in a similar way to anorexia nervosa, at least 90 to 95 percent of cases of bulimia nervosa are female. This is evident in Kjelsas and colleagues' study (2004) which reports the lifetime prevalence rate among adolescent boys (14–15 years) to be 0.4 percent.

Clinical features

Rapid consumption of large quantities of high-caloric food ('bingeing') followed by food elimination ('purging') and a stable over-concern with weight and body shape characterize bulimia nervosa (American Psychiatric Association, 1994). During a binge, these individuals feel unable to control their eating. When they become too distended to continue, feel stomach pain, run out of food or are interrupted, they stop bingeing and focus on getting rid of the food they have just eaten. Most commonly this is accomplished by self-induced vomiting, although they also use laxatives or diet pills, do vigorous exercise, or fast in order to counteract the effects of a binge. Many have a favored method of purging, though others will combine approaches.

Like patients with anorexia nervosa, those with bulimia nervosa fear gaining weight. The adolescent who becomes bulimic has generally tried dieting, or other methods of weight control, with limited success. She may learn about purging through friends or other sources. Most are of normal weight, although individuals with AN, or who are obese, can develop the disorder.

The precise nature of individuals' binges varies widely. Some plan their binges, shopping extensively and selecting particular foods. Others eat whatever is available in the house. Some binge regularly at certain times, such as late at night, while others maintain a more erratic habit. Patients who live with others frequently orchestrate their binges around family or roommates' schedules to guarantee privacy. Vomiting is also preferably done in utmost privacy, episodes taking as long as thirty minutes in some cases. Most patients regurgitate several times to ensure that all food comes up. Vomiting is induced by inserting fingers or hands or an implement. A significant minority have acquired voluntary control of the gag reflex.

Eating behavior apart from binge-eating also varies among adolescents with BN. Some eat regular meals without purging, some purge independent of bingeing, and some diet or eat irregularly. In one study, one-third of a sample of women with BN reported regurgitating and ruminating their food, and spitting out food to avoid absorbing calories (Fairburn and Cooper, 1984).

Although an adolescent may start out bingeing and purging with a girl-friend, more often she develops and sustains the behavior in secrecy. Unlike patients with anorexia nervosa, those with bulimia nervosa are aware that their eating behavior is abnormal and are embarrassed and ashamed. They will often go to great lengths to maintain secrecy, curtailing social activities that might involve eating with others or interfere with opportunities to binge. On the other hand, adolescents with bulimia nervosa may leave intentional or unconscious clues for their families, such as immediately excusing themselves after meals, hiding bags of vomitus under the bed, leaving the refrigerator bare, and so on.

Unlike patients with anorexia nervosa, whose skeletal appearance makes them stand out among their peers, those with bulimia nervosa are often superficially indistinguishable from most adolescents in that they usually present with a body weight in the normal range. Physically they appear healthy, with only an occasional puffiness around the face following a recent binge–purge episode. They appear to be socially outgoing, heterosexually interested, and they do well in school. Beneath the surface, however, these teenagers are lonely and tormented and report substantial difficulties with interpersonal relationships (Herzog *et al.*, 1987). Individuals with BN frequently report that when they seek professional help, a therapist is the first person they have talked to about their problem. In a study by Grissett and Novell (1992), subjects with BN were rated by outside observers as less socially effective than healthy controls. Additionally, these patients scored lower than controls on perceived social support and social competence. The lack of communication about themselves with family and friends contributes to a sense of isolation and unworthiness. Depressive symptoms are common, and studies have found that over half of patients with BN have a lifetime history of a mood disorder, with MDD as the most common diagnosis. Sim and Zeman (2004) found that adolescent girls with BN were more reluctant to express emotions and took longer to recall information relating to an emotional state, when compared to depressed girls in the community. Alcohol and drug abuse have often been found to be elevated in this patient population (Bulik et al., 1994). A subgroup engage in other impulsive behaviors, such as sexual promiscuity, suicidal gesturing and shoplifting.

Adolescents with bulimia nervosa report frequent weight fluctuations and menstrual irregularities, including amenorrhea (Fairburn and Cooper, 1984; Abraham and Beumont, 1982). Researchers have hypothesized that the chaotic diet, excessive exercise and fluctuations in weight all play a role in the menstrual disturbance.

Course and outcome

Bulimia nervosa appears to have an episodic course, with high rate of relapse (Keller et al., 1989; Keel and Mitchell, 1997) often within one to two years of recovery (Herzog et al., 1996). The majority of adolescents and adults with BN improve over time, with recovery rates from 35 to 75 percent at five or more years of follow-up (Fairburn et al., 2000; Fichter and Quadflieg, 1999; Herzog et al., 1999). In a review by Keel and Mitchell (1997), the authors found that within five to ten years following presentation about 50 percent of women initially diagnosed with bulimia nervosa fully recovered, 20 percent continued to meet criteria for the disorder, and about 30 percent relapsed into bulimic symptoms.

Mortality is a rare outcome in BN, with mortality rates as low as 0.5 percent (Keel et al., 1999). Few prognostic factors in BN have been consistently reported across studies, but low self-esteem, longer duration of illness prior to presentation, higher frequency or severity of binge-eating, substance abuse history, and a history of obesity have been reported to be associated with poor outcome (Bulik et al., 1998; Fairburn et al., 2003; Keel et al., 1999).

Depressive syndromes in patients with BN also appear to follow an episodic course, although it is not clear how recovery from the eating disorder is related to recovery and relapse from depressive disorders. In our study, 83 percent of the patients with BN met standardized criteria for a lifetime affective disorder, and 57 percent met criteria for a concurrent affective disorder. Fifty-nine percent of those with concurrent mood disorder at presentation recovered from the mood disorder, but 43 percent went on to relapse into a second, and in some cases, a third, episode of mood disorder (Keller et al., 1989). Four subjects also developed affective disorders during the follow-up period. Recovery from one disorder did not precede or follow recovery from another in any systematic pattern. Other studies of treated samples have reported substantial reductions in depressive symptoms (Fairburn *et al.*, 1986; Norman and Herzog, 1986; Mitchell *et al.*, 1985) at follow-up. However, one study found that 64 percent of fifty-six patients treated with behavioral therapy were dysphoric at 12–35 months' follow-up, with 20 percent exhibiting at least four additional symptoms of depression (Hsu and Holder, 1986).

Many factors have been assessed as predictors of recovery and relapse in bulimia nervosa. Reports on prognostic factors in BN have yielded few consistent findings. Some studies found a history of different psychiatric symptoms, such as alcohol abuse (Lacey, 1983), suicide attempts (Abraham *et al.*, 1983) and increased depression at follow-up (Swift *et al.*, 1985), to predict poor outcome. We found that lower scores at baseline on an index measuring eating symptomatology and self-image predicted positive outcome from BN three years later, as did having satisfactory social support at follow-up (Keller *et al.*, 1998). Age at presentation, duration of illness, a past history of anorexia nervosa, comorbid affective disorder and frequency of binge–purge episodes have been found to be unrelated to outcome from bulimia nervosa.

Medical complications

Pediatricians and primary health care professionals play a particularly vital role in the detection of bulimia nervosa, because the illness is not obvious and patients typically try to conceal it. Common complaints of these patients, including swelling in the hands, feet and cheeks, abdominal fullness, fatigue, headaches, dental problems, chest pain, constipation, rectal bleeding or fluid retention, may furnish clues to the presence of the disorder. However, three physical signs of the disorder can also be identified from a routine physical examination, and are useful in aiding diagnosis.

The first sign is hypertrophy of the salivary glands, particularly of the parotid glands. The hypertrophy is usually bilateral, painless and quite apparent. Hypertrophy occurs in 20 to 30 percent of patients with BN, and it is thought to be secondary to binge-eating and vomiting. Hypertrophy of the salivary glands does normalize with resumption of regular eating behavior.

A second diagnostic indicator is the evidence of skin changes over the dorsum of the hand (Russell's sign), secondary to the trauma to the skin caused by using the hand to stimulate the gag reflex. Lesions can vary from elongated, superficial ulcerations to hyperpigmented calluses or scarring. These lesions can be seen anywhere over the dorsal surfaces of the hands, particularly at the metacarpal phalangial joint of each finger.

The presence of dental erosion is a third marker of possible bulimia nervosa. Classically, the erosion involves decalcification of the lingual, palatal and posterior occlusal surfaces of the teeth. This pattern indicates that the acid is coming from the back of the mouth, which it would do in the case of frequent vomiting.

Medical complications of bulimia nervosa stem mainly from chronic vomiting or laxative abuse. Vomiting disturbs fluid and electrolyte balance, and can lead to a hypokalemic, hypochloremic alkalosis. Total body potassium may be depleted, despite a normal serum potassium, leading to dangerous symptoms in the face of a normal laboratory examination. Chronic vomiting can also lead to complaints of frequent sore throat, abdominal pain, esophagitis and mild hematemesis.

Laxative use, another relatively common form of purging, is also potentially dangerous. Electrolyte depletion can lead to metabolic acidosis. Prolonged use of laxatives can also reduce calcium and magnesium absorption. As with anorexia nervosa, dehydration can cause renal calculi to develop.

Some patients with bulimia nervosa, as well as those with anorexia nervosa who purge, resort to the use of ipecac syrup to induce vomiting. These patients are at risk for emetine poisoning, which can cause irreversible myocardial damage and even death.

Medical complications as a result of bingeing and vomiting or using purgatives tend to normalize with the resumption of regular eating behavior.

Risk factors in eating disorders

Various factors have been identified as putting an adolescent at increased risk for developing an eating disorder. These include personality and developmental factors, socio-cultural pressures, family relations, biological predispositions, family history of psychopathology and psychiatric disorders (Johnson et al., 2002). Some of these factors are particular to the developmental phase of adolescence and may be one reason why eating disorders predominantly originate in adolescence and early adulthood.

The high incidence of eating disorders among females compared to males points clearly to girls and women being at much higher risk than boys and men for developing anorexia nervosa or bulimia nervosa, perhaps because of the greater societal stress placed on a slender appearance for females (Garner et al., 1980; Thompson and Chad, 2002). Within the adolescent female population, those girls who are preoccupied with weight and body-related concerns to an extreme degree, with most of their self-esteem resting on achieving and maintaining a certain 'look', may be at particular risk for developing an eating disorder, as may be those who grow up in a family that stresses the importance of slenderness, particularly in women (Striegel-Moore et al., 1986). The greater the disparity between actual weight and desired weight, and the greater the emphasis placed on appearance as an index of self-worth, presumably the higher the risk of an adolescent resorting to extreme measures in order to control and manage her weight. This is particularly the case when a teenager has tried several diets without success.

Participation in certain activities and professions also appears to foster increased risk for the development of eating disorders. Ballet participation has received substantial attention (Klump *et al.*, 2001) due to the high levels of exercise required and pressures for thinness and athletic excellence (Garner and Garfinkel, 1980; Vaisman *et al.*, 1996; Weeda-Mannak and Drop, 1985). One study found a sixfold increase in the prevalence rate of anorexia nervosa among professional dance students compared to non-professional high school students (Garner and Garfinkel, 1980). Ballet dancers are similar with respect to their eating habits and concerns about body weight and shape to those with eating disorders. In a study by Khan *et al.* (1996), these disturbed eating attitudes and behaviors persisted among ballet dancers after retirement, a finding not seen among other athlete groups, including gymnasts (O'Connor *et al.*, 1996). Achievement motivation may also play an interactive role with the emphasis on body shape: twice the rate of students at highly competitive dance schools developed anorexia nervosa during the course of their training compared to students in a less rigorous program, while students in a competitive music program, on the other hand, had minimal concerns about weight compared to the dancing students (Garner and Garfinkel, 1980). These results suggest that while achievement pressures alone may not put one at risk for an eating disorder, these pressures in conjunction with weight concerns can increase the risk.

Just as not all women who worry about weight develop an eating disorder, neither do the majority of professionals in competitive careers that emphasize body shape. Clearly, other factors are also important in elevating risk. Studies have linked anorexia nervosa to a cluster of personality attributes such as negative self-evaluation, low self-esteem, extreme compliance, obsessionality, perfectionism, neuroticism, and harm avoidance (Anderluh *et al.*, 2003; Bulik *et al.*, 1995, 2003; Fairburn *et al.*, 1999). These traits continue to characterize individuals with anorexia nervosa even after recovery (Bulik *et al.*, 2000; Kaye *et al.*, 1993), suggesting that they preceded the onset of the disorder and represent vulnerability factors.

Several potential biological and genetic risk factors have also been identified (see Chapter 8). These include being overweight or having a family history of obesity (Garfinkel *et al.*, 1987), or having a family member with an eating disorder. Twins studies have found a substantially higher concordance rate for anorexia nervosa amongst monozygotic twins than amongst dizygotic twins (Holland *et al.*, 1984, 1988), suggesting that a vulnerability to anorexia nervosa is at least partially inherited. Family history studies, which trace the psychiatric pedigrees of eating disordered individuals, show elevated rates of anorexia nervosa and bulimia nervosa in first-degree female relatives compared to relatives of controls (Gershon *et al.*, 1983; Hudson *et al.*, 1987; Kassett *et al.*, 1989; Stern *et al.*, 1984; Strober *et al.*, in press). Additionally, relatives of individuals with anorexia nervosa and bulimia nervosa have significantly increased rates of eating disorders that do not meet full diagnostic criteria, suggesting a broad spectrum of eating pathology in families (Lilenfeld *et al.*, 1998; Strober *et al.*, 2000).

Many family studies have also shown a link between anorexia nervosa and affective disorders, with first-degree relatives of eating disordered patients manifesting a higher rate of affective disorder than relatives of controls (Rivinus *et al.*, 1984; Winokur *et al.*, 1980). Some studies of families of patients with bulimia nervosa have found a similar association (Bulik, 1987; Hudson *et al.*, 1983) but others did not (Blouin *et al.*, 1986; Stern *et al.*, 1984). The relationship between a family history of affective disorder and the levels of mood disturbance at presentation is discussed in Chapter 8. Higher rates of substance abuse, particularly alcohol, have also been found in relatives of women with anorexia nervosa (Rivinus *et al.*, 1984) and bulimia nervosa (Bulik, 1987), compared to normal controls. Although the evidence is not conclusive, it appears that family propensity to depression and alcoholism may represent additional risk factors for the development of an eating disorder, at least in patients who themselves have affective disorders.

Diabetes mellitus, which requires attention to eating and diet, may create yet another situation conducive to the development of an eating disorder in adolescents. A study of female adolescents and young adults with insulin-dependent diabetes mellitus found prevalence rates of 6.5 percent for both anorexia nervosa and bulimia nervosa, considerably higher than those of the general population (Rodin *et al.*, 1986). In this study another 6 percent manifested subclinical syndromes. Ten percent (3/30) of our own sample of adolescent patients with bulimia nervosa were diabetic, at least one of whom purged by not taking her insulin. Other chronic conditions have been linked with the development of eating disorders in adolescents, but thus far the evidence is largely anecdotal.

Males at higher risk for developing eating disorders include those whose profession or subculture put great emphasis on having a lower weight or a more slender body type. Jockeys and wrestlers, whose professions demand set weights, have higher rates of disturbed eating (Silberstein *et al.*, 1989). Being homosexual may put men at greater risk for developing disordered eating. Some have observed that contemporary gay male culture stresses the importance of physical appearance to a greater extent than does heterosexual male culture; however, studies have yielded mixed findings.

Conclusion

Anorexia nervosa and bulimia nervosa, the two eating disorders of adolescence, affect mainly females from across socioeconomic strata. Both disorders constitute disturbances in attitudes toward weight and body shape and manifest themselves in maladaptive eating behavior. Adolescents with anorexia nervosa starve themselves due to their fears of becoming fat, while maintaining a distorted body image and denying that their behavior is abnormal. Normal-weight young women with bulimia nervosa engage in repeated sessions of binge-eating, followed by vomiting or other means of purging. Feelings of isolation, depression, and personality traits of compliance and perfectionism accompany both disorders, but those with anorexia nervosa tend to be more socially withdrawn and ritualistically obsessive, while those with bulimia nervosa tend to be more impulsive, sexually active and have higher rates of alcoholism and drug use. The course of anorexia nervosa tends to be steady, with a major proscribed period of illness followed by recovery or deteriorating chronicity. Mortality rates are relatively high. Bulimia nervosa takes a more episodic course. Its mortality rate is unknown.

Medical complications are those that result from malnutrition and semi-starvation, in the case of anorexia nervosa, and from bingeing and purging for bulimia nervosa. Although most major systems of the body are negatively affected by anorexia nervosa, most recover fully when adequate weight is restored. However, some patients never regain menses and some go on to develop osteoporosis.

Risk factors for the development of an eating disorder in adolescence include sociological, familial, psychological and biological variables. Girls who place a high value on a slender appearance, who have family histories of obesity and eating disorders, who diet frequently and who are themselves overweight, are at particularly high risk. Subcultures that emphasize the importance of weight and body shape also appear to foster eating pathology. Personality traits of perfectionism, low self-esteem, obsessionality and dependence appear to represent additional predisposing factors.

Pediatricians play a vital role in the detection and prevention of anorexia nervosa and bulimia nervosa. By understanding the nature of eating disorders in adolescents, by paying close attention to patients who seem particularly concerned about their weight and by inquiring into their dietary habits, pediatricians can educate their patients about the dangers of eating disorders, and recommend psychiatric and nutritional treatment. In this way, pediatricians represent the 'front line' in the combat against these destructive disorders.

References

Abraham, S. F. and Beumont, P. J. V. (1982) How patients describe bulimia or binge-eating. *Psychological Medicine*, 12, 625–635.

Abraham, S. F., Mira, M. and Llewellyn-Jones, D. (1983) Bulimia: a study of outcome. *International Journal of Eating Disorders*, 2, 175–180.

Adler, A. G., Watinsky, P., Krall, R. A. and Cho, S. Y. (1980) Death resulting from ipecac syrup poisoning. *Journal of the American Medical Association*, 243, 1927–1928.

American Psychiatric Association (1980) *Diagnostic and Statistical Manual of Mental Disorders* (3rd edition). Washington, DC: American Psychiatric Association.

American Psychiatric Association (1987) *Diagnostic and Statistical Manual of Mental*

Disorders (3rd edition. Revised). Washington, DC: American Psychiatric Association.

American Psychiatric Association (1994) *Diagnostic and Statistical Manual of Mental Disorders* (4th edition). Washington, DC: American Psychiatric Association.

Anderluh, M. B., Tchanturia, K., Rabe-Hesketh, S. *et al.* (2003) Childhood obsessive-compulsive personality traits in adult women with eating disorders: defining a broader eating disorder phenotype. *American Journal of Psychiatry*, 160(2), 242–247.

Beck, D., Casper, R. and Andersen, A. (1996) Truly late onset of eating disorders: a study of 11 cases averaging 60 years of age at presentation. *International Journal of Eating Disorders*, 20(4), 389–395.

Becker, A. E., Grinspoon, S. K., Klibanski, A. and Herzog, D. B. (1999) Eating disorders. *New England Journal of Medicine*, 340(14), 1092–1098.

Beresin, E. V., Gordon, C. and Herzog, D. B. (1989) The process of recovering from anorexia nervosa. *Journal of the American Academy of Psychoanalysis*, 17(1), 103–130.

Biller, B. M., Saxe, V., Herzog, D. B., Rosenthal, D. I., Holzman, S. and Klibanski, A. (1989) Mechanisms of osteoporosis in adult and adolescent women with anorexia nervosa. *Journal of Clinical Endocrinology and Metabolism*, 68(3), 548–554.

Blouin, J., Blouin, A., Perez, E., Seidel, B. and Bushnik, T. (1986) Family history factors in bulimia (abstract). The Second International Conference on Eating Disorders. New York.

Bowers, T. K. and Eckert, E. (1978) Leukopenia in anorexia nervosa. *Archives of Internal Medicine*, 138, 1520–1523.

Bruch, H. (1973) *Eating Disorders*. New York: Basic Books.

Bruch, H. (1978) *The Golden Cage*. Cambridge, MA: Harvard University Press.

Bulik, C. M. (1987) Drug and alcohol abuse by bulimic women and their families. *American Journal of Psychiatry*, 144, 1604–1606.

Bulik, C. M., Sullivan, P. F., Mckee, M., Weltzin, T. E. and Kaye, W. H. (1994) Characteristics of bulimic women with and without alcohol-abuse. *American Journal of Drug and Alcohol Abuse*, 20(2), 273–283.

Bulik, C. M., Sullivan, P. F., Weltzin, T. E. and Kaye, W. H. (1995) Temperament in eating disorders. *International Journal of Eating Disorders*, 17(3), 251–261.

Bulik, C. M., Sullivan, P. F., Joyce, P. R., Carter, F. A. and McIntosh, V. V. (1998) Predictions of 1-year treatment outcome in bulimia nervosa. *Comprehensive Psychiatry*, 39(4), 206–214.

Bulik, C. M., Sullivan, P. F., Fear, J. L. and Pickering, A. (2000) Outcome of anorexia nervosa: eating attitudes, personality, and parental bonding. *International Journal of Eating Disorders*, 28(2), 139–147.

Bulik, C. M., Tozzi, F., Anderson, C., Mazzeo, S. E., Aggen, S. and Sullivan, P. F. (2003) The relation between eating disorders and components of perfectionism. *American Journal of Psychiatry*, 160(2), 366–368.

Cantwell, D. P., Sturzenberger, S., Burroughs, J., Salkin, B. and Green, J. K. (1977) Anorexia nervosa. An affective disorder? *Archives of General Psychiatry*, 34(9), 1087–1093.

Casper, R. C., Elke, E. D., Halmi, K. A., Goldberg, S. C. and Davis, J. M. (1980) Bulimia: its incidence and clinical importance in patients with anorexia nervosa. *Archives of General Psychiatry*, 37, 1030–1035.

Castro, J., Gila, A., Gual, P., Lahotiga, F., Saura, B. and Toro, J. (2004) Perfectionism dimensions in children and adolescents with anorexia nervosa. *Journal of Adolescent Health*, 35(5), 392–398.

Cooper, P. J. and Fairburn, C. G. (1983) Binge-eating and self-induced vomiting in the community: a preliminary study. *British Journal of Psychiatry*, 142, 139–144.

Cooper, P. J., Charnock, D. J. and Taylor, M. J. (1987) The prevalence of bulimia nervosa. *British Journal of Psychiatry*, 151, 684–686.

Cooper, P. J., Watkins, B., Bryant-Waugh, R. and Lask, B. (2002) The nosological status of early onset anorexia nervosa. *Psychological Medicine*, 32(5), 873–880.

Crisp, A. (1970) Premorbid factors in adult disorders of weight, with particular reference to primary anorexia nervosa (weight phobia). A literature review. *Journal of Psychosomatic Research*, 14, 1–22.

Crisp, A. H. and Toms, D. A. (1972) Primary anorexia nervosa or weight phobia in the male: report on 13 cases. *British Medical Journal*, 1, 334–338.

Crisp, A. H., Palmer, R. L. and Kalucy, R. S. (1976) How common is anorexia nervosa? A prevalence study. *British Journal of Psychiatry*, 128, 549–554.

Crisp, A., Hsu, R. L. and Stonehill, L. (1979) Personality, body weight and ultimate outcome in anorexia nervosa. *British Journal of Psychiatry*, 40, 335–352.

Cullberg, J. and Engstrom-Lindberg, M. (1986) Prevalence and incidence of eating disorders in a suburban population. *Acta Psychiatrica Scandinavica*, 78, 314–319.

Eddy, K. T., Keel, P. K., Dorer, D. J., Delinsky, S. S., Franko, D. L. and Herzog, D. B. (2002) Longitudinal comparison of anorexia nervosa subtypes. *International Journal of Eating Disorders*, 31(2), 191–201.

Eliot, A. O. and Baker, C. W. (2001) Eating disordered adolescent males. *Adolescence*, 36(143), 535–543.

Fairburn, C. G. and Cooper, P. J. (1984) The clinical features of bulimia nervosa. *British Journal of Psychiatry*, 144, 238–246.

Fairburn, C. G. and Harrison, P. J. (2003) Eating disorders. *Lancet*, 361(9355), 407–416.

Fairburn, C. G., Cooper, P. J., Kirk, J. and O'Conner, M. (1986) A comparison of two psychological treatments for bulimia nervosa. *Behavioral Research and Therapy*, 24, 629–643.

Fairburn, C. G., Cooper, Z., Doll, H. A., *et al.* (1999) Risk factors for anorexia nervosa – three integrated case-control comparisons. *Archives of General Psychiatry*, 56(5), 468–476.

Fairburn, C.G., Cooper, Z., Doll, H.A., *et al.* (2000) The natural course of bulimia nervosa and binge eating disorder in young women. *Archives of General Psychiatry*, 57(7), 659–665.

Fairburn, C. G., Stice, E., Cooper, Z., *et al.* (2003) Understanding persistence in bulimia nervosa: a 5-year naturalistic study. *Journal of Consulting and Clinical Psychology*, 71(1), 103–109.

Fichter, M. M. and Quadflieg, N. (1999) Six-year course and outcome of anorexia nervosa. *International Journal of Eating Disorders*, 26(4), 359–385.

Fries, H. (1977) Studies on secondary amenorrhea, anorectic behavior and body-image perception: importance for the early recognition of anorexia nervosa. In *Anorexia Nervosa* (ed. R. A. Vigersky). New York: Raven Press.

Garfinkel, P. E. and Garner, D. M. (1982) *Anorexia Nervosa: A Multidimensional Perspective*. New York: Brunner/Mazel.

Garfinkel, P. E., Garner, D. M. and Goldbloom, D. S. (1987) Eating disorders: implications for the 1990s. *Canadian Journal of Psychiatry*, 32, 624–630.

Garner, D. M. and Garfinkel, P. E. (1980) Socio-cultural factors in the development of anorexia nervosa. *Psychological Medicine*, 10(4), 647–656.

Garner, D. M., Garfinkel, P. E., Schwartz, D. and Thompson, M. (1980) Cultural expectations of thinness in women. *Psychological Reports*, 47, 483–491.

Gershon, E. S., Hamovit, J. R., Schreiber, J. L., Dibble, E. D., Kaye, W., Nurnberger, J. I., Andersen, A. and Ebert, M. (1983) Anorexia nervosa and major affective disorders associated in families: a preliminary report. In *Childhood Psychopathology and Development* (ed. S. B. Guze, F. J. Earls and J. E. Barrett). New York: Raven Press.

Gershon, E. S., Schreiber, J. L., Hamovit, J. R., Dibble, E. D., Kaye, W., Nurnberger, J. L., Andersen, A. E. and Ebert, M. (1984) Clinical findings in patients with anorexia nervosa and affective illness in their relatives. *American Journal of Psychiatry*, 141, 1419–1422.

Golden, N. H. (2003) Osteopenia and osteoporosis in anorexia nervosa. *Adolescent Medicine State of the Art Reviews*, 14(1), 97–108.

Gordon, C., Beresin, E. and Herzog, D. B. (1989) The parents' relationship and the child's illness in anorexia nervosa. *Journal of the American Academy of Psychoanalysis*, 17, 29–42.

Gottdiener, J. S., Gross, H. A., Henry, W. L., Borer, J. S. and Ebert, M. H. (1978) Effects of self-induced starvation on cardiac size and function in anorexia nervosa. *Circulation*, 58, 426–433.

Gowers, S. G. and Shore, A. (2001) Development of weight and shape concerns in the aetiology of eating disorders. *British Journal of Psychiatry*, 179, 236–242.

Grinspoon, S., Miller, K., Coyle, C., Krempin, J., Armstrong, C., Pitts, S. *et al.* (1999) Severity of osteopenia in estrogen-deficient women with anorexia nervosa and hypothalamic amenorrhea. *Journal of Clinical Endocrinology and Metabolism*, 84(6), 2049–2055.

Grinspoon, S., Thomas, E., Pitts, S., Gross, E., Mickley, D., Miller, K. *et al.* (2000) Prevalence and predictive factors for regional osteopenia in women with anorexia nervosa. (See comment.) *Annals of Internal Medicine*, 133(10), 790–794.

Grissett N. I. and Norvell, N. K. (1992) Perceived social support, social skills, and quality of relationships in bulimic women. *Journal of Consulting and Clinical Psychology*, 60(2), 293–299.

Hall, A., Slim, E., Hawker, F. and Salmond, C. (1984) Anorexia nervosa: long-term outcome of 50 female patients. *British Journal of Psychiatry*, 145, 407–413.

Hall, R. C., Tice, L., Beresford, T. P., Wooley, B. and Hall, A. K. (1989) Sexual abuse in patients with anorexia nervosa and bulimia. *Psychosomatics*, 30, 73–79.

Halmi, K. A., Casper, R. C., Eckert, E. D., Goldberg, S. C. and Davis, J. M. (1979) Unique features associated with the age of onset of anorexia nervosa. *Psychiatry Research*, 1, 209–215.

Halmi, K. A., Falk, J. R. and Schwartz, E. (1981) Binge-eating and vomiting: a survey of a college population. *Psychological Medicine*, 11, 697–706.

Halmi, K. A., Eckert, E. D., Marchl, P. and Cohen, J. (1988) Ten year follow-up of anorexia nervosa. Third plenary session: Outcome studies of anorexia nervosa and bulimia nervosa. Third International Conference of Eating Disorders, New York.

Halmi, K. A., Sunday, S. R., Strober, M., Kaplan, A., Woodside, D. B., Fichter, M.,

Treasure, J., Berretini, W. H. and Kaye, W. H. (2000) Perfectionism in anorexia nervosa: variation by clinical subtype, obsessionality and pathological eating behavior. *American Journal of Psychiatry*, 157(11), 1799–1805.

Hatsukami, D. K., Mitchell, J. E. and Eckert, E. D. (1984) Eating disorders: a variant of mood disorders? *Psychiatric Clinics of North America*, 7, 349–365.

Herpertz-Dahlmann, B. M., Wewetzer, C., Schulz, E. and Remschmidt, H. (1996) Course and outcome in adolescent anorexia nervosa. *International Journal of Eating Disorders*, 19(4), 335–345.

Herpertz-Dahlmann, B., Muller, B., Herpertz, S., Heussen, N., Hebebrand, J. and Remschmidt, H. (2001) Prospective 10-year follow-up in adolescent anorexia nervosa – course, outcome, psychiatric comorbidity, and psychosocial adaptation. *Journal of Child Psychology and Psychiatry and Allied Disciplines*, 42(5), 603–612.

Herzog, D. B. (1984) Are anorectics and bulimics depressed? *American Journal of Psychiatry*, 141, 1594–1597.

Herzog, D. B. and Copeland, P. M. (1985) Medical progress: eating disorders. *New England Journal of Medicine*, 313, 295–303.

Herzog, D. B., Norman, D. K., Gordon, C. and Pepose, M. (1984) Sexual conflict and eating disorder in 27 males. *American Journal of Psychiatry*, 141, 989–990.

Herzog, D. B., Pepose, M., Norman, D. K. and Rigotti, N. A. (1985) Eating disorders and social maladjustment in female medical students. *Journal of Nervous and Mental Disease*, 173, 734–740.

Herzog, D. B., Keller, M. B., Lavorl, P. W. and Ott, I. L. (1987) Social impairment in bulimia. *International Journal of Eating Disorders*, 6, 741–747.

Herzog, D. B., Keller, M. B. and Lavorl, P. W. (1988) Outcome in anorexia nervosa and bulimia nervosa: a review of the literature. *Journal of Nervous and Mental Disease*, 176, 131–143.

Herzog, D. B., Nussbaum, K. M. and Marmor, A. K. (1996) Comorbidity and outcome in eating disorders. *Psychiatric Clinics of North America*, 19(4), 843–859.

Herzog, D. B., Dorer, D. J., Keel, P. K., *et al.* (1999) Recovery and relapse in anorexia and bulimia nervosa: a 7.5-year follow-up study. *Journal of the American Academy of Child and Adolescent Psychiatry*, 38(7), 829–837.

Herzog, D. B., Newman, K. L., Yeh, C. J. and Warshaw, M. (1991) Body image satisfaction in homosexual and heterosexual females. *Journal of Nervous and Mental Disease*, 179(6), 356–359.

Hoek, H. W. and van Hoeken, D. (2003) Review of the prevalence and incidence of eating disorders. *International Journal of Eating Disorders*, 34(4), 383–396.

Hoek, H. W., van Harten, P. N., van Hoeken, D. and Susser, E. (1998) Lack of relation between culture and anorexia nervosa – results of an incidence study on Curacao. *New England Journal of Medicine*, 338(17), 1231–1232.

Holland, A. J., Hall, A., Murray, R., Russell, G. F. M. and Crisp, A. H. (1984) Anorexia nervosa: a study of 34 twin pairs. *British Journal of Psychiatry*, 145, 414–419.

Holland, A. J., Sicotte, N. and Treasure, J. (1988) Anorexia nervosa: evidence for a genetic basis. *Journal of Psychosomatic Research*, 32, 561–571.

Hsu, L. K. G. and Holder, D. (1986) Bulimia nervosa: treatment and short-term outcome. *Psychological Medicine*, 16, 65–70.

Hsu, L. K. G., Crisp, A. H. and Harding, B. (1979) Outcome of anorexia nervosa. *Lancet*, 1, 61–65.

Hudson, J. I., Pope, H. G., Jonas, J. M. and Yurgelun-Todd, D. (1983) Family history study of anorexia nervosa and bulimia. *Psychiatry Research*, 142, 133–138.

Hudson, J. I., Pope, H. G., Jonas, J. M., Yurgelun-Todd, D. and Frankenburg, F. R. (1987) A controlled family history study of bulimia. *Psychological Medicine*, 17, 883–890.

Huon, G. F., Mingyi, Q., Oliver, K. and Xiao, G. (2002) A large-scale survey of eating disorder symptomatology among female adolescents in the People's Republic of China. *International Journal of Eating Disorders*, 32(2), 192–205.

Inagaki, T., Horiguchi, J., Tsubouchi, K., Miyaoka, T., Uegaki, J. and Seno, H. (2002) Late onset anorexia nervosa: two case reports. *International Journal of Psychiatry in Medicine*, 32(1), 91–95.

Johnson, J. G., Cohen, P., Kotler, L., Kasen, S. and Brook, J. S. (2002) Psychiatric disorders associated with risk for the development of eating disorders during adolescence and early adulthood. *Journal of Consulting and Clinical Psychology*, 70(5), 1119–1128.

Jones, D. J., Fox, M. M., Babigian, H. M. and Hutton, H. E. (1980) Epidemiology of anorexia nervosa in Monroe County, New York: 1960–1976. *Psychosomatic Medicine*, 42(6), 551–558.

Kassett, J. A., Gershon, E. S., Maxwell, M. E., Guroff, J. J., Kazuba, D. M., Smith, A. L., Brandt, H. A. and Jimerson, D. C. (1989) Psychiatric disorders in the first-degree relatives of probands with bulimia nervosa. *American Journal of Psychiatry*, 146, 1468–1471.

Kaye, W. H., Weltzin, T. and Hsu, L. K. (1993) Relationship between anorexia nervosa and obsessive and compulsive behaviors. *Psychiatric Annals*, 23, 365–373.

Keel, P. K. and Klump, K. L. (2003) Are eating disorders culture-bound syndromes? Implications for conceptualizing their etiology. *Psychological Bulletin*, 129(5), 747–769.

Keel, P. K. and Mitchell, J. E. (1997) Outcome in bulimia nervosa. *American Journal of Psychiatry*, 154(3), 313–321.

Keel, P. K., Mitchell, J. E., Miller, K. B., *et al.* (1999) Long-term outcome of bulimia nervosa. *Archives of General Psychiatry*, 56(1), 63–69.

Keel, P. K., Dorer, D. J., Eddy, K. T., Franko, D., Charatan, D. L. and Herzog, D. B. (2003) Predictors of mortality in eating disorders. *Archives of General Psychiatry*, 60(2), 179–183.

Keller, M. B., Herzog, D. B., Lavorl, P. W., Ott, I. L., Bradburn, I. S. and Mahoney, E. M. (1989) High rates of chronicity and rapidity of relapse in patients with bulimia nervosa. *Archives of General Psychiatry*, 46, 480–481.

Keller, M. B., Herzog, D. B., Lavorl, P. W. and Bradburn, I. S. (1991) The naturalistic history of bulimia nervosa: extraordinarily high rates of chronicity, relapse, recurrence and psychosocial morbidity. *International Journal of Eating Disorders*, 12, 1–9.

Khan, K. M., Green, R. M., Saul, A., *et al.* (1996) Retired elite female ballet dancers and nonathletic controls have similar bone mineral density at weightbearing sites. *Journal of Bone and Mineral Research*, 11(10), 1566–1574.

Killen, J. D., Taylor, B., Teich, M. J., Saylor, K. E., Maron, D. J. and Robinson, T. N. (1986) Self-induced vomiting and laxative and diuretic use among teenagers: precursors of the binge-purge syndrome? *Journal of the American Medical Association*, 255, 1447–1450.

Kjelsas, E., Bjornstrom, C. and Gotestam, K. G. (2004) Prevalence of eating disorders in female and male adolescents (14–15 years). *Eating Behavior*, 5(1), 13–25.

Klump, K. L., Ringham, R. M., Marcus, M. D. and Kaye, W. H. (2001) A family history/family study approach to examining the nature of eating disorder risk in ballet dancers: evidence for gene–environment combinations? Paper presented at the Eating Disorder Research Society Annual Meeting, Albuquerque, New Mexico.

Kron, L., Katz, J. L., Gorzynski, G. and Weiner, H. (1978) Hyperactivity in anorexia nervosa: a fundamental clinical feature. *Comprehensive Psychiatry*, 19, 433–440.

Lacey, H. (1983) Bulimia nervosa, binge eating, and psychogenic vomiting: a controlled treatment study and long term outcome. *British Medical Journal*, 286, 1609–1613.

Lilenfeld, L. R., Kaye, W. H., Greeno, C. G., *et al.* (1998) A controlled family study of anorexia nervosa and bulimia nervosa – psychiatric disorders in first-degree relatives and effects of proband comorbidity. *Archives of General Psychiatry*, 55(7), 603–610.

Lucas, A. R., Beard C. M., O'Fallon, W. M. and Kurland, L. T. (1988) Anorexia nervosa in Rochester, Minnesota: a 45 year study. *Mayo Clinic Proceedings*, 63, 433–442.

Lucas, A. R., Beard, C. M., O'Fallon, W. M. and Kurland, L. T. (1991) 50-year trends in the incidence of anorexia nervosa in Rochester, Minn.: a population-based study. *American Journal of Psychiatry*, 148(7), 917–922.

Makino, M., Tsuboi, K. and Dennerstein, L. (2004) Prevalence of eating disorders: a comparison of Western and non-Western countries. *Medscape General Medicine*, 6(3), 49.

Mangweth, B., Pope, H. G., Jr., Hudson, J. I., Olivardia, R., Kinzl, J. and Biebl, W. (1997) Eating disorders in Austrian men: an intracultural and crosscultural comparison study. *Psychotherapy and Psychosomatics*, 66(4), 214–221.

Misra, M., Aggarwal, A., Miller, K. K., Almazan, C., Worley, M., Soyka, L. A. *et al.* (2004) Effects of anorexia nervosa on clinical, hematologic, biochemical, and bone density parameters in community-dwelling girls. *Pediatrics*, 114(6), 1574–1583.

Mitchell, J. E., Davis, L. and Goff, G. (1985) The process of relapse in patients with bulimia. *International Journal of Eating Disorders*, 4, 457–463.

Morgan, H. G. and Russell, G. F. M. (1975) Value of family background and clinical features as predictors of long-term outcome in anorexia nervosa: four year follow-up of 41 patients. *Psychological Medicine*, 5, 355–371.

Munoz, M. T. and Argente, J. (2002) Anorexia nervosa in female adolescents: endocrine and bone mineral density disturbances. *European Journal of Endocrinology*, 147(3), 275–286.

Nobakht, M. and Dezhkam, M. (2000) An epidemiological study of eating disorders in Iran. *International Journal of Eating Disorders*, 28(3), 265–271.

Norman, D. K. and Herzog, D. G. (1986) A three year outcome study in normal-weight bulimia: assessment of psychosocial functioning and eating attitudes. *Psychiatry Research*, 19, 199–205.

O'Connor, P. J., Lewis, R. D., Kirchner, E. M., *et al.* (1996) Eating disorder symptoms in former female college gymnasts: relations with body composition. *American Journal of Clinical Nutrition*, 64(6), 840–843.

O'Dea, J.A, and Abraham, S. (1999) Onset of disordered eating attitudes and behaviors in early adolescence: interplay of pubertal status, gender, weight and age. *Adolescence*, 34(136), 671–679.

Olivardia, R., Pope, H. G., Jr., Mangweth, B. and Hudson, J. I. (1995) Eating disorders in college men. *American Journal of Psychiatry*, 152(9), 1279–1285.

Palla, B. and Litt, I. F. (1988) Medical complications of eating disorders in adolescents. *Pediatrics*, 81, 613–623.

Patton, G. C. (1988) Mortality in eating disorders. *Psychological Medicine*, 18, 947–951.

Piran, N., Kennedy, S., Garfinkel, P. E. and Owens, M. (1985) Affective disturbance in eating disorders. *Journal of Nervous and Mental Disease*, 173, 395–400.

Pope, H. G., Hudson, J. I., Jonas, J. M. and Yurgelun-Todd, D. (1985) Antidepressant treatment of bulimia: a two-year follow-up study. *Journal of Clinical Psychopharmacology*, 5, 320–327.

Pope, H. G., Champoux, R. F. and Hudson, J. I. (1987) Eating disorders and socio-economic class: anorexia nervosa and bulimia in nine communities. *Journal of Nervous and Mental Disease*, 175, 620–623.

Pope, H. G., Jr., Katz, D. L. and Hudson, J. I. (1993) Anorexia nervosa and 'reverse anorexia' among 108 male bodybuilders. *Comprehensive Psychiatry*, 34(6), 406–409.

Pyle, R. L., Mitchell, J. E., Eckert, E. D., Halvorson, P. A., Neuman, P. A. and Goff, G. M. (1983) The incidence of bulimia in a freshman college population. *International Journal of Eating Disorders*, 2, 75–85.

Rathner, G. and Messner, K. (1993) Detection of eating disorders in a small rural town – an epidemiologic study. *Psychological Medicine*, 23(1), 175–184.

Rigotti, N. A., Nussbaum, S. R., Herzog, D. B. and Neer, R. M. (1984) Osteoporosis in women with anorexia nervosa. *New England Journal of Medicine*, 311, 1601–1606.

Rigotti, N. A., Neer, R. M., Skates, S. J., Herzog, D. B. and Nussbaum, S. R. (1991) The clinical course of osteoporosis in anorexia nervosa. A longitudinal study of cortical bone mass. *Journal of the American Medical Association*, 265(9), 1133–1138.

Rivinus, T. M., Biederman, J., Herzog, D. B., Kemper, K., Harper, G. P., Harmatz, J. S. and Houseworth, S. (1984) Anorexia nervosa and affective disorders: a controlled family history study. *American Journal of Psychiatry*, 141, 1414–1418.

Rodin, G., Daneman, D., Johnston, L., Kenshole, A. and Garfinkel, P. E. (1986) Anorexia nervosa and bulimia in insulin-dependent diabetes mellitus. *International Journal of Psychiatric Medicine*, 16, 46–57.

Rodriguez, A., Novalbos, J. P., Martinez, J. M., Ruiz, M. A., Fernandez, J. R. and Jimenez, D. (2001) Eating disorders and altered eating behaviours in adolescents of normal weight in a Spanish city. *Journal of Adolescent Health*, 28(4), 338–345.

Russell, G. F. M. (1979) Bulimia nervosa: an ominous variant of anorexia nervosa. *Psychological Medicine*, 9, 429–448.

Russell, G. F. M. (1988) Twenty year follow-up of anorexia nervosa. Third plenary session: Outcome studies of anorexia nervosa and bulimia nervosa. Third International Conference of Eating Disorders, New York.

Russell, C. J. and Keel, P. K. (2002) Homosexuality as a specific risk factor for eating disorders in men. *International Journal of Eating Disorders*, 31(3), 300–306.

Shafran, R., Cooper, Z. and Fairburn, C. G. (2002) Clinical perfectionism: a cognitive-behavioural analysis. (See comment.) *Behaviour Research and Therapy*, 40(7), 773–791.

Silberstein, L. R., Mishkind, M. E., Striegel-Moore, R. H., Timko, C. and Rodin, J. (1989) Men and their bodies: a comparison of homosexual and heterosexual men. *Psychosomatic Medicine*, 51, 337–346.

Sim, L. and Zeman, J. (2004) Emotion awareness and identification skills in adolescent girls with bulimia nervosa. *Journal of Clinical Child and Adolescent Psychology*, 33(4), 760–771.

Sloan, G. and Leichner, P. (1986) Is there a relationship between sexual abuse or incest and eating disorders? *Canadian Journal of Psychiatry – Revue Canadienne de Psychiatrie*, 31(7), 656–660.

Soyka, L. A., Misra, M., Frenchman, A., Miller, K. K., Grinspoon, S., Schoenfeld, D. A. *et al.* (2002) Abnormal bone mineral accrual in adolescent girls with anorexia nervosa. *Journal of Clinical Endocrinology and Metabolism*, 87(9), 4177–4185.

Steiner-Adair, C. (1986) The body politic: normal female adolescent development and the development of eating disorders. *Journal of the American Academy of Psychoanalysis*, 14, 95–114.

Steinhausen, H. C. (2002) The outcome of anorexia nervosa in the 20th century. *American Journal of Psychiatry*, 159(8), 1284–1293.

Steinhausen, H. C., Winkler, C. and Meier, M. (1997) Eating disorders in adolescence in a Swiss epidemiological study. *International Journal of Eating Disorders*, 22(2), 147–151.

Stern, S. L., Dixon, K. N., Nemzer, E., Lake, M. D., Sansone, R. A., Smeltzer, D. J., Lantz, S. and Schrier, S. S. (1984) Affective disorder in the families of women with normal weight bulimia. *American Journal of Psychiatry*, 141, 1224–1227.

Striegel-Moore, R. H., Silberstein, L. R. and Rodin, J. (1986) Toward an understanding of risk factors for bulimia. *American Psychologist*, 41, 246–263.

Strober, M. (1980) Personality and symptomatological features in young, nonchronic anorexia nervosa patients. *Journal of Psychosomatic Research*, 24, 353–359.

Strober, M., Morrell, W., Burroughs, J., Salkin, B. and Jacobs, C. (1985) A controlled family study of anorexia nervosa. *Journal of Psychiatric Research*, 19, 239–246.

Strober, M., Lampert, C., Morrell, W., Burroughs, J. and Jacobs, C. (1990) A controlled family study of anorexia nervosa: evidence of familial aggregation and lack of shared transmission with affective disorders. *International Journal of Eating Disorders*, 9, 239–253.

Strober, M., Freeman, R. and Morrell, W. (1997) The long-term course of severe anorexia nervosa in adolescents: survival analysis of recovery, relapse, and outcome predictors over 10–15 years in a prospective study. *International Journal of Eating Disorders*, 22(4), 339–360.

Strober, M., Freeman, R., Lampert, C., *et al.* (2000) Controlled family study of anorexia nervosa and bulimia nervosa: evidence of shared liability and transmission of partial syndromes. *American Journal of Psychiatry*, 157(3), 393–401.

Sullivan, P. F. (1995) Mortality in anorexia nervosa. *American Journal of Psychiatry*, 152(7), 1073–1074.

Swift, W. J., Kalin, N. H., Wamboldt, F. S., Kaslow, N. and Ritholz, M. (1985) Depression in bulimia at 2–5 year follow-up. *Psychiatry Research*, 16, 111–122.

Swift, W. J., Rithoiz, M., Kalin, N. H. and Kaslow, N. (1987) A follow-up study of thirty hospitalized bulimics. *Psychosomatic Medicine*, 49, 45–55.

Szabo, P. and Tury, F. (1991) The prevalence of bulimia-nervosa in a Hungarian college and secondary-school population. *Psychotherapy and Psychosomatics*, 56(1–2), 43–47.

Szmukler, G. I. (1983) Weight and food preoccupation in a population of English schoolgirls. In *Understanding Anorexia Nervosa and Bulimia* (ed. G. J. Burgman). Fourth Ross Conference on Medical Research, Ross Laboratories, Ohio, 21–27.

Szmukler, G. I. (1985) The epidemiology of anorexia nervosa and bulimia. *Journal of Psychiatric Research*, 19(2–3), 143–153.

Szmukler, G. I., Eisler, I., Gillies, C. and Hayward, M. E. (1985) The implications of anorexia nervosa in a ballet school. *Journal of Psychiatric Research*, 19(2–3), 177–181.

Theander, S. (1985) Outcome and prognosis in anorexia nervosa and bulimia: some results of previous investigations, compared with those of a Swedish long-term study. *Journal of Psychiatric Research*, 19, 493–508.

Thompson, A. M. and Chad, K. E. (2002) The relationship of social physique anxiety to risk for developing an eating disorder in young females. *Journal of Adolescent Health*, 31(2), 183–189.

Timko, C., Striegel-Moore, R. H., Silberstein, L. R. and Rodin, J. (1987) Femininity/masculinity and disordered eating in women: how are they related? *International Journal of Eating Disorders*, 61, 701–712.

Vaisman, N., Voet, H., Akivis, A. and Sive-Ner, I. (1996) Weight perception of adolescent dancing school students. *Archives of Pediatrics and Adolescent Medicine*, 150(2), 187–190.

Verhulst, F. C., van der Ende, J., Ferdinand, R. F. and Kasius, M. C. (1997) The prevalence of DSM-III-R diagnoses in a national sample of Dutch adolescents. *Archives of General Psychiatry*, 54, 329–336.

Walsh, B. T., Roose, S. P., Glassman, A. H., Gladis, M. and Sadik, C. (1985) Bulimia and depression. *Psychosomatic Medicine*, 47, 123–131.

Weedamannak, W. L. and Drop, M. J. (1985) The discriminative value of psychological characteristics in anorexia-nervosa – clinical and psychometric comparison between anorexia-nervosa patients, ballet dancers and controls. *Journal of Psychiatric Research*, 19(2–3), 285–290.

Wentz, E., Gillberg, C., Gillberg, I. C. and Rastam, M. (2001) Ten-year follow-up of adolescent-onset anorexia nervosa: psychiatric disorders and overall functioning scales. *Journal of Child Psychology and Psychiatry and Allied Disciplines*, 42(5), 613–622.

Wiederman, M. W., Pryor, T. and Morgan, C. D. (1996) The sexual experience of women diagnosed with anorexia nervosa or bulimia nervosa. *International Journal of Eating Disorders*, 19(2), 109–118.

Willi, J. and Grossmann, S. (1983) Epidemiology of anorexia nervosa in a defined region of Switzerland. *American Journal of Psychiatry*, 140, 564–567.

Winokur, A., March, V. and Mendels, J. (1980) Primary affective disorder in relatives of patients with anorexia nervosa. *American Journal of Psychiatry*, 137, 695–698.

WlodarczykBisaga, K. and Dolan, B. (1996) A two-stage epidemiological study of abnormal eating attitudes and their prospective risk factors in Polish schoolgirls. *Psychological Medicine*, 26(5), 1021–1032.

Woods, S. (2004) Untreated recovery from eating disorders. *Adolescence*, 39(154), 361–371.

Yager, J., Kurtzman, F., Landsverk, J. and Wiesmeier, E. (1988) Behaviors and attitudes related to eating disorders in homosexual male college students. *American Journal of Psychiatry*, 145(4), 495–497.

Chapter 8

Genetic factors in anorexia nervosa and bulimia nervosa

Michael Strober, Lisa R. Lilenfeld, Walter Kaye and Cynthia Bulik

Introduction

Anorexia nervosa (AN) and bulimia nervosa (BN) often follow a protracted and disabling course, complicated further by the usual presence of other psychiatric comorbidities. Insights into the complex psychopathology of eating disorders necessarily draw from several, often quite disparate, conceptual vantage points as their core phenotypic elements cross behavioral, cognitive, and biological domains; likewise, etiology is widely assumed to be multiply determined. Even so, in recent decades many workers have avowed that powerful sociocultural factors must figure centrally in the causation of eating disorders as the dieting abnormality of both AN and BN is so evidently impacted by more broadly transmitted, and widely embraced, attitudes toward a thin ideal body weight and slender shape.

In spite of the intuitive appeal of this line of thought, evidence for the overarching importance of a purely environmental-cultural etiology is hardly persuasive. In contrast to the seemingly ubiquitous presence of body dissatisfaction amongst females in industrialized countries, eating disorders affect a relatively small minority of the general population, thus begging the question of the nature of risk and susceptibility in those who are affected with clinical disorder. Moreover, strong evidence now exists that particular dimensions of personality which are known to be moderately heritable play a formative role in risk to eating disorders (see Lilenfeld *et al.*, 1998 for review), suggesting that genetically transmitted behavioral and biological processes might be an important aspect of liability toward developing either AN or BN.

This chapter reviews evidence supporting such a possibility and considers how the application of modern advances in quantitative and molecular genetics to the study of eating disorders offers a firm new scientific footing for pursuing more refined searches for genetic and environmental mechanisms of etiology.

Familial aspects

When familial predisposition to an illness exists, there is, in most cases, resemblance for this particular disorder amongst blood relatives of affected individuals. In simple terms, if eating disorders are transmissible, first-degree relatives of individuals with AN or BN should exhibit a statistically greater lifetime risk of the illness compared to relatives of unaffected control probands. Results from controlled family studies of eating disorders to date appear in Table 8.1. It will be noted that several studies have found increased rates of both eating disorders, that is co-aggregation, in relatives of AN probands, as well as amongst relatives of BN probands, compared to rates amongst relatives of controls (Gershon *et al.*, 1983; Hudson *et al.*, 1987; Kassett *et al.*, 1989), suggesting that AN and BN may conceivably share transmissible vulnerabilities in common.

In the first rigorously conducted case control family-genetic study of anorexia nervosa, Gershon *et al.* (1983) examined 99 first-degree relatives of 24 AN probands and 265 first-degree relatives of 44 nonpsychiatrically ill controls using a structured psychiatric assessment and operationalized diagnostic criteria. Approximately three-quarters of interviews were conducted blind to proband status and 54 per cent of relatives were directly interviewed. The morbid risks for AN and BN amongst first-degree relatives of AN probands were 2 per cent and 4.4 per cent respectively, compared to 0 per cent and 1.3 per cent amongst relatives of control probands.

Hudson *et al.* (1987) conducted lifetime psychiatric assessments on 432 first-degree relatives of 69 BN and 28 control probands, as well as 104 relatives of 24 probands with major depressive disorder. Diagnoses of relatives were based solely on family history information provided by the probands. Eating disorder was completely absent amongst relatives of controls, whereas the combined rate of AN and BN amongst relatives of BN probands was 3.4 per cent.

Kassett *et al.* (1989) studied lifetime risk of eating disorder in 185 first-degree relatives of 40 probands with DSM-III-R bulimia nervosa and 118 relatives of 24 normal controls. Diagnoses were made blind to proband status, and were based on direct interviews for 62 per cent of relatives and family history information for relatives who were unavailable for face-to-face interview. The rate of AN and BN in relatives of probands was over three times that of relatives of controls.

Strober *et al.* (1990), in a family-genetic study of anorexia nervosa, examined nearly 400 first-degree relatives over the age of 12 of nearly 100 AN probands, 269 relatives of 66 affective disorder probands, and 469 relatives of 117 non-mood disorder psychiatrically ill probands. Direct interviews were available for nearly 80 per cent of relatives and diagnoses were rendered blind to proband status. A history of AN was identified in 4.1 per cent of relatives of AN probands, whereas no case of AN was detected amongst relatives of

Table 8.1 Controlled studies of lifetime risk of eating disorders among first-degree relatives of eating disorder probands

Study	Number of probands				Relatives interviewed	Diagnosis in relatives, %			Diagnosis in control relatives, %		
	AN	BN	NC	Other controls		AN	BN	Total	AN	BN	Total
Gershon et al.	24	–	43	–	Y	2.0	4.4	6.4	0	1.3	1.3
Hudson et al.	–	69	28	24	N	1.7	1.7	3.4	0	0	0
Logue et al.	17	13	20	16	Y	0	0	0	0	0	0
Kassett et al.	–	40	24	–	Y	2.2	9.6	11.8	0	3.5	3.5
Strober et al.	97	–	–	183	Y	4.1	2.6	6.7	0	1.1	1.1
Halmi et al.	62	–	62	–	Y	1.2	1.2	2.4	0	0	0
Stern et al.	34	–	34	–	one parent	5.9	2.9	8.8	0	5.9	5.9
Lilenfeld et al.	26	47	44	–	Y	1.1	1.1, 2.3 (relatives of AN and BN probands, respectively)	11.8* and 19.8* (relatives of AN and BN probands, respectively)	0	0	3.7*
Strober et al.	152	171	181	–	Y	3.4, 3.7 (relatives of AN and BN probands, respectively)	3.8, 4.0 (relatives of AN and BN probands, respectively)	7.2 and 7.7 (relatives of AN and BN probands, respectively)	0.9	2.2	3.1

Notes
AN = anorexia nervosa; BN = bulimia nervosa; NC = non-eating disorder control
* Includes anorexia nervosa, bulimia nervosa, and eating disorder not otherwise specified diagnosis

either control group. The lifetime rate of bulimia nervosa was 2.6 per cent among relatives of AN probands, a rate that did not differ substantially from the population risk of this disorder among females.

Lilenfeld *et al.* (1998) studied 93 first-degree relatives of 26 restricting AN probands, 177 first-degree relatives of 47 BN probands, and 190 first-degree relatives of 44 non-eating disordered control women. All interviewers were blind to proband status, and direct interviews were conducted with approximately three-quarters of all relatives. Although familial aggregation of full syndromes of eating disorders was not found, the combined rates of illness, which included subacute cases, were 11.8 per cent and 19.8 per cent amongst the relatives of AN and BN probands, respectively, compared to 3.7 per cent amongst relatives of control women.

Finally, in the largest family study of eating disorders conducted to date, Strober *et al.* (2000) determined lifetime rates of full and partial syndromes of anorexia and bulimia nervosa in over 18,031 first-degree relatives of 152 probands with anorexia nervosa, 171 probands with bulimia nervosa, and 181 never-ill control probands based on direct, structured clinical interview and family history. Diagnoses were rendered blind to proband status and kindred identity using a best-estimate procedure. Full and partial syndromes were highly familial. The rate of full anorexia nervosa was 11.3 times as high in the female relatives of anorexia nervosa probands as in the relatives of never ill controls (3.4 per cent vs 0.3 per cent, respectively), whereas female relatives of probands with bulimia nervosa had a rate of bulimia nervosa that was 4.4 times as high as that for the relatives of never ill control probands (4.0 per cent vs 0.9). Importantly, both syndromes were cross transmitted, with anorexia nervosa diagnosed in 3.7 per cent of the female relatives of bulimia nervosa probands and bulimia nervosa diagnosed in 3.8 per cent of the female relatives of anorexia nervosa probands. The results suggest that there is a continuum of familial genetic liability to eating disorders and that the major syndromes share risk factors in common.

Three studies (Logue *et al.*, 1989; Halmi *et al.*, 1991; Stern *et al.*, 1992) have found no evidence of familial aggregation of eating disorders when considering AN and BN in total. However, two (Logue *et al.*, 1989; Stern *et al.*, 1992) are compromised by extremely small sample sizes, lack of blinding of diagnostic assessments, or reliance on single informants or family history information in diagnosing relatives. Logue *et al.* (1989) compared rates of illness in 132 first-degree relatives of 30 eating disorder probands, including only 6 with restricting AN and 13 with BN, with rates in 107 relatives of non-ill controls and 75 relatives of depressed controls. While the majority of relatives were interviewed directly, diagnoses were not blind to proband status. Halmi *et al.* (1991) obtained lifetime psychiatric history information on 62 AN probands and their 169 first-degree relatives, and 62 control women and their 178 first-degree relatives. The overall case–control difference in risk, 2.4 per cent versus 0 per cent, respectively, was not statistically significant.

Stern *et al.* (1992) studied relatives of 34 anorexic probands and 34 control women, obtaining diagnostic information from only one parent of each proband. Although a history of AN was found only in relatives of probands (5.9 per cent), the case–control difference in risk for total eating disorder did not reach statistical significance. Since AN has a relatively low base rate in the general population the possibility that these negative findings might be accounted for by diminished statistical power or inadequate sensitivity of family diagnostic methods cannot be excluded.

On balance, evidence from family study data suggests an elevation in the lifetime prevalence of eating disorders amongst the relatives of probands with eating disorders. Moreover, suggestive evidence of the co-aggregation of AN and BN found in several studies raises the provocative possibility of shared etiologic factors underpinning these two conditions.

Twin studies

An obvious limitation of the family study is that genetic and environmental sources of variance in liability are perfectly confounded. By contrast, a comparison of concordance for illness in monozygotic (MZ) versus dizygotic (DZ) twin pairs allows for the parsing of variance in liability to illness into independent genetic and environmental sources and for estimation of the magnitude of their effects. Existing reports based on twin data are summarized in Table 8.2. In the first such study of AN, Holland *et al.* (1984) ascertained 16 MZ and 14 DZ twin pairs through referrals to eating disorder treatment programs, and voluntary referrals based on knowledge of the study. Zygosity was established by blood group in 15 of the 16 MZ pairs and 10 of the 14 DZ pairs. They found the concordance rate for AN to be 56 per cent for MZ twins compared to 7 per cent for DZ pairs, suggesting a very strong heritable component to the illness.

Two subsequent reports from this research team provided additional statistical analyses based on larger samples. The first (Holland *et al.*, 1988) reported on a total of 45 twin pairs, including 10 pairs who were part of the earlier study. Again, the ascertainment was unsystematic, with 27 pairs obtained through voluntary referrals and 18 through local hospital clinics. Of note, MZ twins and concordant pairs were overrepresented among volunteers. In these 45 pairs, concordance for AN was found to be 56 per cent in the MZ twin pairs compared to 5 per cent in the DZ twin pairs. In the second report (Treasure and Holland, 1989), analyses were based on 59 twin pairs, including an unspecified number of pairs included in the prior two analyses. The proband-wise concordance for restricting-type AN was substantially higher for MZ twins (66 per cent) than for DZ twins (0 per cent). In contrast, there was no evidence of differential concordance for MZ and DZ twin pairs for BN, where concordance rates were 35 per cent and 29 per cent, respectively.

Table 8.2 Twin studies

Study	Subjects (n)	Concordance rates (no. of concordant twin pairs)	Heritability estimate
Holland et al.	Anorexia nervosa (60)	56% MZ (9 of 16) 7% DZ (1 of 14)	.54*
Holland et al.	Anorexia nervosa (90)	56% MZ (14 of 25) 5% DZ (1 of 20)	.80
Treasure and Holland	Anorexia nervosa (62)	66% MZ (14 of 21) 0% DZ (0 of 10)	.70
	Bulimia nervosa (62)	35% MZ (5 of 14) 29% DZ (5 of 17)	.15
Fichter and Noegel	Bulimia nervosa (42)	83% MZ (5 of 6) 27% DZ (4 of 15)	not estimated
Hsu et al.	Bulimia nervosa (22)	33% MZ (2 of 6) 0% DZ (0 of 5)	not estimated
Kendler et al.	Epidemiological female twin sample (total n=2,163)		.55
	Narrowly defined bulimia nervosa (n=60)	Narrow definition: 23% MZ 9% DZ	
	Broadly defined bulimia nervosa (n=123)	Broad definition: 26% MZ 16% DZ	
Walters and Kendler	Epidemiological female twin sample (total n=2,163)		not estimated
	Narrowly defined anorexia nervosa (n=35)	Narrow definition: not reported	
	Broadly defined anorexia nervosa (n=80)	Broad definition: 10% MZ 22% DZ	

* Broad heritability estimate based on Smith (1974)

Two other small twin studies of BN report evidence of higher concordance for the illness in MZ than in DZ twin pairs; however, sample sizes are too small to be conclusive, and bias from nonsystematic recruitment is a potential confound. Fichter and Noegel (1990) obtained subjects from responses to a survey on BN, from patients in an eating disorders clinic, and from hospitalized patients at a university psychiatric facility. Zygosity was determined only by physical similarity and eating disorder diagnoses were based on responses to self-report questionnaires. Pair-wise concordance was found to be 83 per cent (5 of 6) in MZ twins and 27 per cent (4 of 15) in DZ twins. In a study of 11 twin pairs by Hsu *et al.* (1990), subjects were obtained from patients referred over a three-year period to a university eating disorders clinic. Zygosity was based only on physical similarity and diagnoses were made by direct interviews with the subjects. Two of the 6 (33 per cent) MZ pairs and 0 of the 5 (0 per cent) DZ pairs were concordant for bulimia nervosa.

In sum, while the pattern of differential concordance for AN and BN in twin studies to date suggests the preeminence of genetic factors in their etiopathogenesis, the reliance on physical similarity for determination of zygosity, and poor controls for participation, referral, and reporting biases constrains their interpretation and generalizability.

The Virginia Twin Registry (VTR) study of eating disorders

The VTR studies of heritability of eating disorders are of particular import-ance because of the attention given to the methodology of this project and the rigor and breadth of its quantitative analyses. A series of reports from the VTR pertaining to eating disorders have now been published, based on comprehensive behavioral, psychological, and psychiatric assessments obtained on 2,163 female twins ascertained through the population-based twin registry in the Commonwealth of Virginia. The first report (Kendler *et al.*, 1991) pertaining to genetic aspects and heritability of BN was based on personal, structured interviews conducted with 590 MZ and 440 DZ twin pairs, and 3 pairs of unknown zygosity. All assessments were reviewed blindly and zygosity determinations were based on a series of standard questions concerning similarity and frequency of confusion, shown to be >95 per cent accurate (Walters and Kendler, 1995), and by DNA analysis in cases of uncertain zygosity. The proband-wise concordance for narrowly defined BN (i.e. definite or probable case based on DSM-III-R criteria) was 22.9 per cent in MZ pairs compared to 8.7 per cent in DZ pairs, with the best fitting model attributing familial aggregation of BN solely to additive genetic factors with a heritability of liability of 55 per cent and remaining variance attributable to individual-specific environmental influences. Although the contribution of shared environment to liability to BN was found to be negligible, the power of the statistical analysis to categorically reject a role for family environ-mental factors in twin resemblance was only modest because of the relatively small number of affected twins in the sample. A later report focusing on AN (Walters and Kendler, 1995) found much lower concordance rates among MZ twins than previous studies by Holland and colleagues (Holland *et al.*, 1984, 1988; Treasure and Holland, 1989); however, the number of identified pairs in which one twin had AN was extremely small due to the epidemiological nature of the sample, thereby precluding calculation of traditional herit-ability estimates. On the other hand, the authors found that the risk for a co-twin having AN, given that her twin had the disorder, was between 5 and 50, depending upon the definition of AN used. Of further note, the authors found that the risk of BN was also elevated nearly threefold in the co-twin of a twin with AN, even after controlling for comorbidity with AN. This finding converges with previously discussed family study data in implicating common transmissible factors in liability to develop AN and BN, thereby suggesting that family-genetic factors may contribute jointly to the liability to develop AN or BN.

Several follow-up reports from the VTR have provided more detailed estimates of the contribution of genetic and environmental sources of variance to the liability to BN. First, Kendler *et al.* (Walters and Kendler, 1995) examined interrelationships among genetic and environmental risk factors for six major psychiatric disorders (major depression, panic, generalized anxiety, phobias, alcoholism, and BN) using multivariate twin modeling techniques. BN was found to share a genetic risk in common with panic and phobia, a finding consistent with high rates of comorbid anxiety in women with BN (Bulik *et al.*, 1997) and the phobic avoidance of even minor fluctuations in body weight in many of these patients. Using expanded data from a second, follow-up wave of interviews, Sullivan *et al.* (1998) attempted to dismantle the syndrome of BN into its key component behaviors by using univariate and bivariate twin modeling techniques to estimate the relative contributions of genetic and environmental factors to the lifetime history of binge eating and self-induced vomiting and to determine the extent of overlap of these risk factors. The prevalences in the sample for binge eating and vomiting were 24 per cent and 5 per cent, respectively, with a very strong, albeit expected, association between the two behaviors (odds ratio = 8.8). In the univariate model, heritability of binge eating was estimated at 49 per cent with the remaining variance attributed to individual-specific environmental factors; for lifetime history of vomiting, heritability was estimated at 70 per cent, with individual-specific environmental factors accounting for the remainder of variance. Importantly, the bivariate modeling suggested that additive genes contributing to binge eating and vomiting overlapped considerably, thus supporting, at least from a quantitative genetic vantage point, the bundling together of these behaviors in the diagnosis of BN.

A limitation of parameter estimates in twin studies is the unknown bias accounting for measurement error (i.e. a false positive diagnosis in the purportedly affected twin, or a false negative in the purportedly unaffected twin). Such error can account for underestimation of additive genetic effects and inflated estimates of individual-specific environmental effects in structural equation modeling of twin data. In addressing this problem, Bulik and colleagues (1998) obtained diagnostic information from MZ and DZ twins on two separate occasions separated by five years and included measurement error in the modeling of liability to BN. Doing so resulted in a substantial increase in the estimated heritability of latent vulnerability to 83 per cent.

Thus, it would appear, at least judging from the VTR data, that BN is a disorder with high heritability yet its lifetime diagnosis is beset by the problem of low reliability.

Supporting this conclusion is a recent study by Wade *et al.* (1998) which pooled data from three waves of measurement conducted on a large volunteer sample of twins from Australia. The modeling of latent liability to BN was based on self-report data obtained at the wave 1 interview, a clinical interview at wave 2, and a structured assessment of eating disorder symptoms at wave 3. The best fitting model was found to include additive genetic and individual-specific environmental factors with heritability estimated at 59 per cent. Further recent evidence of substantial additive genetic variance underlying binge eating and bulimic symptoms has been reported in population based twin registries studied in Norway by Reichborn-Kjennerud *et al.* (2004), and as part of the Virginia Twin Study of Adolescent Behavioral Development by Rowe *et al.* (2002).

Twin studies of quantitative traits associated with disordered eating

Several additional contributions have been made by investigators studying the heritability of quantitative traits possibly continuous with eating disorders. Rutherford *et al.* (1993) examined heritability of self-reported eating attitudes and behaviors in 147 MZ and 99 DZ female twin pairs. Heritability estimates were 41 per cent for the total score, 42 per cent for a factor analytically derived index of dieting behavior, 52 per cent for body dissatisfaction, and 44 per cent for drive for thinness. Shared environmental effects were not detected in any of the models, thus suggesting that environmental experiences shared by members of a family play little role in the transmissibility of these particular behavioral traits.

Wade *et al.* (1999) modeled genetic and environmental effects on interview-derived measures of dietary restriction, eating concern, and weight concern in an Australian sample of 325 female twins. For the first two measures, the best fitting model included additive genetic and individual-specific environment effects, with heritability estimates of 58 per cent and 50 per cent, respectively; by contrast, the best fitting model for weight concern included common and individual-specific environment. These differential patterns suggest that distinct causal mechanisms underpin these phenomena and that general weight dissatisfaction in particular may be impacted more strongly by shared cultural environmental experiences.

Finally, Klump *et al.* (2000) studied two twin cohorts, 680 11-year-olds, and 602 17-year-olds, and found greater heritability for abnormal eating attitudes and body dissatisfaction amongst the older twins, pointing up possibly important developmental or age effects on the structure of genetic and environmental sources of liability to eating disorders.

Molecular genetic studies

Several efforts have been made to identify the map position of individual genes conferring susceptibility to AN. To date, the focus has been on genes involved in serotonergic (5HT) neurotransmission. Collier *et al.* (1997) conducted an association study of 81 women with AN and 226 controls, finding a modest increase in the frequency of the $5HT_{2A}$–1438/A allele in AN compared to controls. These results have since been replicated by Sorbi *et al.* (1998), and by Enoch *et al.* (1998). Interestingly, in the Sorbi *et al.* study the increased frequency of this allelic variant was seen only in the subset of non-purging restricting anorexics, whereas in the Enoch *et al.* study this genotype was not found to discriminate BN patients from controls, yet was also more common amongst patients with obsessive compulsive disease.

Two studies have failed to replicate the $5HT_{2A}$ finding. Campbell *et al.* (1998) studied 157 anorexic patients and 150 controls, finding no association of this polymorphism with AN; however, stratification by the presence versus absence of purging was not performed and the frequency of the 1438A genotype in their controls was higher than in other reported control samples. Still, Hinney *et al.* (1998) studied 100 anorexics, with 100 underweight but non-anorexic controls, and 100 obese controls, and found no inter-group differences in the frequency of this genotype.

In the first comprehensive, large scale genetic study of eating disorders, Grice *et al.* (2000) conducted a genome wide allele sharing linkage analysis of 192 families with at least one affected relative pair with anorexia nervosa and related eating disorders ascertained as part of the multi-center Price Foundation Study of the Genetics of Eating Disorders (Kaye *et al.* 2000). Only modest evidence for linkage on chromosome 4 was determined. However, an analysis restricted exclusively to kindreds expressing the more clinically homogenous subgroup of anorexia nervosa without binge eating or purging behaviors produced a multipoint nonparametric linkage score of 3.03 on chromosome 1p, increasing to 3.45 when additional markers in the 1p33-36 linkage region were considered.

A linkage analysis conducted by the Price Foundation Investigators on 308 multiplex families recruited through a proband with bulimia nervosa (Bulik *et al.* 2003) yielded a genomewide significant lod score of 2.92 on chromosome 10p, increasing to 3.39 when the analysis was restricted to a subset of 133 families in which at least two affected relatives reported the symptom of self induced vomiting, an attribute of the bulimic syndrome previously noted (Sullivan *et al.* 1998) to have high heritability.

Several follow-up analyses have expanded upon these initial linkage reports, highlighting the importance of delimiting aspects of heterogeneity among families in the search for susceptibility loci. Given that a wide assortment of behavioral attributes characterize persons with eating disorders, Devlin *et al.* (2002) performed an affected sib pair linkage analysis on 196

Price Foundation kindreds identified through an anorexia nervosa proband incorporating behavioral covariates into the analysis. Two variables, drive for thinness and obsessionality, sorted the families into broad clusters, one in which each affected sibling displayed high and concordant values for these traits, and a second in which the siblings did not exhibit this covariation. The authors suggest that befitting the nature of complex phenotypes, multiple loci are bound to contribute in different ways to eating disorder liability, and to differences among affected individuals in traits associated with such liabilities. Complementing this effort is one further report that described a multilayer decision making process to identify behavioral phenotypes as quantitative traits or covariates in linkage analyses on the anorexia nervosa and bulimia nervosa cohorts (Bacanu et al. 2005; Bulik et al. 2005).

Two linkage analyses exploring specific candidate genes have also been reported by the Price Foundation Group. In the first, Bergen et al. (2003) using single nucleotide polymorphisms for two candidate genes in the 1p33-36 region, the serotonin 1D receptor, and the opioid delta receptor, increased this linkage signal in the restricting anorexia nervosa kindreds to 3.91. And second, Bergen et al. (2005) investigated the dopamine D2 receptor as a candidate susceptibility gene in anorexia nervosa using both a case:control and family transmission disequilibrium design. Significant evidence for the association of this gene to anorexia nervosa was found in case:control, linkage disequilibrium, and transmission distortion analyses.

Family studies of comorbidity

Both AN and BN are often accompanied by other psychiatric symptoms and disorders. While it is apparent that in some patients these comorbidities are merely consequences of malnutrition and pathologic eating behaviors, in others they antedate weight loss or disordered eating or persist after recovery of normal weight or abstinence from binge eating. Whether such symptoms enhance vulnerability to the development of eating disorders, and, if so, through what causal mechanisms, remains uncertain.

One potential strategy for investigating these questions is using the family study to investigate patterns of transmission of psychiatric disorders among first-degree relatives of probands in reference to the presence versus absence of these same conditions in probands. Doing so allows for the testing of different hypotheses regarding the nature of associations between these phenotypically different forms of psychopathology. As summarized by Klein and Riso (1993), covariation amongst phenotypically distinct disorders can arise from several different mechanisms: (a) if the disorders are manifestations of a shared underlying etiology; (b) if one disorder causes the second; (c) if a third independent factor confers risk to each disorder; or (d) if the two disorders stem from an admixture of shared and disorder-specific liabilities.

Depression

A substantial number of family studies have shown elevated lifetime rates of major mood disorders among relatives of individuals with eating disorders compared to relatives of controls (Lilenfeld *et al.*, 1998; Gershon *et al.*, 1983; Hudson *et al.*, 1987; Kassett *et al.*, 1989; Strober *et al.*, 1990; Logue *et al.*, 1989; Winokur *et al.*, 1980; Hudson *et al.*, 1983; Rivinus *et al.*, 1983; Bulik, 1987; Boumann and Yates, 1994). By contrast, two studies (Halmi *et al.*, 1991; Stern *et al.*, 1984) failed to detect familial aggregation of mood disorders among relatives of women with BN. Tables 8.3 and 8.4 give results from these studies.

It can be seen by reference to the estimate of relative risks that relatives of eating disorder probands have lifetime rates of affective illness that are some to 2 to 4.2 times greater than those in relatives of controls. The one noteworthy exception to these findings is the study by Hudson *et al.* (1983), in which a relative risk of over 25 was found for relatives of AN probands. This figure may be spuriously inflated by reliance on hospital chart records for the diagnosis of family members, which may have underestimated the true risk of affective illness among the relatives of psychiatric control probands.

Several studies have determined the effects of proband comorbidity on familial risk for mood disorders. A summary of these findings appears in Table 8.5. In reports by Lilenfeld *et al.* (1998), Strober *et al.* (1990), and Biederman *et al.* (1985), mood disorders were elevated only amongst relatives

Table 8.3 Controlled studies of lifetime risk of mood disorders among first-degree relatives of anorexia nervosa probands

| Study | Number of probands | Relatives interviewed | Diagnosis in relatives (%) | | | Relative risk[a] |
			Unipolar depression	Bipolar illness	Total	
Winokur *et al.*	25	Y	20.4	6.8	27.2	2.1
Gershon *et al.*	24	Y	13.3[b]	8.3[b]	21.6[b]	3.2
Hudson *et al.* (1983)	34	N	14.2	3.0	17.2	25.6[c]
Rivinus *et al.*	40	N	16.1[b]	0.0[b]	16.1[b]	3.4
Logue *et al.*	17	Y	14.7	–	14.7	2.9
Strober *et al.*	97	Y	7.2	1.6	8.8	2.1[d]
Halmi *et al.*	62	Y	6.5	0.6	7.1	1.4
Lilenfeld *et al.*	26	Y	15.1	1.1	16.2	2.2

Notes
[a] Rate of illness in relatives of anorexic probands divided by rate of illness in relatives of normal control subjects.
[b] With age correction
[c] Personality disorder and schizophrenic control subjects, screened for mood and eating disorders
[d] Mood disorder and other psychiatrically ill control subjects, screened for mood and eating disorders

Table 8.4 Controlled studies of lifetime risk of mood disorders among first-degree relatives of bulimia nervosa probands

Study	Number of probands	Relatives interviewed	Diagnosis in relatives (%)			Relative risk[a]
			Unipolar depression	Bipolar illness	Total	
Hudson et al. (1983)	55	N	15.1	1.2	16.3	23.3[b]
Stern et al. (1984)	27	Y (1 parent only)	–	–	9.0	0.9[c]
Hudson et al. (1987)	69	N	15.5	4.2	19.8	4.2[c]
Bulik (1987)	35	N	37.1	–	37.1	2.6
Logue et al.	13	Y	10.5	–	10.5	2.1
Kassett et al.	40	Y	22.0[d]	5.9	27.9[d]	3.2
Boumann and Yates	25	N (reports on parents only)	28.0	–	28.0	2.8
Lilenfeld et al.	47	Y	15.8	0.6	16.4	2.2

Notes
[a] Rate of illness in relatives of bulimic probands divided by rate of illness in relatives of normal control subjects
[b] Personality disorder and schizophrenic control subjects, screened for mood and eating disorders
[c] Unscreened community control subjects
[d] With age correction

of AN probands with concomitant mood disorder, a pattern consistent with independent transmission of liabilities to mood and eating disorder. In Lilenfeld *et al.* (1998), similar findings were obtained for families of BN probands. By contrast, two studies (Gershon *et al.*, 1983; Logue *et al.*, 1989) have reported similarly elevated rates of affective illness in relatives of eating disorder probands with or without affective illness, suggestive of shared liability between these conditions, whereas two others (Hudson *et al.*, 1987; Kassett *et al.*, 1989) failed to yield clear support for either hypothesis. On balance, the weight of evidence at present suggests that mood disorders and eating disorders frequently co-exist, but that this association is not accounted for by a shared family-transmitted liability.

Substance use disorders

It is particularly important to distinguish between AN and BN when studying the relationship between substance use disorders (SUD) and eating disorders, as alcohol and drug use disorders appear to be significantly more common in BN than in AN (Holderness *et al.*, 1994; Lilenfeld and Kaye, 1996).

Table 8.5 Risk of affective illness in first-degree relatives by affective status of probands

Study	Probands		Risk to relatives (%)		
	Affective status	n	Unipolar depression	Bipolar illness	Total
Gershon et al.	AN + MAD	13	13.4[a]	10.1[a]	23.5[a]
	AN – MAD	11	13.1[a]	5.3[a]	18.4[a]
Biederman et al.	AN + MAD	17	17.3	0.0	17.3
	AN – MAD	21	3.3	0.0	3.3
Hudson et al. (1987)	BN + MAD	46	–	–	36.2[a]
	BN – MAD	23	–	–	18.7[a]
Logue et al.	ED + MAD	10	13.0	–	13.0
	ED – MAD	20	12.0	–	12.0
Kassett et al.	BN + MAD	23	29.5[a]	5.3[a]	34.8[a]
	BN – MAD	17	12.5[a]	6.6[a]	19.1[a]
Strober et al.	AN + MAD	28	14.4	3.6	18.0
	AN – MAD	69	4.3	0.7	5.1
Lilenfeld et al.	AN + MDD	12	19.0	–	19.0
	AN – MDD	14	17.1	–	17.1
	BN + MDD	26	20.2	–	20.2
	BN – MDD	21	12.3	–	12.3

Notes
AN = anorexia nervosa; BN = bulimia nervosa; ED = eating disorder (anorexia nervosa and bulimia nervosa combined); MAD = major affective disorder; MDD = major depressive disorder
[a] With age correction

A number of family studies have shown elevated lifetime rates of SUD amongst relatives of individuals with BN compared to relatives of individuals with AN, or relatives of non-eating disordered controls (Holderness *et al.*, 1994). However, few studies have used the family study design to investigate whether patterns of illness in relatives and probands support the hypothesis of either a common transmitted liability underlying eating disorders and SUD, or the existence of independently transmitted risk factors. A summary of the controlled family studies of SUD in AN and BN probands is presented in Tables 8.6 and 8.7.

Bulik (1991) reported that bulimics with comorbid alcohol abuse or dependence were more likely to have one or more relatives with a history of drug or alcohol abuse or dependence compared to bulimics without lifetime alcohol use. Likewise, Mitchell *et al.* (1988) found that bulimic women with positive family histories of SUD were more likely than bulimic women without such histories to have experienced SUD themselves. In a study by Kaye and colleagues (1996), first-degree relatives of 47 women with DSM-III-R

Table 8.6 Controlled studies of lifetime risk of substance use disorders among first-degree relatives of anorexia nervosa probands

Study	Number of probands	Relatives interviewed	Diagnosis in relatives (%)					Relative risk[a]
			Alcohol abuse	Alcohol dependence	Drug abuse	Drug dependence	Total	
Rivinus et al.	40	N	–	–	–	–	11.9[b]	1.7
Logue et al.	17	Y	–	17.0[c]	4.0	–	21.0	0.8
Halmi et al.	62	Y (parents only)	–	5.3[c]	–	1.2[d]	6.5	3.8
Stern et al. (1992)	34	Y (1 parent only)	–	3.0[c]	–	3.0[d]	5.0	0.6
Lilenfeld et al.	26	Y	7.5	12.9	4.3	4.3	23.7	0.8

Notes
[a] Rate of illness in relatives of anorexic probands divided by rate of illness in relatives of normal control subjects
[b] With age correction
[c] Alcohol abuse and/or dependence
[d] Drug abuse and/or dependence

Table 8.7 Controlled studies of lifetime risk of substance use disorders among first-degree relatives of bulimia nervosa probands

Study	Number of probands	Relatives interviewed	Diagnosis in relatives (%)					Relative risk[a]
			Alcohol abuse	Alcohol dependence	Drug abuse	Drug dependence	Total	
Stern et al. (1984)	27	Y (1 parent only)	–	–	–	–	8.2	1.3
Hudson et al. (1983)	69	N	–	16.1[bc]	–	4.0[bd]	19.1[b]	2.1
Bulik (1987)	35	N	–	48.6[c]	–	22.9[d]	–	2.4[c]; 1.3[d]
Logue et al.	13	Y	–	21.0[c]	2.0	–	23.0	0.9
Kassett et al.	40	Y	–	27.6[c]	11.9	–	39.5	2.0
Keck et al.	66	N	–	8.6[bc]	–	3.4[bd]	12.0[b]	1.8
Boumann and Yates	25	N (reports on parents only)	–	10.0[c]	–	–	10.0	2.5
Lilenfeld et al.	47	Y	10.7	19.2	9.6	7.9	36.7	1.2

Notes
[a] Rate of illness in relatives of bulimic probands divided by rate of illness in relatives of normal control subjects
[b] With age correction
[c] Alcohol abuse and/or dependence
[d] Drug abuse and/or dependence

bulimia nervosa, stratified by the presence versus absence of lifetime history of SUD, and 44 non-eating disordered control women, were assessed for lifetime SUD. Rates of SUD were elevated only in first-degree relatives of BN probands with comorbid SUD. Similar findings of a lack of common familial transmission between BN and SUD were obtained from a large study of alcohol-dependent probands and their relatives by Schuckit *et al.* (1996). Structured interviews were conducted with 2,283 women and 1,982 men participating in the Collaborative Study on the Genetics of Alcoholism. Lifetime rates of AN and BN were compared in alcohol-dependent probands and their relatives, and control probands and their relatives. Eating disorders were not found to aggregate in relatives of alcoholic probands. The authors concluded that any relationship that might exist between eating disorders and alcohol dependence is not likely to be due to a strong genetic link between the two disorders.

These family study findings converge with multivariate genetic modeling of the large population-based twin study database from the VTR. Investigating the genotypic structure of six major psychiatric disorders, Kendler and colleagues (1991) demonstrated that genes influencing liability to BN were separate from those underlying alcoholism.

Anxiety disorders

Little data presently exists regarding the rate or patterns of transmission of anxiety disorders in families of probands with eating disorders, despite the fact that anxiety disorders are quite common comorbidities in AN and BN probands themselves. The one exception is obsessive-compulsive disorder (OCD), in which three family studies (Lilenfeld *et al.*, 1998; Halmi *et al.*, 1991; Pasquale *et al.*, 1994) reported elevated rates of OCD among the relatives of probands with eating disorders. Halmi *et al.* (1991) reported a rate of OCD of 11 per cent in mothers of probands with AN, compared to 2 per cent in mothers of control women. Pasquale *et al.* (1994) assessed lifetime rates of OCD among the first-degree relatives of three proband groups: OCD, eating disorders, and mood disorder. First-degree relatives of probands with AN had a threefold elevation in lifetime risk for OCD. Similarly, Lilenfeld and colleagues (1998) found a fourfold increased risk for OCD in relatives of AN probands and a threefold elevation in relatives of BN probands compared to relatives of non-eating disordered control women. However, OCD aggregated only in relatives of eating disorder probands with comorbid OCD, thus arguing against a shared genetic liability. Thus, although OCD and eating disorders frequently co-occur within individuals and within families, the results of this study argue against the existence of a single shared etiologic factor. Other anxiety disorders with increased rates of occurrence in relatives of AN and BN probands compared to relatives of normal controls reported by Lilenfeld *et al.* (1998) were generalized anxiety, panic, and, in relatives of AN probands only, social phobia. Due to limitations of the sample size in this study, analysis of familial transmission controlling for proband comorbidity was not feasible. Thus, the question of whether or not eating disorders and these particular forms of anxiety disorder share transmissible risk factors remains unexplored.

Personality disorders

Little data exists regarding the rates and patterns of transmission of personality disorders in families of probands with eating disorders, despite the fact that certain traits or temperaments are common among individuals with eating disorders: in particular, obsessionality in restricting anorexia nervosa, and impulsivity, rejection sensitivity, and mood lability in bulimia nervosa (Sohlberg and Strober, 1994; Vitousek and Manke, 1994). To our knowledge, only two studies have assessed personality disorders among the family members of individuals with eating disorders.

Carney *et al.* (1990) assessed personality disorders among women with BN, normal controls, and first-degree relatives of both groups using a personality disorder questionnaire. Few differences of note were found among the first-degree relatives of these groups. In contrast, Lilenfeld *et al.* (1998) found elevated lifetime rates of obsessive-compulsive personality disorder amongst the relatives of AN probands compared to relatives of BN probands and relatives of normal controls, whether or not this personality disorder was present or absent in the proband herself. One interpretation of this pattern is that obsessional traits may constitute a familially determined vulnerability factor for restricting-type AN, and that obsessive-compulsive personality disorder and restricting-type AN may represent a continuum of phenotypic expressions of a similar genotype.

Conclusion

An increasing body of evidence supports the notion that AN and BN have a strong familial component, and that this liability is independent from those contributing to other transmissible psychiatric disorders often associated comorbidly with eating disorders. Twin data add further credence to evidence of familiality and heritability, suggesting, as well, that additive genetic effects on eating attitudes may strengthen from childhood to mid-adolescence. Moreover, both family and twin data suggest at least a moderate familial-genetic correlation between AN and BN, in keeping with the common presence of weight phobia in both disorders and the not infrequent development of binge eating during the natural course of AN.

That available twin study data have failed to identify common environment – those events to which family members are exposed equally – as a robust influence of liability to either BN or AN is of particular theoretical significance. There are several plausible explanations. First, environmental experiences that are shared in common by members of a family may have little bearing on risk to eating disorders. Second, the statistical power of twin data to detect such effects in the presence of genetic influences may be inadequate. Third, if familial factors exert effects in concert with an individual's genetic propensities, main effects of familial environment will be weak but effects operating in gene–environment interaction might be considerable. Finally, the effects of shared environment may be more robust at earlier ages but decrease in magnitude with aging.

An obvious critical question that ensues from these findings is the nature of a purported inherited diathesis, as it is improbable that specific genes exist that code for body weight phobia or dietary restraint. Indeed, critical to future studies of etiology will be efforts at defining the risk spectrum phenotype and identifying those specific components that are most heritable and, through covariation with symptoms of the disorder, candidates for mediation of genetic risk. Incorporating a focus on certain quantitative temperamental or personality traits in future genetic studies of eating disorders may be of great promise in this regard. For example, restricting-type AN in particular is characterized by a remarkably consistent cluster of heritable behavioral traits, including emotional restraint, avoidance of novelty, anxious worry and self-doubt, compliancy, perfectionism, and perseverance in the face of nonreward (Strober 1995). In this regard, the current focus on candidate genes regulating serotonergic neurotransmission as a risk factor for AN derives intuitively and empirically on the one hand from preclinical data linking serotonergic neurotransmission to restraint of reward motivation for exploring novel environments, inhibitory modulation of feeding and sexual behavior, and enhanced sensitivity of neurobehavioral systems to stimulus events (Kaye *et al.*, 1993), and on the other from evidence adduced from clinical studies (Kaye *et al.*, 1991) of impaired regulation of serotonergic activity in AN patients well after restoration to normal weight levels. Thus, a convergence of preclinical and clinical data implicates abnormalities of serotonergically mediated brain and behavioral systems in the pathogenesis of AN by conferring extreme propensities toward behavioral rigidity, obsessiveness, perfectionism, and constraint.

Although the presentation of BN is less stereotypic than that of restricting-type AN, a role for heritable personality and behavioral traits as indices of a biologically mediated etiologic mechanism in the development of this disorder is also heuristically and theoretically defensible. In contrast to AN, women with BN more often display traits of thrill seeking and excitability, and are more dysphoric in response to rejection or nonreward (Strober, 1995). These features may militate against sustained dietary restriction, thereby predisposing to periodic lapses in control and eventual dietary chaos under setting conditions of stress or threats to self-esteem. In this same vein, possible heritable variations in the sensitivity of brain emotional systems to the reward properties of feeding behavior may constitute a diathesis for the development and reinforcement of dysregulated appetitive behavior at times of emotional despair or life stress. These models of 'genetic' risk are easily reconciled with prevailing psychological theories of BN which view binge eating as a compensatory modulation of dysphoric states linked to deeply entrenched negative self schemas.

In closing, we believe that the search for susceptibility genes in eating disorders is an exciting and valid research agenda. It may well hold forth the promise of bringing resolution to the continuing uncertainty over whether AN and BN are truly separate entities, or have risk and vulnerability factors in common. Given the body of research reviewed in this chapter, future empirical investigation bridging the behavioral and biological sciences and exploiting the rapidly advancing science of molecular and family-genetic epidemiology may yield keys to refining our knowledge of the etiology, nosology, and therapeutics of the eating disorders.

References

Bacanu, S.-A., Bulik, C. M., Klump, K., Fichter, M., Halmi, K. A., Keel, P., Kaplan, A. S., Mitchell, J. E., Rotondo, A., Strober, M., Treasure, J., Woodside, V. A., Xie, W., Bergen, A., Berrettini, W. H., Kaye, W. H., Devlin, B. (2005). Linkage analysis of anorexia and bulimia nervosa cohorts using selected behavioral phenotypes as quantitative traits or covariates. *American Journal of Medical Genetics (Neuropsychiatric Genetics)* 139B, 61–68.

Bergen, A. W., van den Bree, M. B., Yeager, M., Welch, R., Ganjei, J. K., Haque, K., Bacanu, S.-A., Berrettini, W. H., Grice, D. E., Goldman, D., Bulik, C. M., Klump, K., Fichter, M., Halmi, K. A., Kaplan, A. S., Strober, M., Treasure, J., Woodside, D. Blake, Kaye, W. H. (2003). Candidate genes for anorexia nervosa in the 1p33-36 linkage region: serotonin 1D and delta opioid receptor loci exhibit significant association to anorexia nervosa. *Molecular Psychiatry*, 8, 397–406.

Bergen, A. W., Yeager, M., Welch, R., Haque, K., Ganjei, J. K., van den Bree, M. B., Mazzanti, C., Nardi, I., Fichter, M., Halmi, K. A., Kaplan, A. S., Strober, M., Treasure, J., Woodside, D. Blake, Bulik, C. M., Bacanu, S.-A., Devlin, B., Berrettini, W. H., Goldman, D. and Kaye, W. H. (2005). Association of multiple DRD2 polymorphisms with anorexia nervosa. *Neuropsychopharmacology*, 30, 1703–1710.

Biederman, J., Rivinus, T., Kemper, K., Hamilton, D., MacFadyen, J., and Harmatz, J. (1985) Depressive disorders in relatives of anorexia nervosa patients with and without a current episode of nonbipolar major depression. *American Journal of Psychiatry*, 142, 1495–1496.

Boumann, C. E. and Yates, W. R. (1994) Risk factors for bulimia nervosa: a controlled study of parental psychiatric illness and divorce. *Addictive Behaviors*, 19, 667–675.

Bulik, C. M. (1987) Drug and alcohol abuse by bulimic women and their families. *American Journal of Psychiatry*, 144, 1604–1606.

Bulik, C. (1991) Family histories of bulimic women with and without comorbid alcohol abuse or dependence. *American Journal of Psychiatry*, 148, 1267–1268.

Bulik, C., Sullivan, P., Feat, J., and Joyce, P. (1997) Eating disorders and antecedent anxiety disorders. *Acta Psychiatrica Scandinavica*, 96, 101–107.

Bulik, C. M., Sullivan, P. F., and Kendler, K. S. (1998) Heritability of binge eating and broadly defined bulimia nervosa. *Biological Psychiatry*, 44, 1210–1218.

Bulik, C. M., Bacanu, S.-A., Klump, K., Fichter, M., Halmi, K. A., Keel, P., Kaplan, A. S., Mitchell, J. E., Rotondo, A., Strober, M., Treasure, J., Woodside, V. A., Xie, W., Bergen, A., Berrettini, W. H., Kaye, W. H. and Devlin, B. (2005). Selection of behavioral phenotypes for linkage analysis. *American Journal of Medical Genetics (Neuropsychiatric Genetics)* 139B, 81–87.

Bulik, C. M., Devlin, B., Bacanu, S.-A., Thornton, L., Klump, K., Fichter, M., Halmi, K. A., Kaplan, A. S., Strober, M., Woodside, D. Blake, Bergen, A., Ganjei, J. K., Crow, S., Mitchell, J. E., Rotondo, A., Mauri, M., Cassano, G., Keel, P., Berrettini, W. H., and Kaye, W. H. (2003). Significant linkage on chromosome 10p in families with bulimia nervosa. *American Journal of Human Genetics*, 72, 200–207.

Campbell, D. A., Sundaramurthy, D., Markham, A. F., and Pieri, L. F. (1998) Lack of association between 5-HT2A gene promoter polymorphism and susceptibility to anorexia nervosa. *Lancet*, 351, 499.

Carney, C. P., Yates, W. R., and Cizaldo, B. (1990) A controlled family study of personality in normal-weight bulimia nervosa. *International Journal of Eating Disorders*, 9, 659–665.

Collier, D. A., Arranz, M. J., Li, T., Mupita, D., Brown, N., and Treasure, J. (1997) Association between 5-HT2A gene promoter polymorphism and anorexia nervosa. *Lancet*, 350, 412.

Devlin, B., Bacanu, S.-A, Klump, K., Bulik, C. M., Fichter, M., Halmi, K. A., Kaplan, A. S., Strober, M., Treasure, J., Woodside, D. Blake, Berrettini, W. H., Kaye, W. H. (2002). Linkage analysis of anorexia nervosa incorporating behavioral covariates. *Human Molecular Genetics*, 11, 689–696.

Enoch, M. A., Kaye, W. H., Rotondo, A., Greenberg, B. D., Murphy, D. L., and Goldman, D. (1998) 5-HT2A promoter polymorphism-1438G/A, anorexia nervosa, and obsessive-compulsive disorder. *Lancet*, 351, 1785–1786.

Fichter, M. M. and Noegel, R. (1990) Concordance for bulimia nervosa in twins. *International Journal of Eating Disorders*, 9, 255–263.

Gershon, E. S., Schreiber, J. L., Hamovit, J. R., Dibble, E. D., Kaye, W. H., Nurnberger, J. I., Jr., Andersen, A., and Ebert, M. (1983) Anorexia nervosa and major affective disorders associated in families: a preliminary report. In *Childhood Psychopathology and Development* (ed. S. B. Guze, F. G. Earls, and J. E. Barrett). New York: Raven Press, pp. 279–284.

Grice, D. E., Halmi, K. A., Fichter, M., Strober, M., Woodside, D. Blake, Treasure, J., Kaplan, A. S., Magistretti, P. J., Goldman, D., Bulik, C. M., Kaye, W. H., and Berrettini, W. H. (2002). Evidence for a susceptibility gene for anorexia nervosa on chromosome 1. *American Journal of Human Genetics*, 70, 787–792.

Halmi, K. A., Eckert, E., Marchi, P., Sampugnaro, V., Apple, R., and Cohen, R. (1991) Comorbidity of psychiatric diagnoses in anorexia nervosa. *Archives of General Psychiatry*, 48, 712–718.

Hinney, A., Ziegler, A., Nothen, M., Remschmidt, H., and Hebebrand, J. (1998) 5-HT2A receptor gene polymorphisms, anorexia nervosa, and obesity. *Lancet*, 350, 1724–1725.

Holderness, C. C., Brooks-Gunn, J., and Warren, W. P. (1994) Co-morbidity of eating disorders and substance abuse: review of the literature. *International Journal of Eating Disorders*, 16, 1–34.

Holland, A. J., Hall, A., Murray, R., Russell, G. F. M., and Crisp, A. H. (1984) Anorexia nervosa: a study of 34 twin pairs. *British Journal of Psychiatry*, 145, 414–419.

Holland, A. J., Sicotte, N., and Treasure, J. (1988) Anorexia nervosa: evidence for a genetic basis. *Journal of Psychosomatic Research*, 32, 561–571.

Hsu, L. K. G., Chesler, B. E., and Santhouse, R. (1990) Bulimia nervosa in eleven sets of twins: a clinical report. *International Journal of Eating Disorders*, 9, 275–282.

Hudson, J. I., Pope, H. G., Jonas, J. M., and Yurgelun-Todd, D. (1983) A family history study of anorexia nervosa and bulimia. *British Journal of Psychiatry*, 142, 133–138.

Hudson, J. I., Pope, H. G., Jonas, J. M., Yurgelun-Todd, D., and Frankenburg, F. R. (1987) A controlled family history study of bulimia. *Psychological Medicine*, 17, 883–890.

Kassett, J. A., Gershon, E. S., Maxwell, E. M., Guroff, J. J., Kazuba, D. M., Smith, A. L., Brandt, H. A., and Jimerson, D. C. (1989) Psychiatric disorders in the first-degree relatives of probands with bulimia nervosa. *American Journal of Psychiatry*, 146, 1468–1471.

Kaye, W. H., Gwirtsman, H. E., George, D. T., and Ebert, M. H. (1991) Altered serotonin activity in anorexia nervosa after long-term weight restoration. *Archives of General Psychiatry*, 48, 556–562.

Kaye, W. H., Weltzin, T., and Hsu, L. K. G. (1993) Relationship between anorexia nervosa and obsessive and compulsive behaviors. *Psychiatric Annals*, 23, 365–373.

Kaye, W. H., Lilenfeld, L. R., Plotnicov, K., Merikangas, K. R., Nagy, L., Strober, M., Bulik, C. M., Moss, H., and Greeno, C. G. (1996) Bulimia nervosa and substance dependence: association and family transmission. *Alcoholism: Clinical and Experimental Research*, 20, 878–881.

Kaye, W. H., Lilenfeld, L. R., Berrettini, W. H., Strober, M., Devlin, B., Klump, K., Goldman, D., Bulik, C. M., Halmi, K. A., Fichter, M., Kaplan, A. S., Woodside, D. Blake, Treasure, J., Plotnicov, K. H., Pollice, C., and McConaha, C. (2000). A search for susceptibility loci for anorexia nervosa: Methods and sample description. *Biological Psychiatry*, 47, 794–803.

Keck, P. E., Pope, H. G., Jr., Hudson, J. I., McElroy, S. L., Yurgelun-Todd, D., and Hundert, E. M. (1990) A controlled study of phenomenology and family history in outpatients with bulimia nervosa. *Comprehensive Psychiatry*, 31, 277–283.

Kendler, K. S., MacLean, C., Neale, M., Kessler, R., Heath, A., and Eaves, L. (1991) The genetic epidemiology of bulimia nervosa. *American Journal of Psychiatry*, 148, 1627–1637.

Kendler, K. S., Walters, E. E., Neale, M. C., Kessler, R., Heath, A., and Eaves, L. (1995) The structure of the genetic and environmental risk factors for six major psychiatric disorders in women. *Archives of General Psychiatry*, 52, 374–383.

Klein, D. N. and Riso, L. P. (1993) Psychiatric disorders: problems of boundaries and comorbidity. In *Basic Issues in Psychopathology* (ed. C. C. Costello). New York: Guilford Press, pp. 19–66.

Klump, K., McGue, M., and Iacono, W. (2000) Age differences in genetic and environmental influences on eating attitudes and behaviors in adolescent female twins. *Journal of Abnormal Psychology*, 109, 239–251.

Lilenfeld, L. R. and Kaye, W. H. (1996) The link between alcoholism and eating disorders. *Alcohol Health and Research World*, 20, 94–99.

Lilenfeld, L. R., Kaye, W. H., Greeno, C. G., Merikangas, K. R., Plotnicov, K., Pollice, C., Rao, R., Strober, M., Bulik, C. M., and Nagy, L. (1998) A controlled family study of anorexia nervosa and bulimia nervosa: psychiatric disorders in first-degree relatives and effects of proband comorbidity. *Archives of General Psychiatry*, 55, 603–610.

Logue, C. M., Crowe, R. R., and Bean, J. A. (1989) A family study of anorexia nervosa and bulimia. *British Journal of Psychiatry*, 30, 179–188.

Mitchell, J., Hatsukami, D., Pyle, R. L., and Eckert, E. D. (1988) Bulimia with and without a family history of drug abuse. *Addictive Behaviors*, 13, 245–251.

Pasquale, L., Sciuto, G., Cocchi, S., Ronshi, P., and Billodi, L. (1994) A family study of obsessive compulsive, eating, and mood disorders. *European Psychiatry*, 9, 33–38.

Reichborn-Kjennerud, T., Bulik, C. M., Tambs, K., and Harris, J. R. (2004). Genetic and environmental influences on binge eating in the absence of compensatory behaviors: A population-based twin study. *International Journal of Eating Disorders*, 36, 307–314.

Rivinus, T. M., Beiderman, J., Herzog, D. B., Kemper, K., Harper, G. P., Harmatz, J. S., and Houseworth, S. (1984) Anorexia nervosa and affective disorders: a controlled family history study. *American Journal of Psychiatry*, 141, 1414–1418.

Rowe, R., Pickles, A., Siminoff, E., Bulik, C. M., and Silberg, J. L. (2002). Bulimic symptoms in the Virginia Twin Study of Adolescent Behavioral Development: Correlates, comorbidity, and genetics. *Biological Psychiatry*, 51, 172–182.

Rutherford, J., McGuffin, P., Katz, R., and Murray, R. (1993) Genetic influences on eating attitudes in a normal female twin population. *Psychological Medicine*, 23, 425–436.

Schuckit, M. A., Tipp, J. E., Anthenelli, R. M., Bucholz, K. K., Hesselbrock, V. M., and Nurnberger, J. I., Jr. (1996) Anorexia nervosa and bulimia nervosa in alcohol-dependent men and women and their relatives. *American Journal of Psychiatry*, 153, 74–82.

Smith, C. (1974) Concordance in twins – methods and interpretation. *American Journal of Human Genetics*, 26, 4, 454–466.

Sohlberg, S. and Strober, M. (1994) Personality in anorexia nervosa: an update and theoretical integration. *Acta Psychiatrica Scandinavica*, 89, 1–15.

Sorbi, S., Nacmias, B., Tedde, A., Ricca, V., Mezzani, B., and Rotella, C. (1998) 5-HT2A promoter polymorphism in anorexia nervosa. *Lancet*, 351, 1785.

Stern, S. L., Dixon, K. N., Nemzer, E., Lake, M. D., Sansone, R. A. (1984) Affective disorder in the families of women with normal weight bulimia. *American Journal of Psychiatry*, 141, 1224–1227.

Stern, S. L., Dixon, K. N., Sansone, R. A., Lake, M. D., Nemzer, E., and Jones, D. (1992) Psychoactive substance use disorder in relatives of patients with anorexia nervosa. *Comprehensive Psychiatry*, 33, 207–212.

Strober, M. (1995) Family-genetic perspectives on anorexia nervosa and bulimia nervosa. In *Eating Disorders and Obesity* (ed. K. D. Brownell and C. G. Fairburn). New York: Guilford Press, pp. 212–218.

Strober, M., Lampert, C., Morrell, W., Burroughs, J., and Jacobs, C. (1990) A controlled family study of anorexia nervosa: evidence of familial aggregation and lack of shared transmission with affective disorders. *International Journal of Eating Disorders*, 9, 239–253.

Strober, M., Freeman, R., Lampert, C., Diamond, and Kaye, W. H. (2000). Controlled family study of anorexia nervosa: Evidence of shared liability and transmission of partial syndromes. *American Journal of Psychiatry*, 157, 393–401.

Sullivan, P., Bulik, C., and Kendler, K. S. (1998) The genetic epidemiology of bingeing and vomiting. *British Journal of Psychiatry*, 173, 75–79.

Treasure, J. and Holland, A. J. (1989) Genetic vulnerability to eating disorders: evidence from twin and family studies. In *Child and Youth Psychiatry: European Perspectives* (ed. H. Remschmidt and M. H. Schmidt). New York: Hogrefe and Huber, pp. 59–68.

Vitousek, K. and Manke, F. (1994) Personality variables and disorders in anorexia nervosa and bulimia nervosa. *Journal of Abnormal Psychology*, 1, 137–147.

Wade, T., Martin, N., and Tiggemann, M. (1998) Genetic and environmental risk factors for the weight and shape concerns characteristic of bulimia nervosa. *Psychological Medicine*, 28, 761–771.

Wade, T., Martin, N., Neale, M., Tiggemann, M., Trealor, S., Heath, A., Bucholz, K., and Madden, P. (1999) The structure of genetic and environmental risk factors for three measures of disordered eating characteristic of bulimia nervosa. *Psychological Medicine*, 29, 925–934.

Walters, E. E. and Kendler, K. S. (1995) Anorexia nervosa and anorexic-like syndromes in a population-based twin sample. *American Journal of Psychiatry*, 152, 64–71.

Winokur, A., March, V., and Mendels, J. (1980) Primary affective disorder in relatives of patients with anorexia nervosa. *American Journal of Psychiatry*, 137, 695–698.

Chapter 9

Management of early onset anorexia nervosa

Bryan Lask and Rachel Bryant-Waugh

Introduction

Early onset anorexia nervosa is a serious disorder with a high rate of continuing morbidity after treatment and in the longer term a significant mortality (Steinhausen, 2002). With such a potentially poor prognosis an intensive and comprehensive treatment programme is indicated. The NICE (National Institute for Clinical Excellence) guidelines for the treatment of eating disorders contain recommendations based on a rigorous and comprehensive review of research evidence and expert consensus, including recommendations specific to children and adolescents (NICE, 2004). The guidelines are intended to provide 'systematically developed statements that assist clinicians and patients in making decisions about appropriate treatment' (p. 8). Some of the key NICE recommendations regarding the management of children with anorexia nervosa are summarised in Table 9.1, although clinicians working with such patients have a responsibility to refer to the original document. The current chapter aims to describe in more detail an approach to the management of anorexia nervosa, which should preferably be initiated early, before the illness is consolidated. We recommend, consistent with NICE guidance, that such a programme should include:

1 Provision of information and education
2 Ensuring that the adults (parents and care-givers) rather than the child are in charge
3 A decision about in-patient care
4 Calculation of a target weight range
5 Weight restoration
6 Medication where indicated
7 The use of family therapy and/or parental counselling
8 The use of motivational techniques and individual therapy (in some instances)
9 Group therapy (in some instances)
10 Attention to schooling issues

Table 9.1 Main recommendations in the NICE guidelines regarding the management of children and adolescents with anorexia nervosa

- Treatment should normally involve family members (including siblings) and the effects of AN on other family members should be recognised.
- Patients should be offered family interventions that directly address the eating disorder.
- Parents/carers should be included in dietary education or meal planning.
- Patients should also be offered individual appointments separate from those with their family members or carers, and their right to confidentiality should be respected.
- The need for in-patient treatment and the need for urgent weight restoration should be balanced alongside educational and social needs.
- In-patient treatment should be provided within reasonable travelling distance to enable the involvement of the family, to maintain social links and to facilitate continuity of care.
- Admission should be to age-appropriate facilities, able to provide appropriate educational and related activities.
- Feeding against the will of the patient should only be done in the context of the Mental Health Act 1983 or the Children Act 1989.
- When a young person refuses treatment considered essential, consider using the Mental Health Act 1983 or the right of those with parental responsibility to override the young person's refusal.
- Following weight restoration, ensure that children and adolescents have the increased energy and necessary nutrients available in their diet to support continued growth and development.
- Oestrogen administration should not be used to treat bone density problems due to risk of premature fusion of the epiphyses.

The emphasis needs to be on integrating these aspects of treatment into a comprehensive approach rather than using them as possible alternatives (Lask, in Lask and Bryant-Waugh, 2000, pp. 167–186).

Information and education

It is important to make a clear statement to the parents about the diagnosis, its implications, course and prognosis. We find it better to do this before discussing treatment since such discussion often leads to debate within the family, which can prevent the parents from learning about the illness. We find it helpful to use an almost ritualistic method of conveying the seriousness of the situation, which includes a statement along the following lines:

As you probably realise, your daughter has anorexia nervosa. This is uncommon in children but by no means unknown, and we have now seen large numbers of such children. It is a serious illness which can be difficult to overcome. Indeed, less than one-half make a full recovery. It can impair growth and the onset of puberty, may ultimately have adverse effects on fertility and can lead to osteoporosis. Some children become desperately ill, and a few die. If your child is to recover, she will need you to take full control of her health care which includes eating. The children who are most likely to recover fully are those whose parents are able to work together to ensure their child's health. I should warn you that it is going to be a long, hard struggle, and that even if she appears to be eating well, she may actually not gain weight. People with anorexia nervosa are so desperate to avoid gaining weight that they often resort to a wide range of other means to try to prevent this.

At this point, it is best to encourage questions and discussion and refer to appropriate sources of useful, factual information before moving on to tackling issues of control.

Adults in charge

One of the central themes in anorexia nervosa, and no less so in pre-pubertal anorexia nervosa, is control. The child frequently feels controlled by others and lacking control in her own life. Two areas in which she feels she can have control are her food intake and her weight. In consequence she often reactively over-controls her food intake, with the subsequent sense of achievement, mastery and well-being rapidly becoming positive reinforcers. In principle it is perfectly reasonable for a child to have some control over her life, but unfortunately in anorexia nervosa this takes on pathological and life-threatening proportions.

For this reason, it is essential that the adults responsible for the child take charge of her eating in the early stages of treatment. Very often parents either collude with the child or completely relinquish control. Many parents find their child's distress around eating too difficult to bear and so continue to allow minimal amounts to be eaten. Sometimes parents may have eating and weight concerns of their own. The child's ill-health can exacerbate the parents' tendency not to be firm with regard to eating or other aspects of health care.

From the first moment of contact the clinician needs to establish that adults are in charge. Clear statements to this effect should be made to the parents thus encouraging and empowering them to take control. By now the child has usually challenged the professional's authority and either manages to create anxiety in her parents as to whether they are really doing the right thing, or states that she will not do whatever it is that is being suggested. Both may involve dissolving into (often angry) tears. At this point it is necessary to demonstrate to the parents the 'battle for control' and help them recognise the necessity for them to win. This does not mean that they must or even should take control of all aspects of their child's life, but specifically those concerning health and safety. This conflict may be expressed over a number of related issues, such as food intake, frequency of weighing, or the need for hospitalisation. It is wise to advise parents that the child should be allowed control in other areas less important than health.

Related issues include the frequent tendency for the parents to be in conflict, with each taking an opposing view of how to handle the problem. Usually one feels unsupported by the other or that the other is handling the situation badly. Commonly, the child sides with one parent against the other, the latter feeling undermined, helpless and resentful.

Having made a clear statement about the need for adults to be in charge, the clinician can at this stage point out how the parents cannot be in charge so long as they disagree on management. They are then helped to reach an agreement on such vital issues as whether or not they wish to accept treatment, where this should be and whether this should be on an in-patient or out-patient basis. It is important here that the clinician does not take sides, but rather offers advice and helps the parents to reach an agreement. Throughout this process the child is likely to interrupt either by word or deed, and the parents are encouraged to ignore or disallow the interruptions, to show that they are in charge, and that at this stage they are making decisions as parents in the best interests of their child.

Having set the tone, the clinician continues to support the parents in working together and regaining control. The child's protestations may make this process difficult, and every effort should be made to show her that her problems are recognized, but will not be allowed to dominate or take over. It may be useful to say something along these lines:

> I can see that you are angry/upset about things just now, and that you probably think everyone is making a ridiculous fuss. On the other hand I guess you are also a bit frightened, and wondering whether everything has got out of control. I am going to help your parents to get you better. We won't let you get any more ill, or let you die, and nor will we let you get overweight, which might be another fear you have. Do you want to ask me any questions about what I have just said?

Often at this point the child tearfully or angrily denies that she has any problems and turns to her parents for support. It is useful then to remind the parents of the appropriateness of their concerns and of the necessity to work together and to regain control. We have found the concept of 'externalisation' particularly helpful. This involves referring to the illness as separate from the child. We refer to it by name, e.g. the anorexia, describe its motivation to control the child and threaten her health, its determination to succeed and its deviousness – speaking through the child, denying its own existence – and its secretiveness. Parents seem to find this helpful as it does make sense of their child's behaviour and distinguishes between their previously healthy child and the child consumed by the illness. They appear to be empowered by the concept of us all joining together to help their daughter fight the illness.

Parents also value written information (e.g. Bryant-Waugh and Lask, 2004) to guide them through the trauma of realising their child has anorexia nervosa and then through the dramatic course of the illness.

In-patient or out-patient treatment

A number of factors will determine whether or not a child should be admitted to hospital, including the child's physical and mental state, bed availability and the parents' wishes. As a general rule we recommend admission be given serious consideration under any of the following circumstances:

1 The child's weight has dropped to less than 70 per cent weight for height by age or below the 2nd percentile for BMI (based on standard growth monitoring charts – see references).
2 The child is markedly dehydrated or there is severe electrolyte imbalance.
3 There are signs of circulatory failure such as hypotension, bradycardia or severely impaired peripheral circulation.
4 There is persistent vomiting.
5 The illness is complicated by marked depression or other major psychiatric disturbance.

The relative scarcity of child psychiatric units and specialist eating disorder units for children frequently makes it difficult to find a suitable placement. If urgent hospitalisation is indicated then the child should preferably be admitted to a paediatric unit under the joint care of a paediatrician and child mental health specialist until a more suitable placement becomes available. The management of children with anorexia nervosa requires highly skilled treatment and nursing which may not be available on a busy general paediatric unit.

Parents are often loath to have their child admitted, particularly if she is adamantly resisting the idea. The clinician's responsibility here is to advise the parents whether out-patient treatment would be adequate. If this option is pursued with a very ill child, its success will depend very much on the active, committed input from parents. If unsuccessful, in-patient admission must be swiftly reconsidered before further deterioration takes place.

Target weights and ranges

Children with anorexia nervosa are excessively preoccupied with their weight and it is sensible to discuss with them and their parents as soon as possible what is a recommended satisfactory weight. We prefer to use a range rather than a specific weight, and refer to this as their target range. We explain that any weight within that range should be safe and healthy. Given the reality that no such children will want to be overweight, it is not unreasonable to offer as a lowest safe weight a 95 per cent weight for height ratio (above 25th percentile BMI), with a highest ratio of 100 per cent (50th percentile BMI). This would place these children between the 25th and 50th percentile for weight. Thus, a girl of 11 of average height would have a target range of 33.5 to 35 kg; while a girl of 13 of average height would have a target range of 43 to 45 kg.

We find it worth emphasising to children and parents that, while there are individual differences, in our experience menstruation is unlikely to occur at less than about 42 kg, and that fertility, bone density and growth can be impaired if weight remains too low for lengthy periods. We also know that target weights set between 95 per cent and 100 per cent tend to achieve higher rates of onset or resumption of menses (Key et al., 2002). One of the best indicators of satisfactory weight is the age-appropriate appearance of the ovaries and uterus on pelvic ultrasound. If these are of the correct shape, size and content for age then the weight is probably satisfactory. Once we have explained the reasoning behind the setting of the target weight range, and how we have derived the values, we find it best not to engage in further endless negotiation around this.

Graded weight restoration

Inevitably an essential component of the treatment is a refeeding programme involving rehydration, remedying any electrolyte imbalance and nutritional deficiency, and gradual restoration of the child's weight. Opinions differ as to whether refeeding should commence gradually or whether full portions should be instituted immediately. Children whose intake has been minimal should be started on small amounts (around 1,000 kcal, which should be increased within a few days, assuming it is tolerated) to avoid the risk of refeeding syndrome – a potentially fatal complication. Children who have eaten inadequately for long periods and are frightened of weight gain may find it easier to eat if initially offered small portions. It also helps for these to be served on a large plate. Size of portions can be gradually increased every few days. Children whose weight loss is not too marked and who are being treated on an out-patient basis should be expected to eat normal portions immediately.

Children with anorexia nervosa will invariably argue about the amounts given, insisting that these are excessive in the same way that they will insist that their weight is adequate and that the scales are wrong. The parents' or care-takers' task is to avoid these arguments and to ensure, kindly but firmly, that the meals are consumed.

As part of the 'relentless pursuit of thinness', characteristic of those with anorexia nervosa, additional means of avoiding weight gain are frequently adopted. The most common are hiding food, self-induced vomiting, laxative abuse and excessive exercising. Parents need to be aware that not only are these strategies a possibility, but some of them are very likely to occur. Indeed, our experience of the more seriously ill children is that self-induced vomiting is very common; and, if they appear to be eating normally but not gaining weight, secretive vomiting and exercising are the most likely causes. Appropriate precautions need to be taken including insisting on close supervision for a couple of hours after meals, and accompanying the child to the toilet.

In situations where a child adamantly refuses to eat and drink and where there is a deterioration in physical state, artificial feeding, usually by means of nasogastric tube, may be necessary. This should not be delayed because of fears that it is too drastic a measure. Many children with other illnesses require nasogastric feeding and in anorexia nervosa it can be a life-saving measure. The advice of a paediatrician or dietician should be obtained with regard to the content of the feeds. The child should be told that nasogastric feeding will continue for as long as necessary, and that the amount of feed will be reduced in proportion to what she takes by mouth. Nasogastric feeding can be terminated once satisfactory amounts of food and fluids can be taken.

Medication

Medication has only a small part to play in the management of children with anorexia nervosa. When such a child is depressed, with psychomotor retardation and feelings of guilt and worthlessness, an antidepressant such as fluoxetine, 20 mg daily, can be used. Treatment may need to be continued for several weeks before an effect is noticed, and checks should be made, if possible, that the therapeutic range has been reached. If effective, the antidepressant should be continued for at least three to four months after improvement has been noted.

There is no place for tranquillisers or appetite stimulants and any vitamin, zinc or iron deficiency is usually rapidly reversed once a normal diet is resumed. If constipation is troublesome this is best treated by dietary means rather than starting the child on a laxative career!

Family therapy

The essence of family therapy is the focus on the whole family rather than the individual patient (Honig, in Lask and Bryant-Waugh, 2000, pp. 187–204). Attention is paid to family function and communication rather than individual psychopathology. The most common areas for attention are: the effectiveness of the parental subsystem, parental relationship difficulties, parent–child over-involvement and over-protectiveness, and communication dysfunction. While each of these factors is distinct, there tends to be considerable overlap. In consequence, dealing with them separately is somewhat artificial and misleading.

Characteristically the family is in turmoil and despair. Attention is often almost exclusively focused on the sick child. The parents commonly adopt different attitudes to the management of the problem, with one parent finding it hard not to give in, while the other is firm and even punitive. This leads to conflict and inconsistency, with the child splitting the parents and often accentuating the tension between the two. There is often closer involvement of one parent with the child, while the other is peripheral or alienated. The more involved parent is likely to take a highly protective stance. Consistency, communication and cooperation are conspicuous by their absence. Parental relationship tensions are almost always present, if only as a result of the child's problem. More often, however, such conflict is long-standing and in some cases the illness may have emerged in that context.

There are many different schools of family therapy, and there are many contributions to the literature from these schools on the family treatment of anorexia nervosa. There is no evidence that one treatment is more effective than another. With regard to early onset anorexia nervosa, it is self-evident that there should be a focus on the competence and effectiveness of the parental subsystem in addressing the child's eating difficulties. Dysfunction is often evident from the outset, when a decision may need to be made with regard to whether or not the child should be admitted to hospital. Other areas of disagreement include how much pressure should be placed on the child to eat, and what quantities she should eat.

The family therapist's task here is not to make these decisions for the parents but rather to help them to reach an agreement themselves. In this respect the therapist functions rather like a go-between in a negotiating process. It is wise to avoid taking sides as much as possible, for in so doing one parent is alienated and therefore likely to be less cooperative.

Conflict within the parental relationship, if not already evident at commencement of therapy, often becomes apparent fairly quickly. It can be unhelpful, however, to tackle this too soon unless the parents make a specific request to do so. Otherwise there is a danger of confronting an issue that is too emotionally fraught for the parents at that point and does not relate to what they see as being the main problem. It is more useful to make a statement along the following lines:

> It would be surprising if the two of you did not from time to time get cross with each other under the circumstances. Having a child so ill is very upsetting and you obviously both want to do what is best for her. I can see that your relationship is not as comfortable as either of you would like at present. However it may be that you would rather focus on

trying to get your daughter better first and then we can think about whether the two of you want help for yourselves.

Most couples are relieved that the problem has been acknowledged but not directly confronted. When the parental relationship has irretrievably broken down it is still important to work on parenting issues and it is useful to make the point that although their relationship as a couple may be at an end they still have to work together as parents.

It can be helpful to encourage each parent to say in what ways each would like the other to handle the situation differently. Such a technique has several advantages. It promotes a more open communication within the family, initiates a process of compromise and cooperation and demonstrates to the child that her parents are trying to work together. Inappropriate alliances may become evident at this point and the therapist can point these out and help the family to adjust accordingly. For example, as the parents are discussing management, the child may interrupt with some form of protest which leads to one parent taking the child's side against the other. It is the occurrence of such sequences that validates the family approach. Without the child present these dysfunctions cannot be observed, and therefore cannot be so readily remedied. Similarly such issues as over-involvement and over-protectiveness can be directly tackled.

A common feature of children with anorexia nervosa is their tendency to block or deny feelings. Their body posture, facial expression and general behaviour indicate considerable emotional arousal, but they seem unable to acknowledge their distress with words. One aspect of the family therapy is the promotion of a more appropriate expression of feelings within the family, by the therapist acknowledging and accepting each person's feelings. This process of validation rather than denial or disqualification of feelings has considerable therapeutic benefit.

There are very many different techniques available to the family therapist besides those discussed here. The choice of techniques seems to be a matter of personal preference. What seems to be becoming increasingly clear is that family therapy is an essential component of the treatment of anorexia nervosa in the younger patient (NICE, 2004).

The use of motivational techniques and individual therapy

Recent years have seen an increasing emphasis on the use of motivational strategies to promote and facilitate change in people with eating disorders. Much of this work has been developed with adult patient populations (see e.g. Treasure and Bauer, 2003). We know that people with anorexia nervosa tend to be ambivalent about 'getting better' often because they have difficulty recognising that they have a problem, and because the anorexia seems to bring some benefits with it. These positive aspects of anorexia nervosa can serve as reinforcers that maintain the disorder and act as barriers to change. Children, like adults, are often confused and uncertain about whether to engage in treatment, and this is where the use of motivational techniques comes in. Essentially, this involves talking through with the child what the current advantages and disadvantages of having anorexia nervosa are for them, how they might feel about making changes, whether they feel ready and able to make changes, etc. This acknowledgement of the perceived positive aspects of the illness and exploration of less destructive ways to achieve the same effects can greatly increase the child's willingness to participate in therapy, and move towards sustained change. Children will rarely have chosen to initiate treatment as they are almost always brought to treatment by parents or other concerned adults, and this type of conversation can reassure them that you are trying to work with, rather than against, them. Often the use of motivational techniques precedes a course of individual therapy.

Two main forms of individual therapy are commonly used, psychodynamic psychotherapy (Magagna, in Lask and Bryant-Waugh, 2000, pp. 227–264) and individual work involving cognitive behaviour therapy techniques (Christie, in Lask and Bryant-Waugh, 2000, pp. 205–226). Clinical experience indicates that each has a part to play. The prime indications seem to be in those situations where the family dysfunction is such that there is little likelihood of sufficient change to allow the child to recover, or when the child's psychopathology is so severe and entrenched that family therapy is unlikely to have any sufficient effect. With older children – i.e. adolescents – individual therapy can be very useful in terms of focusing on age-appropriate separation and independence issues.

Individual psychotherapy needs to be offered in the context of a comprehensive treatment programme including the support of the physician involved, the school (if therapy occurs during school hours) and parental counselling or family therapy. It should be remembered that during acute starvation such children can be so preoccupied with food and weight that they may be emotionally inaccessible. In consequence, refeeding is one essential prerequisite for individual therapy. Embarking on therapy involves experiencing denied and conflictual feelings, thus necessitating considerable support for the child during a difficult time. Gradually therapy enables the child to develop an inner emotional space in which feelings can be experienced, named and discussed, problems identified and solutions sought. A better-developed inner psychic structure enables the child to sustain healthy dependent relationships as well as to pursue independent development outside the family.

There is no empirical evidence that one form of individual therapy is superior to another, and it is more likely that some children are better able to use one rather than the other. The skill of the therapist is paramount.

Group therapy

There is very little published literature on the use of group therapy for children with anorexia nervosa. The main indication for its use would be for children who have difficulties in their peer group relationships, but groups may also be used to help shift the focus from food, weight and appearance. Acknowledgement, acceptance and appropriate expression of feelings may also be promoted through the group.

The type of group will depend on the experience and inclinations of the therapist. On specialist units it is possible to have groups specifically for children with eating disorders, although it may be more appropriate to have groups for children with a wider range of problems. Groups do not necessarily have to be psychodynamically orientated. Such children's apparent inability to acknowledge or directly express feelings can be addressed in psycho-educational groups which are helpful for teaching the language of emotions. Social skills groups, as well as those using art or drama as modes of communication, all have clinical value and relevance (Wright, in Lask and Bryant-Waugh, 2000, pp. 307–322).

For in-patients the ward milieu is often of considerable value. Through close relationships with key worker and peer group, children can learn new and healthier ways of communicating and relating. Support groups for parents also seem to have considerable value (Nicholls and Magagna, 1997). Parents soon become involved in the group, and value meeting others in similar circumstances, and providing and receiving support.

Schooling

Many children with anorexia nervosa are intelligent, conscientious, and perfectionist. In consequence they usually do very well at school, and often continue working hard, long after the illness has become well established. Parents and teachers commonly confuse such diligence with the child being basically well, whereas it may actually represent an accentuation of the child's conscientiousness and inner struggle. The internal drive to achieve at a high standard can operate to impose greater pressures on the child.

Once the illness has been diagnosed, a decision should be made about whether education should temporarily be suspended. By doing so pressure is removed, but the child may resent such action and feel more distressed. A sensible compromise may be to allow schooling only if the child has resumed eating, and is gaining weight. Otherwise attendance at school should be restricted and closely supervised.

Teachers need to have some awareness of the child's emotional difficulties as well as her eating problems, so that they can manage the child appropriately. It is important that they do not collude with either the child's excessive conscientiousness or her tendency to split adults. In consequence, teachers should be considered as part of the therapeutic team, whether education is being provided in or out of hospital (Tate, in Lask and Bryant-Waugh, 2000, pp. 323–348).

Conclusions

Full recovery from early-onset anorexia nervosa appears to be dependent upon three main factors:

1   adoption of a comprehensive approach to treatment such as the one outlined;
2   the parental relationship and the relationship between the parents and the therapy team being characterised by cooperation, consistency and clear communication;
3   the child going through three phases as outlined in Figure 9.1.

Phase 1 is characterised by the expression of the presenting problems and normally persists for approximately one month after the commencement of treatment.

Phase 2 gradually replaces phase 1 and is characterised by an increasing amount of negative behaviour, including the direct expression of anger, sadness and resentment. This is a difficult phase for parents to accept because, although their child may have started eating and gaining weight, she appears to have undergone a dramatic personality change. In fact she is learning to express everyday feelings in a more direct and vigorous way than

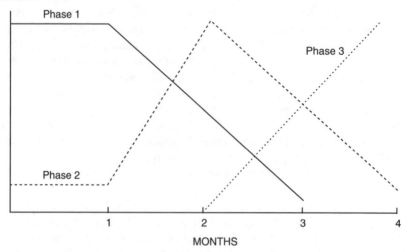

Figure 9.1 Phases of the illness.

previously. This seems to be an essential part of recovery and the parents need considerable support to tolerate such a change. It is wise to warn them in advance of this process which tends to peak after about one month. Finally, phase 3 is one of recovery in which a more normal eating pattern develops, and the child learns to express feelings in a more appropriate manner.

References

Bryant-Waugh, R. and Lask, B. (2004) *Eating Disorders: A Parents' Guide*. Revised edn. Hove: Brunner Routledge.

Growth Monitoring Products (Four in One charts, BMI charts, etc). Child Growth Foundation. Available from Harlow Printing Ltd. www.harlowprinting.co.uk

Key, A., Mason, H., Allen, R. and Lask, B. (2002) Restoration of ovarian and uterine maturity in adolescents with anorexia nervosa. *International Journal of Eating Disorders*, 32, 319–325.

Lask, B. and Bryant-Waugh, R. (eds) (2000) *Anorexia Nervosa and Related Eating Disorders in Childhood and Adolescence*. Hove: Psychology Press.

NICE (2004) Eating Disorders: Core Interventions in the treatment and management of anorexia nervosa, bulimia nervosa and related eating disorders. National clinical practice guideline. Number CG9. London: The British Psychological Society and Gaskell.

Nicholls, D. and Magagna, J. (1997) A group for the parents of children with eating disorders. *Clinical Child Psychology and Psychiatry*, 2, 565–578.

Steinhausen, H.-C. (2002) The outcome of anorexia nervosa in the 20th century. *American Journal of Psychiatry*, 159, 1284–1293.

Treasure, J. and Bauer, B. (2003) Assessment and motivation. In J. Treasure, U. Schmidt and E. van Furth (eds) *Handbook of Eating Disorders*. 2nd edn. Chichester: Wiley, pp. 219–232.

Chapter 10

Outpatient management of anorexia nervosa

Kelly M. Vitousek* and Jennifer A. Gray

Introduction

Outpatient treatment for anorexia nervosa is often discussed as an alternative to inpatient care for mild cases of recent onset or as a follow-up phase of treatment after hospital discharge. Some experts have suggested contraindications for outpatient management that are so inclusive (e.g. weight 15 per cent below expected level, hypotension, suicidal ideation) that few individuals with the diagnosis would be eligible to remain at home. While hospitalization is clearly essential for some patients and may be beneficial for others, biases toward inpatient care as standard treatment for anorexia nervosa are unfortunate for a number of reasons.

Why outpatient therapy is crucial in the treatment of anorexia nervosa (and likely to become more so)

1 Outpatient therapy is needed by all patients

Every anorexic patient requires outpatient management; the relevant question is whether an individual case may, in addition, benefit from hospitalization at one or more points over the course of treatment. Anorexia nervosa is seldom an acute condition that resolves completely through intensive intervention; rather, it is an 'illness of unusual tenacity' whose successful resolution usually spans years rather than months, even after extended inpatient treatment has been provided (Strober *et al.*, 1997). Therefore, patients, families, and care providers must expect to contend with the disorder outside the hospital for most of its total duration.

---

* The former name of the first author is Kelly M. Bemis.

2 Outpatient therapy may have more influence on eventual outcome

Many experts have emphasized that although refeeding in the hospital is a crucial phase of medical management in severe cases, it rarely determines eventual outcome. An impressive short-term response is not difficult to obtain on the ward (Russell, 1977). The challenge arises in transferring gains to the patient's daily life, where clinicians lack control over environmental contingencies. In most instances, inpatient care should be viewed as a temporary intervention that is sometimes necessary to preserve the patient's life or to prepare them for the more important phases of treatment that follow. Learning to manage eating and weight at the dining-room table, in the school cafeteria, at work, in friends' homes, and on holiday is considerably more predictive of recovery than finishing trays of food in a hospital bed in hope of securing release.

3 Routine or extended inpatient treatment may be unnecessary

According to some experts, weight restoration can be accomplished in a majority of cases through outpatient treatment alone (e.g. Dare and Eisler, 1992; Fairburn et al., 1999; Palmer, 2000). Clinic-based care has distinct advantages over hospitalization, including reduced risk of iatrogenic complications and the assumption of greater responsibility for change by the patient herself. More controversially, some commentators note the absence of clear evidence that intensive treatment deflects the natural history of the disorder – and there are a few troubling indications that it may do so in the wrong direction. Correlational data suggest that hospitalization is linked to negative outcomes (Ben-Tovim et al., 2001; Gowers et al., 2000; Meads et al., 2001), although it is impossible to rule out alternative explanations for the association, even when initial severity is controlled statistically. On the clinical level, all specialists can readily furnish instances in which anorexic patients appear to have been 'saved' by timely admissions or 'killed' when these were evaded or denied. Such anecdotes illustrate only that forceful intervention can influence the disorder at some points in time for some patients. They provide no information about whether inpatient care represents optimal treatment for most patients, or how long it should last, or what form it should take.

Two direct comparisons of cases randomly assigned to inpatient versus outpatient treatment have failed to detect strong differences favoring either. One of these investigations, however, was weakened by a high attrition rate, principally due to treatment refusal by patients allocated to hospital care (Crisp et al., 1991); the other remains unpublished (Freeman et al., 1990, in Freeman and Newton, 1992). In view of the clinical and economic implications of recommending inpatient care as a routine or frequent component of treatment for anorexia nervosa, experts agree that stronger data are urgently needed (Agras *et al.*, 2004; Vandereycken, 2003).

Still less information is available to guide decisions about how long inpatient treatment should persist, as no studies have randomly assigned anorexic patients to different periods in hospital. In the absence of such data, several kinds of correlational research have been cited in support of extended stays. One design involves comparing the subsequent status of patients who completed full inpatient regimens with that of patients who were discharged against medical advice and/or at subnormal weight levels (Baran *et al.*, 1995; Commerford *et al.*, 1997; Howard *et al.*, 1999; Woodside *et al.*, 2004). Other studies have examined outcomes for patients treated before and after budget cutbacks forced a sharp reduction in the length of inpatient stays (Cairns *et al.*, 1999), or have compared readmission rates as the average duration of stay decreased over time (Wiseman *et al.*, 2001). Each of these analyses has identified at least some trends toward poorer outcome in patients who were treated briefly or incompletely. These findings have been used to support the argument that extended inpatient treatment actually conserves resources over the course of this severe disorder (Crow and Nyman, 2004; Kaye *et al.*, 1996; Litt, 1999; Zerbe, 1996). While suggestive, however, correlational data provide an insufficient basis for this conclusion, as a number of extraneous factors may have contributed to the pattern of results obtained. Once again, only controlled trials can provide more satisfactory answers through random assignment of patients to varying planned lengths of inpatient treatment and/or different discharge criteria.

4 Routine or extended inpatient treatment is unaffordable

Until research demonstrates the superiority of inpatient treatment (and quite possibly thereafter), private and governmental health programs will be increasingly reluctant to fund such services in an era of dwindling resources. Figures from several national health care systems suggest that anorexia nervosa generates one of the highest average costs by diagnosis, and yields long inpatient stays more consistently than any other psychiatric condition, including schizophrenia and organic brain syndrome (McKenzie and Joyce, 1992). Inpatient episodes have been reported to average 26, 62, 64, and 96 days in different English-speaking countries (Beumont *et al.*, 1993; Robinson, 1993; Striegel-Moore *et al.*, 2000). One register-based study determined that patients spent a mean of 139 days in hospital over the five-year period beginning with their initial admission; almost two-thirds of adolescent cases were hospitalized more than once (McKenzie and Joyce, 1992).

Even if the suspected linkage between early discharge and negative outcome were confirmed, it is unlikely that medical economics would support the extraordinary lengths of stay that have been reported to reduce subsequent relapse. A review of records in one specialized treatment program in the

United States found a dramatic decrease in the average duration of inpatient care over a fifteen-year period, from 149 days in 1984 to 23 days in 1998 (Wiseman *et al.*, 2001). Similar trends have been noted in the United Kingdom, with substantial variability across districts (Meads *et al.*, 2001). The six- to twenty-four-month periods of residential care once recommended as standard practice in some facilities (Story, 1982; Strober and Yager, 1985) appear increasingly fanciful to clinicians forced to document the need for each inpatient day. It is striking that the forty-six-day average stay of the 'prematurely' discharged patients who fared poorly in one of the correlational studies cited above (Baran *et al.*, 1995) exceeds the allowable limit of many private reimbursement plans; the 116-day regimen of Baran *et al.*'s more successful completers is more than four times the typical length of stay provided by most health care systems.

What works in outpatient therapy?

All of these factors suggest that outpatient management is likely to become an increasingly prominent part of total care for anorexia nervosa. Dozens of alternative models have been proposed for the form that psychotherapy should take with this patient population.

Psychodynamic approaches (e.g. Bemporad and Herzog, 1989; Bruch, 1973; Crisp, 1980; Dare and Crowther, 1995; Goodsitt, 1985, 1997) focus on ego deficits and developmental conflicts concerning identity, autonomy, and emotional experience. Although family dynamics may be a prominent part of the content of psychotherapy, treatment is usually conducted on an individual basis, sometimes supplemented by process-oriented family and/or group therapy sessions. These approaches tend to focus less on strategies for remediating specific anorexic symptoms and more on basic aspects of the self that the disordered behaviors are believed to represent. In some psychodynamic models, therapists deliberately minimize the attention paid to weight status and eating behavior, delegating the management of these issues to other elements of a comprehensive treatment program.

Interpersonal psychotherapy assumes that problems arise from social deficits, interpersonal disputes, role transitions, and/or grief (Fairburn, 2002; McIntosh *et al.*, 2000; Wilfley *et al.*, 2003). Like many of the variant forms of psychodynamic treatment, this approach does not address disordered eating or low weight directly, but concentrates on exploring the interpersonal patterns that may contribute to symptom expression and on helping patients develop more satisfying relationships.

Both nutritional management and behavioral approaches emphasize the provision of psychoeducational information, self-monitoring of intake, and meal planning (e.g. Beumont *et al.*, 1997; Touyz and Beumont, 1997). Behavioral models also conduct functional analyses of the environmental variables that elicit or reinforce disordered eating behavior, using strategies such as contingency management and/or exposure and response prevention to modify target symptoms. Cognitive-behavioral therapy (CBT) (e.g., Fairburn *et al.*, 1999, 2003; Garner and Bemis, 1982, 1985; Garner *et al.*, 1997; Vitousek, 2002) usually includes all of these elements, but assigns particular importance to examining distorted ideas about eating, weight, and shape and their implications for the self. All three approaches are typically conducted on an individual basis, although some group applications have been described; in addition, family counseling consonant with these models is recommended for younger patients (Garner *et al.*, 1997).

Structural and strategic family therapy approaches (e.g. Dare and Eisler, 1992; Lask, 1992; Lock *et al.*, 2001; Minuchin *et al.*, 1978; Palazzoli, 1978) work with the family system as a whole, using active and directive techniques to alter the transactional patterns that support anorexic symptoms in one member. In most of these approaches, parents are encouraged to assume total control over the child's eating behavior until she has demonstrated the ability to make appropriate decisions on her own. Family therapy has been recommended for patients in all age ranges, although for obvious reasons the parental control model must be adapted when it is applied to families with older adolescent or adult patients.

Feminist therapy encourages patients to construe their symptoms within the broader cultural context, rather than seeking individual or familial determinants of pathology (e.g. Brown and Jasper, 1993; Fallon *et al.*, 1994; Kearney-Cooke and Striegel-Moore, 1997; Lawrence, 1984; Orbach, 1985). Instead of focusing on the modification of symptoms or the adjustment of family dynamics, these approaches seek to empower women to 'take up more space' with their bodies, needs, and emotions. The therapeutic relationship is more egalitarian and more nurturant than in traditional forms of psychotherapy. Consistent with the emphasis on self-determination, patients are given responsibility for managing their own dietary intake and weight. These approaches emphasize expressive and experiential techniques such as art and movement therapy, guided imagery, and healing from traumatic abuse. They often include participation in both individual and group therapy, and encourage political action that extends beyond the consulting room.

Thumbnail sketches such as these clearly oversimplify the complex interventions they summarize, and misrepresent some of the variant forms subsumed under each general heading. A number of prescriptive models blend concepts and techniques from two or more of these categories. For example, cognitive analytic therapy (CAT) combines elements of cognitive and psychodynamic approaches (Bell, 1999; Tanner and Connan, 2003; Treasure and Ward, 1997a); behavioral family systems therapy (BFST) conjoins the family control model with cognitive and behavioral techniques (Robin *et al.*, 1996); Orbach's (1985) approach is characterized as 'feminist psychoanalytic.' Moreover, as is generally true in the untidy world of psychotherapeutic practice, it is probable that few clinicians implement either the 'pure' or 'blended' protocols precisely as described by their proponents, relying instead on eclectic approaches that combine elements in unsystematic ways.

Unfortunately, the empirical literature offers almost no guidance in choosing from this array of treatment models (Agras *et al.*, 2004; Hay *et al.*, 2003; Vitousek and Gray, 2005; Wilson and Agras, 2001). Some of the most influential approaches have never been tested in any form. Fewer than twenty studies have compared two or more outpatient treatments using random assignment (Ball and Mitchell, 2004; Channon *et al.*, 1989; Crisp *et al.*, 1991; Dare *et al.*, 1990, 2001; Eisler *et al.*, 2000; Geist *et al.*, 2000; Hall and Crisp, 1987; Halmi, 2000; le Grange *et al.*, 1992; McIntosh *et al.*, 2005; Pike *et al.*, 2003; Robin *et al.*, 1994; Russell *et al.*, 1987; Serfaty *et al.*, 1999; Treasure *et al.*, 1995a). Most of these report essentially equivalent – and often rather disappointing – outcomes for patients allocated to different conditions. It is not even clear that treatments designed and delivered by experts outperform services provided by the general professional community. In two studies, patients referred back to standard care have fared poorly compared to those receiving specialized treatments (Crisp *et al.*, 1991; Dare *et al.*, 2001). In one report, however, unspecified 'treatment as usual' appeared equal to two targeted approaches that had been expected to prove superior (Channon *et al.*, 1989); in another, supportive clinical management appeared more effective than specialized therapies (McIntosh *et al.*, 2005).

Together with the data discussed earlier on inpatient versus outpatient care, it might appear that it makes no difference where, how, or by whom anorexic patients are treated. At present, this conclusion would be as premature as the insistence that any one approach is superior. A number of studies have used such small sample sizes that clinically important group differences would have been difficult to detect statistically (e.g. Channon *et al.*, 1989). In others, so many patients refused or dropped out of some treatment conditions that a comparison of results for those who remained is misleading (e.g. Crisp *et al.*, 1991; Halmi, 2000; Serfaty *et al.*, 1999). Most of the controlled trials have provided truncated, attenuated forms of therapy, allocating the same numbers of sessions to the treatment of anorexia nervosa that are specified for disorders such as depression or bulimia nervosa. Some of the tested treatments have no constituency; for example, an 18–25 session course of CBT (Ball and Mitchell, 2004; Channon *et al.*, 1989; McIntosh *et al.*, 2005) – when CBT experts typically recommend 40–60 sessions for established cases of anorexia nervosa (Fairburn *et al.*, 2003; Garner *et al.*, 1997; Pike *et al.*, 2003) – or individual therapy for adolescents that bars all contact between therapists and patients (Russell *et al.*, 1987). Clearly, it is impossible to assess the merits of an intervention that specialists recommend by examining one they do not. Some of these problems are difficult to avoid when studying a rare disorder that requires extended participation by ambivalent patients, but most could be remedied with stronger designs and more adequate funding.

Sorting out what we know about outpatient therapy is also complicated by the heterogeneity of the treatments and patients studied. Even when a positive finding that Treatment X outperforms Treatment Y is obtained, it is hazardous to generalize this conclusion to other circumstances and populations. For example, it may be that Treatment X is superior only with younger patients, while Treatment Y would produce a better response in chronic or adult patients; it may be that Treatment X has the edge in preventing relapse after discharge in patients who are already fully weight-restored, while Treatment Y would have been more effective in promoting weight gain for those treated solely on an outpatient basis. The meager literature available to date hints that some of these interactions are to be anticipated. Family therapy appears to be indicated for young patients with recent onset, but produces unimpressive results in more established cases (Dare *et al.*, 1990; Eisler *et al.*, 2000; Russell *et al.*, 1987); antidepressants seem to provide little or no benefit in promoting weight gain but may reduce the risk of relapse after weight restoration (Ferguson *et al.*, 1999). Therefore, it appears particularly important in this area to avoid drawing broad conclusions on the basis of individual studies.

Family therapy is the most extensively researched treatment for anorexia nervosa, contributing at least one cell to half of all controlled trials of psychotherapy. For adolescent patients, the results are generally positive, although there have been few direct comparisons between family and individual therapies. Only one study (Russell *et al.*, 1987) found family therapy clearly superior to a comparison treatment, and the effect was limited to patients who carried particularly favorable prognoses by virtue of their young age and brief duration of illness.

Subsequent research confirmed the importance of short duration as a predictor of response to family therapy. In a project carried out by the same investigators, all participants had been anorexic for just 2 to 36 months, with an average duration of 12.9 months and a mean age of 15.5 years (Eisler *et al.*, 2000). Even within this extremely restricted range, there was a significant correlation between how recent onset had been and treatment outcome in either of two forms of family therapy. Patients who were doing well at one year had been anorexic for a mean of eight months at the inception of treatment, compared to sixteen months for those with intermediate or poor outcomes. When patients who had received repeated prior treatment on an inpatient or outpatient basis were compared to those obtaining therapy for the first time, the contrast was again sharp: 73 per cent of the treatment veterans did poorly in family therapy, while only 19 per cent of the novices failed to improve. This pattern could have a number of plausible explanations, and the possibilities hold different implications for how we should view the results of family therapy (Vitousek and Gray, 2005). It is not clear that family therapy is contraindicated for established cases, as there is little evidence to suggest that alternative treatments are more effective; however, on the basis of current data, positive statements about its benefits must be restricted to the subgroup of young, recent-onset patients who respond well to this mode of therapy.

The specific variant of family therapy that is most widely recommended is the 'Maudsley model,' in which all family members are seen together for conjoint family therapy sessions (Dare and Eisler, 1992; Lock *et al.*, 2001). Interestingly, the originators of this approach have twice determined that the conjoint format may be less effective than treating patients and parents in separate sessions, particularly for the subset of families showing high levels of expressed emotion (Eisler *et al.*, 2000; le Grange *et al.*, 1992). In spite of this replicated finding, proponents of the Maudsley approach continue to advocate whole-family sessions as the preferred mode of treatment (Lock *et al.*, 2001). Based on the available evidence (as well as common-sense clinical practice), it seems desirable to involve the family when treating young anorexic patients; as yet, however, the data provide little guidance about optimal means of doing so.

Can outpatient treatment become more effective?

With the partial exception of family therapy for at least a subgroup of patients, advocacy of any one treatment model for anorexia nervosa remains 'special pleading,' based on theoretical allegiance and familiarity rather than demonstrated effectiveness. Although research provides some basis for concluding that medication alone and nutritional counseling alone are contraindicated (Halmi, 2000; Pike *et al.*, 2003; Serfaty *et al.*, 1999), there is scant empirical justification for claiming that one brand name of 'talking therapy' is superior to modalities based on contrasting theories and using radically different techniques. Because it is unclear whether therapists should spend their time restructuring family dynamics, revisiting childhood experiences, exploring beliefs about eating and weight, or heightening awareness of the disempowerment of women, we will not attempt to specify the 'correct' content for psychotherapy with anorexic patients. What does seem apparent is that as outpatient services begin to absorb more of the total burden of care, they must be adapted in some predictable ways to fulfill more of the functions previously provided through hospital treatment.

In our opinion, such efforts are likely to fail to the extent that clinicians attempt to transfer the same strategies that can be effective in hospital to the dramatically different circumstances of outpatient care. When therapists try to impose the aggressive tactics sustainable in the controlled environment of the ward to clinic-based therapy, they usually fail – often leading to admissions that the outpatient treatment was intended to prevent. At the same time, it is obvious that some conventional outpatient approaches cannot continue doing 'business as usual' when they must assume more responsibility for overall case management. The therapeutic models outlined above will need to change in different ways to adjust to these conditions. Clinicians who prefer to exclude the minutiae of food and weight from psychotherapy will less often have the luxury of relying on hospital staff to manage these issues without their active participation. On the other hand, therapists who expect to spend their time imparting strategies for symptom control to patients already motivated to recover must become more skilled at engaging resistant patients in treatment.

To a considerable extent, inpatient treatment has remained a prominent part of the management of anorexia nervosa because it shelters the involved parties – if only temporarily – from the most fundamental problems posed by this disorder. Anorexic patients are difficult to treat principally because they want to remain anorexic, while care providers feel morally and medically bound to try to prevent them from doing so. Anorexia nervosa is much more than a 'matter of personal choice,' but patients often defend it passionately as if it were. As the disorder progresses, the desire to become thin is augmented (and sometimes replaced) by fear of change, hopelessness, and the debilitating secondary effects of starvation. In most cases, however, restrictive eating and weight loss continue to be viewed by patients as potential solutions to their distress, rather than its causes. Intense ambivalence about the prospect of change is not a complicating feature of anorexia nervosa – it is built into the nature of the disorder (Vitousek et al., 1998).

In this context, it is not difficult to see why inpatient programs are appealing to clinicians who work with these fragile, frightened, and resistant patients. Admission to hospital suspends the difficulties of contending with dishonest self-report, reluctance to change diet and weight, and the need to coordinate multiple services. Moreover, many therapists find these patients unsympathetic and annoying. As the former anorexic Sheila MacLeod observed, 'It is difficult not to gain the impression from the literature that individual therapy has been devalued because (among other reasons) psychotherapists do not like anorexics, and anorexics do not like psychotherapists' (MacLeod, 1982, p. 121). Inpatient programs also provide some respite to family members strained by concern about the patient's well-being and exhausted from daily struggles to induce her to eat. To many families, as well as clinicians, the availability of a system that allows close supervision of the patient's medical status while promoting rapid and substantial weight gain is welcome indeed. In some cases, the patient herself may prefer hospitalization because it allows external attribution of responsibility for changes she will not attempt on her own.

In spite of these potential advantages, both the frequency of relapse after discharge and the economic considerations outlined above suggest that the systematic study of alternatives is overdue. Clearly, it will never be possible to eliminate hospital treatment as an essential element of comprehensive care for these difficult and sometimes imperiled patients; however, there is no basis for assuming that a shift away from routine or extended inpatient treatment is inherently disadvantageous. For the remainder of this chapter, we will focus on a review of the problems outpatient therapies must address as they assume increased responsibility for the care of anorexic patients – as well as on some of the distinct advantages outpatient therapy can offer. Our general approach is cognitive-behavioral, but we will not be outlining theory-specific techniques such as cognitive restructuring (see Garner and Bemis, 1982, 1985; Garner *et al.*, 1997). Instead, we will summarize strategies for outpatient management that should be consonant with a wide range of models for conducting psychotherapy.

Common problems in outpatient therapy – and some possible solutions

The problem of crisis situations

Because hospital admissions are often triggered by crises, clinic-based programs must work to prevent their occurrence whenever possible. Sometimes the circumstances that prompt decisions to admit are mislabeled 'emergencies' through ignorance, anxiety, or irritation. In other instances, genuine crises might have been averted if appropriate action had been taken earlier.

The following factors frequently contribute to crisis admissions of patients who could be managed successfully on an outpatient basis:

- Panic over abnormal but predictable results from laboratory tests that required interpretation by a more experienced consultant (or need not have been ordered at all). Risk is difficult to calculate in anorexia nervosa, since alarming indices can be consistent with stability at low weight levels while fatal outcomes may occur in patients with normal laboratory values (De Zwaan and Mitchell, 1999; Vandereycken, 1987b).
- Guilt over delayed recognition of symptoms that could have been decoded earlier. For example, in one case we treated recently, the parents of a 15-year-old girl had taken her to the pediatrician because of their concern about her rapid 20 lb. weight loss. The physician reassured them that their daughter was fine – in fact, he commented, approvingly, at 5' 7" and 105 lbs., she looked 'just like a model.' When her parents brought her back one month later and 10 lbs. lighter, the pediatrician hospitalized her immediately. Many preventable admissions seem to be precipitated by a similar sequence: weight loss is initially minimized as normal (or even desirable) – and then triggers a compensatory overreaction when its significance is belatedly appreciated.
- A sense of being backed into a corner when patients fail to comply with contracts that established inappropriate goals and contingencies. Clinicians often agree to a trial of outpatient therapy on the condition that patients demonstrate specified changes in eating and weight. Clearly, some contingent relationships should be defined between weight status and treatment setting, and the terms cannot be subject to renegotiation with frightened patients who are unable to make rational assessments of

risk. Problems often arise, however, when outpatient contracts specify *unrealistic* rates of progress (such as a weekly gain of 2 lbs.) or set *absolute* criteria for hospitalization (such as a 2 lb. loss on any weighing occasion). Such standards are inconsistent with the recognized difficulty of sustaining rapid weight gain outside the hospital and fail to accommodate expected weight variability or predictable periods of retrenchment. Clinicians who institute a faulty contract put themselves in a no-win situation: they risk losing credibility if they suspend its provisions, or bringing about unnecessary admissions if they enforce ill-considered threats.

- Anger over the deception and resistance through which many patients defend their symptoms. In fact, these characteristic features of anorexia nervosa are no more appropriately viewed as the patient's 'fault' than the attempts an obsessive-compulsive individual might make to conceal handwashing rituals (Vitousek *et al.*, 1998). Deplorably, unprofessional elements of retaliation can sometimes be discerned in decisions to admit anorexic patients to hospital – as if their failure to comply with the terms of outpatient treatment is justly punished by the loss of liberty and stringent regimens involved in institutional care.

If clinicians should avoid hasty decisions based on fear or frustration, they should not become complacent about the serious risks associated with this disorder. Concern about the possibility of an adverse outcome is warranted when treating a condition with a 5 to 10 per cent mortality rate (Neumarker, 1997; Sullivan, 2002). Forceful intervention is sometimes necessary to prevent death or deterioration; a degree of pressure for change is always indicated to counter patients' attachment to the status quo. Outpatient management, however, requires that clinicians play a longer hand. They must accept higher levels of ambiguity, slower rates of change, and a diminished degree of professional control in trade for allowing the patient (and in some instances her family) greater responsibility for change.

The problems of expertise and the coordination of services

Inpatient care facilitates the delivery of the expert and multidisciplinary services these complex cases require. Specialists can be concentrated in a central location, drawing patients from a wider geographic region than feasible for an outpatient facility. Physicians, nurses, psychologists, social workers, and dieticians report to work in the same place and convene regularly for staff meetings. Both the team model and the established hierarchical authority in hospital settings promote consistency of care. A 'party line' can be established and, to some extent, enforced across treatment personnel. Uniformity benefits staff through reducing the risk of 'splitting' (a pejorative term used to describe patients' variable success in convincing care providers of their point of view). Consistency benefits patients to the extent that it spares them exposure to incompatible advice on matters they consider of great moment, such as target weight.

Outpatient treatment should devise ways to replicate these theoretical advantages. The first problem to be addressed is the question of 'Who's in charge?' In addition to 'the patient' and/or 'the family,' the best answer is usually 'the care provider who is most knowledgeable about the psychopathology and treatment of the eating disorders.' If a specialty outpatient program is available in the community, it will ordinarily assume that role. In many cases, however, this decision must be sorted out amongst professionals working in separate locations, in different capacities. In a rational world, it would matter less what degree each held and more what expertise he or she possessed. If a psychotherapist has more knowledge and experience with this population, he should define the principles of treatment; if a physician has more specific relevant background, she should take that responsibility. In most instances, the basic parameters defined by the designated 'expert' should be endorsed and implemented by other care providers, regardless of their relative ranking in the conventional health care hierarchy. In turn, the principal care provider should seek regular input from other professionals in their respective domains of practice. Whenever possible, disagreements should be resolved through direct discussions amongst the care providers, rather than passed along through the patient or her family.

In our experience, conflicting messages from professionals contribute substantially to setbacks in treatment (although we are not convinced that these problems occur much more frequently in clinic-based care than in inpatient units). One of our clients had made remarkable progress in outpatient therapy despite a fourteen-year history of anorexia nervosa that included five hospitalizations totaling more than 400 inpatient days. For the first time, she had voluntarily gained to within 2 lbs. of the 'magic weight' she had always feared (approximate BMI of 18) and had decided to cross this psychologically significant boundary. At just that point, her physician advised her during a routine appointment that he 'saw no reason [for her] to gain any additional weight,' since the patient was now within what he defined generously as a normal range. The patient immediately cut back on her intake, and at the next therapy session tearfully announced her intention to lose weight. It took several weeks to restore her confidence in the correctness of her original decision.

Another partially recovered patient panicked after she stepped on the scale (still at least 15 lbs. underweight) and a pediatric nurse commented: 'Well, in spite of what it says here on your chart, you obviously aren't anorexic any more.' Other patients have become confused when health care providers advised them to 'just follow your natural appetite,' told them to avoid sweets and fats while regaining because 'junk food will put on unhealthy weight,' or expressed admiration for their daily three-hour exercise regimens.

Even in domains within which physicians clearly command more general competence, non-medical experts may possess more accurate specialized knowledge about the physical effects of eating disorders. For example, on the basis of an elevated cholesterol level (a common if counterintuitive finding in anorexia nervosa (Feillet *et al.*, 2000; Pomeroy and Mitchell, 2002)), one of our patients was instructed by her physician to cut down on dietary fat and take regular exercise. At a BMI of 16.5, it should not have been difficult to guess that she was getting very little of the former and rather too much of the latter. Hormone replacement therapy is routinely prescribed to 'prevent complications from amenorrhea,' although the evidence indicates that exogenous hormones do not increase bone density in patients with anorexia nervosa (Golden *et al.*, 2002).

Professional pride is misplaced when dealing with serious disorders that require extensive background knowledge. In general, matters related to eating, weight, and the complications of starvation and purgative tactics should be referred to the best available expert – or thoroughly researched if his or her recommendations are disputed. At a minimum, professionals who are not assuming the primary role in the management of an anorexic case should take pains not to undermine the efforts of the responsible clinician.

The problem of motivation for change

As noted earlier, the principal reason for the traditional reliance on inpatient care is that anorexic individuals do not wish to gain weight. The hospital allows clinicians to bypass the patient as an agent of change by setting up conditions that sharply limit her ability to choose. For a period of time, we can guarantee that she will do the right things, whatever she thinks, feels, wants, and fears.

Motivational issues are certainly active at the time of admission if patients need to be convinced to enter the hospital voluntarily. This objective is usually accomplished through a blend of persuasion, coercion, and compulsion by care providers and significant others. The campaign often has the quality of storming the vulnerable position of a weaker opponent – it is bloody but brief, and the assault team usually wins. Thereafter, motivational issues become subordinate to management issues for the duration of inpatient care. In contrast, the ongoing attempt to secure cooperation during outpatient treatment can seem more like a protracted war of attrition. Because such campaigns rarely have a satisfactory outcome for either side, less adversarial tactics should be adopted from the outset. The patient must become an ally, and this is more likely to occur through diplomatic negotiation and recognition of common interests than through combat. As Palmer (2000) emphasizes, 'outpatient management is, and indeed should always be, a matter of cooperation' (p. 141).

Because outpatient therapy cannot bypass the patient's choices to bring about change, it must focus on affecting her own decision-making. Because it is more dependent on the veracity of her self-report, it must increase her comfort and investment in telling the truth. In outpatient therapy, the statement that the patient 'must do the right things, whatever she thinks, feels, wants, and fears' would be absurd. If she does not decide that new behaviors might be in her own best interest, they will simply not occur.

In recent years, motivation for change in anorexia nervosa has received far more research and clinical attention – no doubt in part because of the general trend away from extended inpatient treatment. Research has been directed toward understanding patients' ambivalence about change and their perceptions of the motives for their eating disorder. Several recent articles have outlined explicit clinical strategies for enhancing motivation for change in anorexia nervosa (e.g. Geller, 2002; Goldner *et al.*, 1997; Treasure and Schmidt, 2001; Treasure and Ward, 1997b; Vitousek *et al.*, 1998).

Some of these models have concentrated on the initial challenge of engaging patients in treatment. In particular, Treasure and Ward (1997b) describe the application of motivational interviewing principles to the eating disorders. The motivational interviewing approach was developed by Miller and Rollnick (1991, 2002) as an alternative to confrontational models for the treatment of alcoholism. Miller and Rollnick make a persuasive case – supported by the convergence of research evidence, clinical experience, and old-fashioned common sense – that adversarial tactics typically backfire when directed toward individuals who are ambivalent about change. Indeed, such techniques are particularly contraindicated with the very patients who regularly provoke their use, such as alcoholics, drug abusers, and anorexics. Treatment degenerates into arguments between frustrated professionals who are determined to convince patients of the error and danger of their ways and patients who are increasingly committed to defending the status quo. Miller and Rollnick (2002) note that when clinicians assume the responsibility for advocating change, they force clients to argue for the opposite side of their own ambivalence – paradoxically increasing their investment in the problem behavior. Motivational interviewing uses specific strategies to avoid the escalation of confrontation and denial, while heightening the salience of patients' own concerns about their symptoms.

These principles should be generalizable to work with any individuals in whom ambivalence is marked or whose active cooperation is required for the implementation of complex and aversive treatment regimens, such as diabetics (e.g. Smith *et al.*, 1997). Anorexic clients in outpatient therapy certainly meet both of these criteria. Preliminary trials of motivational interviewing with anorexic patients are encouraging (Feld *et al.*, 2001; Gowers and Smyth, 2004), and more systematic tests of its contribution to treatment engagement are currently underway.

Other clinical recommendations stress that since motivational issues recur across all phases of treatment, they should be considered in designing each of its elements (Vitousek *et al.*, 1998). Because many anorexic individuals value their symptoms, the difficulties are not resolved merely by success in persuading them to enter treatment. Changes in the meaning and function of anorexic behavior must be accomplished through patient, systematic work over an extended period of time. In many cases, central concerns about change emerge only after substantial progress has been made. For example, some patients are more easily persuaded to increase their weight from 75 lbs. to 118 lbs. than to increment it the additional 5 or 10 lbs. that would restore them to a normal weight range. In these cases, the most basic dread of being 'average' can remain concealed while patients are substantially underweight, triggering heightened resistance to change when they reach the brink of full recovery.

The approach outlined by Vitousek *et al.* (1998) incorporates elements of motivational interviewing and CBT, with emphasis on four themes (psycho-educational, experimental, functional, and philosophical) that seem strongly linked to the promotion of change in this population. Although the treatment method as a whole was designed as a framework for intensive individual therapy, the basic themes it identifies can be stressed to advantage by physicians, nurses, and dieticians in their work with these patients.

Across all content areas, empathy for and validation of the patient's experience should be the starting point of all efforts to foster change. Professionals are encouraged to approach patients with warmth, gentleness, and sympathetic recognition of their predicament. Statements such as the following affirm the difficulty of the patient's position without either endorsing or challenging her beliefs:

> It must be frustrating to want so keenly to keep your weight loss, while everyone else seems to have very different ideas about what you ought to be feeling and doing. Tell me about what that has been like for you.

The clinician should convey genuine interest in the patient's own perception of her dilemma and listen respectfully to her answers – while beginning to introduce alternative considerations:

> What do you think things would be like if other people *did* just leave you alone to make your own decisions? What do you anticipate happening after you reach the weight you want to be? What sorts of concerns might make it difficult to *stop* losing weight at that point? Is it ever worrisome to you that you've already gone far below the goal weight you thought you'd like at the outset? What are your hunches about why that occurred?

Psychoeducational

The first theme that should be prominent in work with anorexic patients involves the presentation of factual material about the eating disorders and, more generally, the regulation of eating and weight. Because the anorexic individual must become the agent of change in outpatient therapy, it is not enough for the clinician to be knowledgeable about why normal eating and weight are desirable. Patients are also entitled to know facts relevant to their own decision-making – and accurate information can play a major role in building and sustaining motivation for change.

Some of the material that should be imparted to patients addresses misconceptions on specific points such as the utility of laxatives as a weight control tactic. Other material may have more profound implications for the ways patients conceptualize the disorder itself. In our experience, for example, a detailed review of the findings of the Minnesota experimental study of semi-starvation (Keys *et al.*, 1950) may be more influential than any form of interpersonal support or coercive control in changing a patient's 'set' about her symptoms. Ironically, this remarkable research project was carried out more than fifty years ago with normal male subjects – but its implications for anorexia nervosa encapsulate some of the most critical messages we can offer our patients.

The study exposed thirty-six healthy male volunteers, who were conscientious objectors during World War II, to six months of semi-starvation. On a regimen averaging 1570 calories, the men lost a targeted 25 per cent of original body weight. They were carefully observed before and during the period of caloric restriction, as well as a subsequent period of refeeding. In addition to the host of physical symptoms associated with starvation (including cold intolerance, hair loss, sleep disturbance, and changes in multiple physiological indices), participants showed pronounced deterioration in psychological and social functioning. They became obsessively preoccupied with food and displayed stereotypic changes in eating behavior, including dawdling over meals, increased use of salt and spices, 'souping' of food through the addition of liquid, and the collection of recipes. All experienced symptoms of depression, ranging from mild to severe; many became anxious, irritable, and obsessional. Social isolation was marked, and there was a dramatic decline in sexual interest and activity. The psychological changes were so striking that the investigators coined the term 'semi-starvation neurosis' to describe the constellation of symptoms they observed. Through much of the refeeding phase, participants remained keenly interested in food and often ate massive quantities with no sense of satisfaction or satiety. For some, disturbances in the experience of hunger and fullness and a heightened interest in food persisted after the completion of the year-long project.

The provision of material from this study can be an invaluable means of reframing anorexic symptoms as predictable responses to extreme dietary restriction and weight loss (Garner, 1997; Garner and Bemis, 1985; Vitousek *et al.*, 1998). Its findings underscore the fact that starvation is the unifying cause of distressing experiences that patients may perceive as unrelated. Individuals with anorexia nervosa are cold because they are starving; their hair is falling out because they are starving; they are preoccupied with food because they are starving; they are moody and withdrawn because they are starving; they are inefficient and perseverative because they are starving.

The consistency of the starvation syndrome has both reassuring and disturbing implications for anorexic patients. The voracious appetite that terrifies them does not signify moral weakness (as patients often believe) or 'emotional hunger' (as many therapists suggest). It is an inevitable consequence of restriction, and will abate only after deprivation stops. At the same time, the experience of being 'special' and 'unique' through the disorder is belied by its predictability. Many of the secret things anorexic individuals feel and do were felt and done by male volunteers who were not given enough food to eat half a century ago. Anorexic patients often react to anecdotal material from the Minnesota study with confusion and chagrin. It may evoke the first sense of dissonance required to develop a disposition to change.

Obviously, clinicians must be conversant with a great deal of information on nutrition, weight control, and the effects of eating disorders in order to present psychoeducational material accurately and convincingly. Fortunately, excellent summary articles are available, notably Garner's (1997) concise overview of topics relevant to anorexic and bulimic patients and Fairburn and Brownell's (2002) handbook of basic information on metabolism, weight, and eating disorders. Knowing how to present such information is just as important as knowing what to say. Consistent with the principles of motivational interviewing, clinicians should offer facts respectfully for the patient's consideration, rather than using such material to display their own credentials or to frighten patients into compliance (Vitousek et al., 1998).

Experimental

The second core theme is an emphasis on an experimental model of treatment. From the first meeting with an anorexic patient, the clinician should stress that each step of therapy will be undertaken with an attitude of 'Let's test this out, and see what happens.' The patient need not commit herself to abandoning her accustomed patterns before venturing to try a new course. She need only consent to make graduated changes in deliberate, systematic ways, so that she can gauge the effect of alternative behaviors.

The strategy of *collaborative empiricism* is the cornerstone of cognitive-behavioural therapy for all disorders, but seems especially well suited to this wary population (Garner and Bemis, 1982) – and particularly crucial to successful treatment on an outpatient basis. The promise that patients need only *experiment* with doing things differently is often all that induces anorexic individuals to make the tentative changes that begin dismantling the closed system of their disorder. Casting change in experimental terms is not merely a strategic ploy, however; it reflects reality. For all but the youngest or most medically imperilled anorexics, the entire therapeutic enterprise truly is an experiment from which patients can choose to withdraw. The option of retreating into the disorder remains available to those who still prefer it after examining its implications and exploring other options. From a clinical perspective, there is no advantage to be gained in bluffing about who has the power to determine the patient's choices. It is more persuasive to acknowledge the individual's control over her own destiny because it is both more respectful *and* more accurate.

Functional

The third theme crucial to the development of motivation for change is an emphasis on the functional effects of symptoms. Rather than talking with patients about what is right or wrong, healthy or unhealthy, sensible or silly, clinicians should frame their discussions around the question: 'From your perspective, how well is that working out?'

We usually spend much of the first session with a new anorexic patient developing and discussing a list of the advantages and disadvantages of anorexia nervosa, according to *her* point of view (Vitousek and Gray, 2005; Vitousek and Orimoto, 1993; Vitousek *et al.*, 1998). We do not assume that she is being fully candid, as she has little basis for trusting us as yet; we do not assume that she is even aware of many of the determinants of her disorder. But we think it is important to ask for her opinions in any case, and to listen attentively to her answers. It is disarming when a professional shows keen interest in what the patient thinks she is getting from her disorder – and immediately distinguishes the person who does so from family members and other care providers who have been pushing the patient's face into what is wrong with her behavior.

For example, the opening statement of one 16-year-old made her position quite clear, in the form of a challenge to the name of our clinic:

> Why do you call this the 'Center for Cognitive-*Behavioral* Therapy'? I hate it when people focus on my *behavior* – that means making me eat things I don't want to eat, and trying to get me fat. No one can make me do anything I don't want to do – at least not for very long.

The therapist's response was not deliberately paradoxical, but direct and truthful:

> We call it 'Cognitive-Behavioral' because we care both about what you think *and* what you do. But you are quite right – in the long run, what happens about food and weight is totally in your hands. So let's start talking about what you *do* want. What matters to *you*?

The clinician should always begin by inquiring about the *advantages* of being anorexic. This order of inquiry has a disinhibiting effect on patients' subsequent willingness to divulge the more guarded *disadvantages* of their disorder. When not forced into a corner by a confrontational or condescending expert, most patients are surprisingly forthcoming about their own reservations. Their disclosures help us map out some common ground, as we identify a subset of issues (such as depression, food preoccupation, and fear of losing control) that we can already agree it would be desirable to change.

Within the list generated by the patient, internal inconsistencies are always evident. For example, the patient may identify 'indifference to food' as an asset of her disorder, while nominating food preoccupation and episodes of binge eating as some of its most distressing symptoms. Discrepancies can be juxtaposed by the clinician without editorial commentary:

> So on the one hand, you find thinness desirable in part because people pay more attention to you when you are skinny, and (at least at first) you received a lot of compliments on your weight loss. Yet on the other hand, you also wish that people would stop bothering you about this issue, and you've noticed that you no longer care whether they admire or disapprove of the way you look.

Again, the clinician must be careful not to sound smug or challenging. There should be no sense that the patient has been trapped into contradicting herself; rather, the tone should be one of genuine interest in trying to understand her own predicament from the inside. Very gently, the clinician can begin encouraging the patient to consider the possibility that the 'pros' and 'cons' of her eating disorder are inextricably linked. She will never be able to attain the benefits she attributes to her eating disorder without incurring its significant liabilities. In fact, the ratio of positive and negative effects tends to grow less favorable over time.

The functional emphasis also involves prompting clients to consider the short-term versus long-term consequences of their behavior by projecting the status quo into the future (Garner and Bemis, 1982; Pike et al., 1996). Clients are encouraged to begin exploring the possibility that different coping mechanisms might yield the same or better benefits at lower price. Most of the patient's goals – such as self-control, emotional stability, and respect from others – are separable from the means she has relied on to achieve them; it is the means of food restriction and low weight that cannot be detached from their aversive consequences. The clinician can affirm the appropriateness of the patient's objectives while encouraging her to broaden and refine her repertoire of techniques for goal attainment.

Philosophical

The fourth emphasis for enhancing motivation is a focus on the relationship between the patient's personal values and her eating disorder. Many anorexic patients associate the symptoms of restrictive eating and weight loss with higher-order beliefs about moral virtue, asceticism, and self-control (Vitousek and Hollon, 1990). Thus, their resistance to change can be principled as well as functional or fear-driven. Clinicians face a different therapeutic problem when patients are saying not only 'I like doing this' or 'I fear doing anything else' or 'I don't know how to do anything else,' as in other psychiatric conditions, but 'It is *right* for me to be anorexic.' Rather than challenging these interpretations directly, clinicians can work within the patient's own system of values to reframe the meaning of her behavior.

For example, one of our anorexic patients expressed pride in her food refusal and compulsive exercise as proofs of her superior strength and self-discipline. The therapist agreed that many people find such behaviors both admirable and exceedingly difficult to practice consistently – but went on to explore a curious paradox for the client as an individual. For her, the acts of eating high-calorie foods and *not* going to the gym actually required considerably more courage and fortitude. In contrast, each time she chose to eat less or exercise more, she was taking the 'easy road,' while crediting herself (and often being credited by others) for virtues she was not entitled to claim through these actions.

Once more, it should be underscored that the therapist did not draw out this contradiction for the purpose of dismissing or disparaging the patient's beliefs. Instead, this conflict was elicited through a series of open-ended questions and summaries that led the patient herself to the conclusion that she was not acting in accordance with her own value system. Up to this point, she had viewed the prospect of recovering from her eating disorder as one of 'giving in' and 'going soft'; recasting the effort to control her symptoms as 'brave' and 'powerful' transformed the meaning of change for this fiercely moralistic client.

Because the central problem in outpatient treatment is converting the work of change into the client's choice, clinicians should be closely attuned to opportunities to invoke her own most cherished values to that purpose. This process is highly idiosyncratic, as it draws on the tenets incorporated into each patient's moral code. For example, one of our clients had a strong allegiance to her identity as a scientist. In most domains, with the notable exception of food/weight concerns, she was committed to being rational and empirically minded. Her therapist repeatedly invoked scientific principles (such as falsifiability, reliability, and avoidance of tautological thinking) when encouraging her to re-examine the premises of her eating disorder. A second patient endorsed a radically different world view, attaching importance to being artistic, 'natural,' and 'in touch with the rhythms of the universe.' For this client, an emphasis on the scientific method would have been alienating rather than persuasive. Instead, her therapist gently focused her attention on the dissonance between the value she attached to being 'natural' and her attempt to impose artificial control over eating and weight.

If the process of enlisting the patient as an active participant in change is the most formidable challenge of outpatient treatment, therapy must not stall out at the level of discussing ideals and beliefs. Preliminary decisions to explore different ways of living must be put into practice, in spite of persistent uncertainty. Ambivalence is best resolved through direct experience rather than abstract discussion. The outpatient treatment of anorexic patients will fail if they do not proceed to *do* that which they find frightening.

The problem of managing eating and weight

Research has established that refeeding in the hospital is a fairly simple technical problem that has been solved. The intervention clearly *works*, at least for the short-term objective of weight restoration. Specific procedures have been established to make it work more consistently and/or more rapidly (e.g. Touyz and Beumont, 1997). Indeed, it works so well that existing protocols can produce rates of weight gain that match or exceed the maximum consistent with responsible and compassionate care (Bemis, 1987).

The fact that the gains produced often begin eroding within a day or two of discharge could be seen as an indictment of hospital-centered models. On the other hand, it holds disturbing implications about the effectiveness of clinic-based care as well, as most patients are participating in outpatient therapy while their relapses unfold (as they may also have been at the time of the decline that first occasioned admission to hospital). If more of the burden of treatment must shift to outpatient settings, better ways of supporting weight gain and maintenance outside the ward are crucial.

In the hospital, nursing staff are largely responsible for the unenviable tasks of monitoring intake, weight, exercise, and compensatory tactics, and for enforcing any contingencies established with reference to these. Meal planning is managed by nutritional services, with measured portions served up on trays from the hospital kitchen. Within the context of clinic-based care, however, the patient must assume responsibility for *self*-monitoring target behaviors, as well as for securing and serving her own food, while the therapist ordinarily takes over the assessment of weight and both parties participate in meal planning. Contingency management is seldom relevant to outpatient treatment of adult cases, as there are none to apply – other than the prospect of hospitalization that always lurks in the background. Patients do not want to eat more or differently; many clinicians lack the training or inclination to devote much time in therapy to discussing fat grams and basic food groups. The frequent failure of outpatient treatment is unsurprising when both parties give into the temptation to avoid dealing with the management of eating and weight (Garner, 1985).

Rate of gain

Both extremely low weight and ongoing weight loss are incompatible with outpatient care. If patients are substantially underweight at treatment entry, clear guidelines for minimum weight and expectations for rate of gain should be defined (Garner *et al.*, 1997). If current weight is stable and at least somewhat above an individually-identified critical level, our own terms for outpatient treatment include an agreement that the patient will eat and drink regularly and a zero-tolerance policy for any weight loss trends. In most cases, we do not define a specific required rate of gain or specify an exact target weight. We do set the expectation that weight will show an upward trend at least until patients have surpassed the threshold for menstruation.

A variety of specific outpatient contracts is defensible. The invariant principle is that because the starved organism is not only medically imperiled but cognitively and affectively impaired, there are sharp limits to the therapeutic progress that can be achieved at low weight. Stability of weight is also an important factor, as the disruption caused by a rapid decline from 105 lbs. to 95 lbs. is greater than that associated with maintenance of a steady 85 lbs. For patients who must gain weight to remain eligible for outpatient therapy, a rate of 8 oz. to 1 lb. per week is usually a reasonable goal (in contrast to the 2 to 3 lbs. that can be achieved in hospital) (American Psychiatric Association, 2000). Even more modest targets may be desirable when working with chronic adult patients, for whom zealous treatment approaches are generally contraindicated (Goldner *et al.*, 1997; Strober, 2004; Yager, 2002).

Target weight

The identification of an eventual target weight range is a tricky business in the context of any inpatient or outpatient treatment for anorexia. Although the construct of 'set point' weight (Keesey, 1993) is excessively deterministic, the evidence suggests that individuals do have different 'settling points' for weight maintenance as a result of interactions between their genes and current environments (Pinel, 2000; Wirtshafter and Davis, 1977). The target weight range for each individual should be broadly consistent with a level she can maintain without excessive dietary restraint. Although it is impossible to predict this zone with any precision while the patient is still restricting and/or over-exercising, it should be stressed that the basic goal of 'normal eating' will certainly result in some gain for these deliberately weight-suppressed individuals. Factors such as premorbid weight levels, menstrual threshold weight, and family weight history all aid in the prediction of probable weight.

Target weight range should be defined as plus or minus 2 lbs. around a central number. Ranges should be established with sensitivity to avoiding spans that subsume a weight of symbolic significance for the patient. The distress occasioned by crossing this line repeatedly in the course of normal weight fluctuation predictably results in a decision to suppress below that level.

Weighing

Weight must be monitored regularly. Although it may be uncomfortable or inconvenient for non-medical therapists, weight checks should occur immediately before each session. As Garner *et al.* (1997) note, the appropriate session agenda for a patient who reports cheerfully that 'Everything is going very well' but has lost several pounds in the past week would be quite different from that indicated for another patient who makes the same comment in the context of weight gain or weight stability.

Since clinic-based treatment requires patients to be participants in the process of change rather than its objects, weighing procedures that imply mistrust are counterproductive. Asking patients to void their bladders or empty their pockets before stepping on the scale is incongruous when patients are being entrusted with so many other critical aspects of their own care. We acknowledge and sympathize with the natural temptation to cheat in defense of symptoms. We tell patients that it would be neither surprising nor consequential if they occasionally found themselves resorting to minor stratagems such as drinking an extra glass or two of water before coming to sessions. But we note that extreme or routine attempts to obscure true weight status are unfortunate – not because they represent betrayals of the therapist, but because they deprive patients of the opportunity to receive more accurate feedback and advice (Garner *et al.*, 1997). When clinicians do suspect that weight is being falsified, they should discuss the issue sympathetically but directly, and ask the patient to problem-solve alternative means for handling the problem.

During the early stages of therapy, when the patient's anxiety about weight gain is high and her sophistication about weight fluctuation is low, it is desirable to schedule appointments at approximately the same time of day, and to suggest that patients wear comparable clothing. Clients need psychoeducational information about the normal variability around essentially stable weight, because of factors such as water retention, hormonal shifts, and time of day. Criteria should be established for detecting interpretable trends (such as three successive occasions on which weight increases or decreases occur or persist) to forestall the tendency for either patients or clinicians to overreact to minor fluctuations.

Patients should be asked to predict their weight before stepping on the scale. The data accumulated on the extent, direction, and correlates of their errors in estimation can be used to illustrate the problem of subjectivity in judging weight. Any comments about weight status or weight change by clinicians or other staff members should be framed with great sensitivity to patients' systematic misinterpretation of these remarks. In particular, care providers should never appear to be gloating about weight gain.

Patients should be strongly discouraged from weighing themselves at home until later in therapy. Eventually, regular but infrequent self-weighing should be recommended. For these individuals, both excessive use and complete avoidance of the scale reveal a persistent, excessive concern with weight and shape (Fairburn, 1995); moreover, in the absence of objective feedback, they simply substitute more subjective standards such as 'feeling fat' to gauge their physical status.

Self-monitoring

Patients are asked to keep records of their food intake using a form similar to that described by Fairburn (1985, 1995) in CBT for bulimia nervosa. Quantities should be described in approximate and colloquial terms such as a 'large soup bowl' or a 'half piece.' Patients are dissuaded from precise measuring or weighing of food and from recording calories or fat grams. In spite of the appeal such specificity holds for both patients and professionals, it should be forsworn in the collection of self-monitoring data because it reinforces rigid patterns of food selection (Wilson and Vitousek, 1999).

Compliance with self-monitoring is often much more difficult to obtain with anorexic patients than with bulimic patients (Garner *et al.*, 1997). Patients' most consistent objection is the claim that recording dietary intake increases their preoccupation with food and weight. It may be useful to propose an experiment in which the patient keeps track of these variables on randomly selected days when she does and does not record her intake (Wilson and Vitousek, 1999). Even if her perception is correct, it should be emphasized that any increase in already high levels of concern will be temporary, while the changed eating patterns that self-monitoring can support offer the ultimate solution to such intrusive thoughts. Careful record-keeping can also provide some immediate benefits that are consonant with the patient's own goals, such as a greater sense of predictability and control during the process of necessary weight gain.

Meal planning

Patients with long histories of restrictive eating need considerable structure and support in planning their dietary intake. In the early stages of treatment, they are encouraged to eat preplanned menus at designated hours regardless of circumstances or appetite. The key to meal planning is the systematic addition of increased quantities and types of food while carefully monitoring weight.

The principles of structured eating for anorexic patients are described in Garner *et al.* (1997). The procedures overlap with those recommended in CBT for bulimia nervosa (Fairburn, 1985, 1995; Wilson *et al.*, 1997), but there are distinct differences driven by the problems faced with this patient population. It is one sort of proposition to persuade a bulimic patient who wants to stop bingeing to rearrange the distribution of her food intake, so that she becomes less vulnerable to overeating while maintaining the same weight level. It is quite a different matter to persuade a restricting anorexic patient to eat larger quantities of foods that she fears and shuns, with the deliberate intent of gaining weight (Garner *et al.*, 1997).

The clinician should work collaboratively with the patient to set up specific plans for what, when, and how she will eat. Her job thereafter is to implement the plan, following it mechanically (indeed, almost ritualistically), without regard to sensations of hunger and fullness that have become distorted by her fears and her history of food deprivation. In the initial stages of treatment, patients require the reassurance of structured eating. Indeed, in view of what is known about the likelihood of overeating in the aftermath of starvation (and the development of bulimia after chronic dieting or anorexia nervosa), patients are correct to fear loss of control over appetite as they take steps toward recovery. They are also entitled to expect help in managing it, and the encouragement of structured eating is an important part of that external support.

In outpatient treatment, meal planning begins gradually, working within the patient's own framework of food choices while systematically intro- ducing larger amounts and avoided food types. If proposed changes are too radical, patients will not put them into practice; if patients are scolded for their lack of compliance, they begin to lie. Anorexic individuals should never be punished for accurate descriptions of undesirable behaviors, as it is well established that in such circumstances most people are more disposed to change what they *say* they have done than to modify what they actually *do* (Wilson and Vitousek, 1999). At that point, the spirit of collaborative experimentation on which successful outpatient treatment depends breaks down. Therefore, the art of meal planning involves finding the appropriate balance between steady pressure for change and the provision of a reassuring context of stability.

The key construct for outpatient care is keeping patients in an intermediate zone of distress in which they are neither comfortable nor panic-stricken. Although anorexia nervosa is more complicated than other avoidance-based disorders such as agoraphobia (Bemis, 1983), it clearly does include phobic elements that should be treated through classic exposure principles. Fears of specific foods and situations are unusual sorts of phobias, because in many cases they were deliberately acquired to support the control of weight; for this reason, some patients may not *wish* to resolve their own anxiety. Secondarily, however, these cultivated fears can become so distressing that they interfere with behavioral changes that patients have decided to attempt.

We often use the graphic shown in Figure 10.1 when explaining the ration- ale for exposure to patients. The 'green zone' in the middle represents the relative safety and comfort provided by the status quo: familiar territory, established patterns, rigid rules for food selection and consumption. There is no hope for change as long as patients stay crouched in the centre, no matter

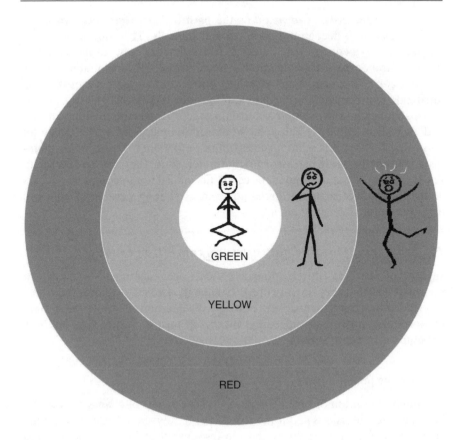

Figure 10.1 Body.

how much insight they may develop about the desirability of living differently. The outer circle or 'red zone' represents intense, sustained exposure to
situations and experiences the patient finds terrifying. The target we strive
for in outpatient therapy is the 'yellow zone' between these extremes. The
patient is on track when she remains in the region that is 'tough but tolerable,'
venturing outside her accustomed habits without triggering the extreme distress that might prompt her to retreat into the false sense of security provided
by her symptoms. Consistent with exposure principles, the good news is
that the accumulation of experience in the 'yellow' zone expands both of the
central circles. To remain in the targeted area over time, patients must take
on progressively more difficult challenges; however, the territory they have
already claimed becomes easier to occupy over time.

The construct depicted in Figure 10.1 catches on well with anorexic individuals, in part because it appeals to many patients' own orientation toward
testing their strength and disdaining choices they regard as 'cheap' or 'easy.'

The exercise reconstrues *anorexia* as the path of least resistance, while the work of *change* is recognized as brave and difficult. The concentric circles diagram is also a concise way to describe the difference between the nature of inpatient and outpatient treatment. For many patients, the hospital represents the 'red zone.' Because of the external control and support it can provide, inpatient treatment makes it possible to sustain high levels of exposure, so that patients can begin eating a normal range of foods almost immediately and experience rapid weight gain. Whatever the merits of that strategy on an inpatient basis, it is seldom successful in outpatient settings. When therapists attempt to push patients into the outer zone, they flee to the safety represented by the status quo in the center (as indeed not uncommonly occurs at the moment of hospital discharge, even after long periods of enforced exposure in the outermost circle).

The problems of insufficient structure, control, and support

In spite of our best efforts, anorexic patients are sometimes so invested in their patterns that they are unwilling to make the choice to change them – or so terrified that they are unable to implement a decision to try. Before settling on hospital admission for refeeding, alternative means of increasing levels of structure, control, or support should be considered.

Involving the family

Although the option of turning parents into the agents of change is available in some cases, decisions about the role of the family should usually be made at the start of treatment rather than in response to difficulties encountered thereafter.

Most family therapy approaches for anorexia nervosa (Dare and Eisler, 1992; Lask, 1992; Lock *et al.*, 2001; Minuchin *et al.*, 1978) advocate that parents unite to take charge of the patient's safety, insisting with 'intransigent but sympathetic firmness' that she must eat (Dare and Eisler, 1992). Although psychological rather than physical force is recommended, during some therapy sessions parents may end up holding the child and pushing food into her mouth, with the clinician's encouragement and support. As noted earlier, there are few data to support (or refute) the view that this *specific* approach is indicated for anorexic patients, although family involvement in some form almost certainly contributes to success in the treatment of non-chronic adolescents.

Our own approach to outpatient therapy is inconsistent with the family control model (although it should be emphasized that we work only with patients who are 14 or older). We share some of the concerns expressed by others (e.g. Vandereycken, 1987a) about the potential for misuse of crisis-inducing methods of family therapy, and concur that family therapy should be viewed as one part of a more comprehensive treatment approach. Advocates of the family control model agree that it is inappropriate for older adolescents and adults, identifying different suggested cut-off ages. No single correct answer is likely to emerge concerning whether it is preferable to direct parents to 'take over' the anorexic child's eating behavior or to stay out of the daily management of intake while providing other forms of support to the work of change. Indications for these alternatives certainly correlate with the child's age, but other factors such as chronicity, the specific dynamics of the case, and the characteristics of the family should also be reviewed. The widely recommended principle of advising parents to 'take control' with reference to younger but not older patients devolves in part from developmental considerations, and in part from pragmatism. As the successful parents of any adolescent usually learn, it is tactically inadvisable to threaten what one cannot deliver; in some instances, more ground may be gained through skillful appeals to maturity and autonomy than through the exercise of external control.

Whatever course is chosen, the clinician, patient, and family should all be clear on which model is being adopted. In our experience, the least successful strategy is a patchwork approach that stitches together bits of coercive control over eating and weight with bits of emphasis on independence in the same domains. If a decision has been made to foster the patient's sense of responsibility for change, the clinician should do everything possible to support and encourage her sense of self-determination and self-efficacy, with strong reinforcement for behaviors consistent with these objectives.

In such instances, families are asked to stay out of the management of food, eating, and weight. With reference to the eating disorder, their job is to get their child into treatment, then do the best they can (with the therapist's and patient's counsel) to provide maximal support and minimal interference. In particular, they are asked to avoid all attempts to micromanage food intake or to police vomiting and exercise (although they are not discouraged from expressions of concern).

Many parents are understandably anxious about ending their close involvement with their child's eating behavior, and need assurances that safety factors will be built in through the clinician's careful attention to weight status. We also remind the parents of older adolescents that in any event the control of these issues will be entirely in the patient's hands within a few years. In our view, it is often preferable to begin treating her accordingly rather than exerting power that all parties realize will soon be unavailable.

The clinician should make clear that he or she is not advocating abdication of parental responsibility over all matters. One mother told us that, in accordance with our recommendation to foster more personal responsibility in her adolescent daughter, she was allowing the 16-year-old to go running at 5:30 in the morning. We asked what the mother's policy would have been if her child were not anorexic. She immediately replied, 'I wouldn't let her do it! I'm worried about her safety, and concerned that she will get too tired before school.' We clarified that these considerations were parental, not therapeutic. If her daughter had *not* developed difficulties in the domains of eating, weight, and exercise, this mother would have vetoed pre-dawn running, without hesitation. To allow the activity *because* her child had become anorexic would be inconsistent with the principles we espouse, on multiple levels.

In fact, our answer to many parental questions that are directly related to eating is also 'What would you be doing if your daughter were *not* anorexic?' If family custom allows individuals to eat at different times, she should be permitted to do so; if it is family practice to alternate who chooses menus, prepares meals, or selects a restaurant, she should take her usual place in the rotation rather than dictating the family's choices through her own fears or preferences. There are a few exceptions. Family members should refrain from all but medically urgent dieting, and should not discuss calories, 'bad foods,' or 'feeling fat' in the patient's presence (or, preferably, anywhere else). They should learn sensitive ways of declining to cooperate with patients' reassurance-seeking behaviors (e.g. interrogating others with variants on the question 'Do you think I'm fat?'). In general, however, the anorexic individual should be treated 'normally' whenever possible, and her symptoms should be neither punished nor rewarded by unnecessary deviations from family rules and customs.

In certain circumstances, it is appropriate and responsible for parents to play a role in the enforcement of contingencies identified by the therapist. Almost without exception, any plans involving negative reinforcement should reflect lawful relationships between the problem behavior and the privilege or activity being withheld. For safety reasons, individuals who are experiencing episodes of dizziness from low weight, vomiting, and/or fasting should not be permitted to drive; significantly underweight patients should not participate in demanding sports regimens unless they are willing to increment their intake and weight sufficiently to protect their physical well-being.

Increased session frequency

Records reviews in the United States (Striegel-Moore *et al.*, 2000) and in one service area of the United Kingdom (Button *et al.*, 1997) suggest that, on average, anorexic patients receive remarkably few outpatient therapy sessions per year, although there is substantial variability across individual cases. Severely ill patients tend to obtain much higher-density outpatient treatment after discharge from hospital (Grigoriadis *et al.*, 2001). In most systems, however, there are economic or structural impediments to seeing patients more frequently than once a week, while many support substantially lower contact levels. Accordingly, the only treatment alternatives may be less than an hour per week of assistance in outpatient therapy – or the giant step up to six to twenty-four hours per day in day hospital or inpatient settings. Although a proportion of patients may respond well to relatively brief courses of treatment with spaced sessions (particularly young, recent-onset cases for whom parental structure and support are available), it is a reasonable guess that others would be best served by options intermediate to these two extremes.

As standard practice, we see anorexic patients two to three times per week for ninety-minute appointments in the early stages of treatment. Extended sessions are especially important if one care provider is responsible for all aspects of treatment. Perhaps we are inefficient – but in our experience, meal planning and weight issues alone require so much focused attention at this point that weekly fifty-minute appointments are inadequate. Inevitably, coverage of either the mechanics of eating or psychological issues crucial to motivation is shortchanged. Moreover, we consider it unrealistic to expect that patients will sustain terrifying changes for seven days in the absence of feedback, encouragement, or reminders of the bases for their decision to experiment. After several months, session frequency shifts down to one to two sessions per week, tapering eventually to every second or third week over an average twelve- to eighteen-month total duration of treatment.

During periods of particular stress, session frequency may increase temporarily. Because the techniques described under the heading of 'motivation for change' are generally successful in promoting patients' investment in treatment, however, there is a risk that concentrated therapy provides some patients with an incentive to do poorly. We tell patients that increased session frequency (and sometimes other extraordinary efforts) are justified as a means of supporting brief, intense periods of *change*, but not for maintenance of the status quo. Therefore, unless patients make use of the opportunity to advance, we will drop back to the usual session spacing or recommend alternative treatments.

This deliberate use of therapeutic contact as leverage for promoting change is similar to the 'blackmail therapy' Linehan (1993) advocates for patients with borderline personality disorder. The practice may seem manipulative, but we concur with Linehan's assertion that it is instead unethical to persist in courses of action that are not working. Moreover, the conventional approach of increasing session density for the duration of 'crises' suggests a disregard for reinforcement principles from which no one is immune.

The same considerations guide other parameters of treatment as well. For example, patients are encouraged to telephone the therapist not only at moments of crisis but also to announce their triumphs or to seek brief support and problem-solving to help them cope with the anxiety caused by the completion of a challenging exercise. We do not bar patients from contacting us at times when they are distressed but have failed to follow through with structured eating. We tell them in advance, however, that on such occasions we will not discuss their distress, as it would be unproductive to devote time to anything other than strategies for getting back on track with the meal plan, in view of the well-established relationship between deprivation and both binge-eating and depression.

In vivo sessions

We make extensive use of *in vivo* therapy in routine work with anorexic patients. Such sessions can be particularly valuable for the provision of extra structure and support during difficult periods. In the very early stages of therapy, these may take the form of supervised meals with patients who are eating irregularly or extremely poorly. The purposes include assuring that the patient is consuming target meals, observing her food choices and eating habits, and assisting with intense anxiety. Clearly, sessions of this kind cannot be scheduled with sufficient frequency to replicate the meal supervision available in day hospital or inpatient settings, and should not be used for more than brief periods of intensive support.

Other types of eating sessions are focused on reintroduction of forbidden foods, exposure to avoided situations (such as fast-food restaurants), and modification of specific eating rituals or concerns (such as eating in the company of someone who appears to be dieting). *In vivo* sessions may also be scheduled for grocery shopping, trying on clothing, or going to the gym. Patients are of course encouraged to experiment with new behaviors on their own; however, *in vivo* sessions can be invaluable when patients are unwilling to make changes or are too anxious to attempt the more difficult exercises that *in vivo* sessions can accommodate.

In vivo therapy requires particular skills and cautions (Vitousek, 1998). The quality of these sessions should fall somewhere between a typical in-office therapy appointment and a social occasion. *In vivo* therapists should be prepared to switch back and forth between modes during the course of a session; however, even when the therapeutic mode is indicated, it is usually a sort of 'therapy lite.' This tone is desirable both because the patient's privacy must be preserved in the public places where sessions typically occur, and because one of the major purposes of this treatment element is the reintroduction of social eating to patients who usually consume their rations in isolation and with deadly seriousness. While it is desirable for primary therapists to have at least a few *in vivo* sessions with their clients, we often select a different clinician as the *in vivo* therapist if such work is a prominent part of treatment, because of the delicacy of shifting between the styles appropriate to therapy versus *in vivo* sessions. *In vivo* therapists should model unrestrained eating, and must be comfortable handling the personal questions about eating and weight that arise in these situations.

The objectives for each session should be outlined collaboratively in advance. Patients are asked to anticipate likely problems and to make predictions about the outcome of the experience. If patients balk or become distraught during sessions, therapists should use 'gentle herding' rather than debate or bullying, reminding patients of their own better judgment outside the frightening situation and reiterating the experimental nature of the approach.

Unfortunately and, we suspect, irrationally, many national and private health care programs will support neither the scheduling of frequent therapy sessions nor the provision of *in vivo* treatment. Creative solutions can sometimes be devised, such as the use of trained student assistants as *in vivo* therapists. Eventually, the collection of data on the contribution of such support to decreased need for inpatient care may be persuasive in modifying such policies, for economic reasons alone. For approximately half the cost of a single month of inpatient care followed by eleven months of weekly therapy, patients could be provided with a year of four outpatient sessions per week, divided equally between psychotherapy and meal-planning or *in vivo* exposure sessions. We do not know whether such intensive support would prevent hospitalization or produce comparable final outcomes, but it is reasonable to test an approach that seems better suited to the well-studied course of this disorder than crisis-driven models of care (Wilson *et al.*, 2000).

Partial hospital

In communities where specialized day hospital programs are available, they offer an appealing alternative to inpatient care in cases where additional structure and support are indicated. The model program of this kind was developed in Toronto (see Chapter 13), and has demonstrated beneficial effects for the majority of anorexic patients eligible for participation (Kaplan and Olmsted, 1997; Piran and Kaplan, 1990). Other pilot programs have been described for community mental health centers, some of which operate during the late afternoon and evening hours so that patients can continue working or attending school (Zastowny *et al.*, 1991). The clinical and financial advantages of such compromise programs seem obvious (Gerlinghoff *et al.*, 1998; Williamson *et al.*, 2001; Zipfel *et al.*, 2002). Little information is available, however, on the longer-term outcomes of anorexic patients treated in these settings (Zipfel *et al.*, 2002); moreover, the population base they require limits their use to patients who are living in metropolitan areas or who are able to afford several-month stays in the vicinity (sometimes in partially subsidized housing arranged through these programs).

Brief hospital admission

Some experts have advocated the use of 'strategic admissions' which are planned to provide brief interruption and redirection for patients who are doing poorly (e.g. Andersen, 1995; Garner and Needleman, 1997; Kennedy *et al.*, 1992; Treasure *et al.*, 1995b). Rather than attempting a full course of refeeding, these hospital stays set modest goals such as halting cycles of intractable vomiting or progressive weight loss, or giving a jump start to more intensive, symptom-focused outpatient treatment. No data are yet available on the effectiveness of *intentionally* short hospital admissions for these purposes, but they seem consistent with the financial realities of health care systems and the therapeutic desirability of clinic-based care.

Advantages of outpatient therapy

The advantages of increased patient autonomy and responsibility for change

By default, as noted earlier, individual outpatient therapy must enlist the patient as the principal agent of change. The approach that we use places strong emphasis on intent, choice, active decision-making, and personal responsibility. Because control issues are so central to anorexia nervosa (e.g. Fairburn *et al.*, 1999; Garner and Bemis, 1982; Lawrence, 1984; Slade, 1982), it is especially important to persuade the patient that she can acquire even more powerful strategies to replace the artificial system of self-regulation she has constructed through her disorder. This approach markedly decreases resistance to change, as therapeutic energy is directed toward transforming the meaning of symptoms so that the patient herself rejects the disorder, rather than toward quashing the expression of patterns she continues to defend. The strategy requires a different set of skills and sometimes considerably more patience than external control models. It should not be confused, however, with a passive approach that listens, reflects, and waits until the patient is 'ready' to change; rather, it is an intense, focused campaign to increase the odds that she will choose to change – and will then follow through.

Our experience has been that behavioral changes accomplished in this way are seldom reversed, as they are viewed as personal decisions rather than temporary defeats. We think it misleading to characterize the common pattern of weight loss after hospital discharge as a 'high rate of relapse.' Patients whose symptoms were momentarily suppressed by environmental contingencies cannot be considered in retreat from 'recoveries' that were never accomplished (Orimoto and Vitousek, 1992). Brief hospitalization is sometimes required for starving patients who are unable to receive or respond to efforts to enlist their participation; however, we always view the imposition of external control as a regrettable interruption of our primary object of helping the patient assume responsibility for her own life. Such suspensions should be kept as minimal and temporary as is consistent with the patient's safety.

The advantage of decreased exposure to the sick role

Outpatient therapy reduces the risk that patients will crystallize their identity as anorexic and, more generally, as disturbed individuals dependent on professional care. Particularly at the age when most patients develop anorexia nervosa, there is strong suggestive evidence that symptomatic behavior such as disordered eating, self-harm, and suicidal ideation can spread through social contagion. These dramatic patterns are also easily romanticized by isolated and unhappy individuals. Most of our patients who engage in self-mutilation acquired this behavior through observation (and during periods of intense distress) while in hospital. It is commonplace for patients to describe the community of other eating-disordered individuals encountered in treatment settings as a secret sorority united by opposition to the oppressor; at the same time, exposure to other patients can inflate the standards for thinness and heighten competitiveness. Hornbacher's personal account describes these dynamics with unusual candor:

> On the surface, you're doing this companionably, you're a friggin' unstoppable dieting army and you'll all go down together. On the underside, you're all competing with one another to be the thinnest, most controlled, least weak, and you have your own private crusade on which no one can join you, lest they be as fucked up as you.
>
> (Hornbacher, 1998, p. 110)

Our concern about these dynamics contributes to reservations about day hospital as well as inpatient programs, although again the need for intensive intervention sometimes trumps these considerations. Clinicians should be aware, however, that hospitalization can be psychologically as well as economically costly, and should remain attentive to the risk of iatrogenic complications (Garner, 1985; Gowers et al., 2000; Vandereycken, 1987b; Zipfel et al., 2002).

The advantage of continuity of care

In many settings, inpatient or partial hospital programs are structurally and functionally separate from outpatient programs. Ongoing therapy is often terminated abruptly at the time of admission. When patients are discharged weeks or months later, there may be little or no carryover of information, treatment principles, or helping relationships from the ward.

Such breaks are disadvantageous for many reasons. One problem is the implication that the management of eating and weight is separable from the 'real work' of psychotherapy. The eating disorder field has long debated the merits of splitting versus integrating these foci (e.g. Beumont et al., 1997; Garner et al., 1997; Powers and Powers, 1984; Rampling, 1978; Wilson and Agras, 2001). Our biases are apparent throughout the chapter. Across outpatient, day hospital, and residential settings, we believe that the obvious interdependence of these issues in patients' own experience should be reflected in the design of cohesive, uninterrupted programs of care. Pragmatically, this is often most easily accomplished when shifting needs for structure and support in the individual case can be accommodated by changes in the intensity of outpatient care, rather than through the wholesale substitution of one treatment program for another.

The advantage of the natural environment

An obvious asset of outpatient treatment is that the changes accomplished do not have to be transferred anywhere – they are already taking place in the context of the patient's real life. Daily experience provides numerous opportunities to identify and cope with stressful situations and to practice new patterns of behavior (Kaye et al., 1996). The clinician and patient need not speculate about whether the skills she is acquiring will generalize. As they collaborate in designing experiments for her to implement, they receive immediate feedback from her successes and failures. While the natural environment is crowded with more pressures and distractions than the enclosed world of the ward, it also offers more opportunities for learning to replace the eating disorder with satisfactions derived from relationships, school or work, and recreational activities.

Conclusion

Outpatient management will never eliminate the need for hospitalization in some cases of anorexia nervosa. We believe, however, that changes in the way outpatient treatment is conceptualized and delivered would yield clinical as well as economic benefits. We do *not* contend that 'less is more' (or even the same) in the management of this condition. Delays in initiating treatment are associated with chronicity (Agras et al., 2004; Steinhausen, 1995); *laissez-faire* approaches can unquestionably contribute to morbidity and mortality. Outpatient programs must learn ways – and be provided with means – to do *more* as resources shift away from routine or extended inpatient care.

The field is years from accumulating the masses of data that would allow us to base decisions about cost-effective treatment on validated stepped-care protocols (Garner and Needleman, 1996, 1997; Wilson et al., 2000). A thoughtful review of existing evidence, however, would aid in the development of research while guiding treatment planning in the interim. Some features of anorexia nervosa provide a rational basis for eliminating lower steps on the continuum of care. Although self-help and guided self-help approaches have proven beneficial in the treatment of bulimia nervosa and binge eating disorder, they have little to offer in the treatment of patients with anorexia nervosa (Wilson et al., 2000). Indeed, self-help programs written for other eating disorders typically caution underweight individuals not to 'try this at home' without professional assistance (Cooper, 1993; Fairburn, 1995). Group and psychoeducational strategies are seldom recommended as stand-alone treatments. Primary care physicians cannot provide patients significant benefit by prescribing medication, as current evidence indicates that drugs contribute minimally to the resolution of this disorder (Agras *et al.*, 2004; Garfinkel and Walsh, 1997; Johnson *et al.*, 1996; Walsh, 2002). Pending the discovery of a dramatically different approach, the treatment of anorexia nervosa is likely to remain a costly proposition requiring specialized medical, psychological, and nutritional services.

We see no ethical or clinical basis, however, for deferring research on the higher levels of the stepped-care hierarchy, including comparisons of inpatient and outpatient care and planned variations in the length and intensity of treatment. Such investigations should be favored both by those convinced of the merits of routine or prolonged residential treatment and by those reluctant to fund it. Because of the severe physical complications associated with anorexia nervosa, there is less incentive for private and governmental agencies to deny costly psychological treatments if these can forestall medical admissions.

Our own experience suggests that many severe or chronic patients for whom hospitalization was automatically recommended in the past do well in the kind of outpatient approach we advocate here: motivational, symptom-focused, intensive individual treatment. Younger, recent-onset patients may respond as well or better to the family therapy models whose effectiveness has already been demonstrated. The optimal approach to treating the range of patients with anorexia nervosa can be identified only on the basis of empirical data that will take years to accumulate. In the meantime, a thoughtful restructuring of outpatient programs to better address the management problems posed by this disorder should yield clinical as well as economic benefits in the majority of cases.

References

Agras, W. S., Brandt, H. A., Bulik, C. M., Dolan-Sewell, R., Fairburn, C. G., Halmi, K. A., *et al.* (2004) Report of the National Institutes of Health workshop on overcoming barriers to treatment research in anorexia nervosa. *International Journal of Eating Disorders*, 35, 509–521.

American Psychiatric Association (2000) Practice guidelines for the treatment of patients with eating disorders (Rev.) *American Journal of Psychiatry*, 157 (Suppl. 1), 1–39.

Andersen, A. E. (1995) Sequencing treatment decisions: cooperation or conflict between therapist and patient. In G. Szmukler, C. Dare, and J. Treasure (eds), *Handbook of Eating Disorders: Theory, Treatment, and Research*. Chichester: Wiley, pp. 363–379.

Ball, J. and Mitchell, P. (2004) A randomized controlled study of cognitive behavior therapy and behavioral family therapy for anorexia nervosa patients. *Eating Disorders: The Journal of Treatment and Prevention*, 12, 303–314.

Baran, S. A., Weltzin, T. E., and Kaye, W. H. (1995) Low discharge weight and outcome in anorexia nervosa. *American Journal of Psychiatry*, 152, 1070–1072.

Bell, L. (1999) The spectrum of psychological problems in people with eating disorders: an analysis of 30 eating disordered patients treated with cognitive analytic therapy. *Clinical Psychology and Psychotherapy*, 6, 29–38.

Bemis, K. M. (1983) A comparison of functional relationships in anorexia nervosa and phobia. In P. L. Darby, P. E. Garfinkel, D. M. Garner, and D. V. Coscina (eds), *Anorexia Nervosa: Recent Developments in Research* (pp. 403–415). New York: Alan R. Liss.

Bemis, K. M. (1987) The present status of operant conditioning for the treatment of anorexia nervosa. *Behavior Modification*, 11, 432–463.

Bemporad, J. R. and Herzog, D. B. (eds) (1989) *Psychoanalysis and Eating Disorders*. New York: Guilford Press.

Ben-Tovim, D. I., Walker, K., Gilchrist, P., Freeman, R., Kalucy, R., and Esterman, A. (2001) Outcome in patients with eating disorders: a 5-year study. *Lancet*, 357, 1254–1257.

Beumont, P. J. V., Russell, J. D., and Touyz, S. W. (1993) Treatment of anorexia nervosa. *Lancet*, 341, 1635–1640.

Beumont, P. J. V., Beumont, C. C., Touyz, S. W., and Williams, H. (1997) Nutritional counseling and supervised exercise. In D. M. Garner and P. E. Garfinkel (eds), *Handbook of Treatment for Eating Disorders* (2nd edn) (pp. 178–187). New York: Guilford Press.

Brown, C. and Jasper, K. (eds) (1993) *Consuming Passions: Feminist Approaches to Weight Preoccupation and Eating Disorders* (pp. 176–194). Toronto: Second Story Press.

Bruch, H. (1973) *Eating Disorders: Obesity, Anorexia Nervosa, and the Person Within*. New York: Basic Books.

Button, E. J., Marshall, P., Shinkwin, R., Black, S. H., and Palmer, R. L. (1997) One hundred referrals to an eating disorders service: progress and service consumption over a 2–4 year period. *European Eating Disorders Review*, 5, 47–63.

Cairns, J. C., Phillips-Ward, C., Johnson, L. L., and Pinzon, J. L. (1999) Paper presented at the 4th London International Conference on Eating Disorders, London.

Channon, S., de Silva, P., Hemsley, D., and Perkins, R. (1989) A controlled trial of cognitive-behavioural and behavioural treatment of anorexia nervosa. *Behaviour Research and Therapy*, 27, 529–535.

Commerford, M. C., Licinio, J., and Halmi, K. A. (1997) Guidelines for discharging eating disorder inpatients. *Eating Disorders*, 5, 69–74.

Cooper, P. J. (1993) *Bulimia Nervosa and Binge Eating: A Guide to Recovery*. New York: New York University Press.

Crisp, A. H. (1980) *Anorexia Nervosa: Let Me Be*. London: Academic Press.

Crisp, A. H., Norton, K., Gowers, S., Halek, C., Bowyer, C., Yeldham, D., Levett, G., and Bhat, A. (1991) A controlled study of the effect of therapies aimed at adolescent and family psychopathology in anorexia nervosa. *British Journal of Psychiatry*, 159, 325–333.

Crow, S. J. and Nyman, J. A. (2004) The cost-effectiveness of anorexia nervosa treatment. *International Journal of Eating Disorders*, 35, 155–160.

Dare, C. and Crowther, C. (1995) Psychodynamic models of eating disorders. In G. Szmukler, C. Dare, and J. Treasure (eds), *Handbook of Eating Disorders: Theory, Treatment, and Research* (pp. 125–140). Chichester: Wiley.

Dare, C. and Eisler, I. (1992) Family therapy for anorexia nervosa. In P. J. Cooper and

A. Stein (eds), *Feeding Problems and Eating Disorders in Children and Adolescents* (pp. 147–160). Chur, Switzerland: Harwood Academic Publishers.

Dare, C., Eisler, I., Russell, G. F. M., and Szmukler, G. I. (1990) The clinical and theoretical impact of a controlled trial of family therapy in anorexia nervosa. *Journal of Marital and Family Therapy*, 16, 39–57.

Dare, C., Eisler, I., Russell, G., Treasure, J., and Dodge, L. (2001) Psychological therapies for adults with anorexia nervosa: randomised controlled trial of out-patient treatments. *British Journal of Psychiatry*, 178, 216–221.

De Zwaan, M. and Mitchell, J. E. (1999) Medical evaluation of the patient with an eating disorder: an overview. In P. S. Mehler and A. E. Andersen (eds), *Eating Disorders: A Guide to Medical Care and Complications* (pp. 44–62). Baltimore, MD: Johns Hopkins University Press.

Eisler, I., Dare, C., Hodes, M., Russell, G., Dodge, E., and le Grange, D. (2000) Family therapy for adolescent anorexia nervosa: the results of a controlled comparison of two family interventions. *Journal of Child Psychology and Psychiatry and Allied Disciplines*, 41, 727–736.

Fairburn, C. G. (1985) Cognitive-behavioral treatment for bulimia. In D. M. Garner and P. E. Garfinkel (eds), *Handbook of Psychotherapy for Anorexia Nervosa and Bulimia* (pp. 160–192). New York: Guilford Press.

Fairburn, C. G. (1995) *Overcoming Binge Eating*. New York: Guilford Press.

Fairburn, C. G. (2002) Interpersonal therapy for eating disorders. In C. G. Fairburn and K. D. Brownell, *Eating Disorders and Obesity: A Comprehensive Handbook* (2nd edn) (pp. 320–324). New York: Guilford Press.

Fairburn, C. G. and Brownell, K. D. (2002) *Eating Disorders and Obesity: A Comprehensive Handbook* (2nd edn). New York: Guilford Press.

Fairburn, C. G., Shafran, R., and Cooper, Z. (1999) A cognitive behavioural theory of anorexia nervosa. *Behaviour Research and Therapy*, 37, 1–13.

Fairburn, C. G., Cooper, Z., and Shafran, R. (2003) Cognitive behaviour therapy for eating disorders: a 'transdiagnostic' theory and treatment. *Behaviour Research and Therapy*, 41, 509–528.

Fallon, P., Katzman, M. A., and Wooley, S. C. (eds) (1994) *Feminist Perspectives on Eating Disorders*. New York: Guilford Press.

Feillet, F., Feillet-Coudray, C., Bard, J. M., Parra, H.-J., Favre, E., Kabuth, B., Fruchart, J.-C., and Vidailhet, M. (2000) Plasma cholesterol and endogenous cholesterol synthesis during refeeding in anorexia nervosa. *Clinica Chimica Acta*, 294, 45–56.

Feld, R., Woodside, D. B., Kaplan, A. S., Olmsted, M. P., and Carter, J. (2001) Pretreatment motivational enhancement therapy for eating disorder: a pilot study. *International Journal of Eating Disorders*, 29, 393–400.

Ferguson, C. P., La Via, M. C., Crossan, P. J., Kaye, W. H. (1999) Are serotonin reuptake inhibitors effective in underweight anorexia nervosa? *International Journal of Eating Disorders*, 25, 11–17.

Freeman, C. P. and Newton, J. R. (1992) Anorexia nervosa: what treatments are most effective? In K. Hawton and P. Cowen (eds), *Practical Problems in Clinical Psychiatry* (pp. 77–92). Oxford: Oxford University Press.

Garfinkel, P. E. and Walsh, B. T. (1997) Drug therapies. In D. M. Garner and P. E. Garfinkel (eds), *Handbook of Treatment for Eating Disorders* (2nd edn) (pp. 372–380). New York: Guilford Press.

Garner, D. M. (1985) Iatrogenesis in anorexia nervosa and bulimia nervosa. *International Journal of Eating Disorders*, 4, 701–726.

Garner, D. M. (1997) Psychoeducational principles. In D. M. Garner and P. E. Garfinkel (eds), *Handbook of Treatment for Eating Disorders* (pp. 145–177). New York: Guilford Press.

Garner, D. M. and Bemis, K. M. (1982) A cognitive-behavioral approach to anorexia nervosa. *Cognitive Therapy and Research*, 6, 123–150.

Garner, D. M. and Bemis, K. M. (1985) Cognitive therapy for anorexia nervosa. In D. M. Garner and P. E. Garfinkel (eds), *Handbook of Psychotherapy for Anorexia Nervosa and Bulimia* (pp. 107–146). New York: Guilford Press.

Garner, D. M. and Needleman, L. D. (1996) Stepped-care and decision-tree models for treating eating disorders. In J. K. Thompson (ed.), *Body Image, Eating Disorders, and Obesity* (pp. 225–252). Washington, DC: American Psychological Association.

Garner, D. M. and Needleman, L. D. (1997) Sequencing and integration of treatments. In D. M. Garner and P. E. Garfinkel (eds), *Handbook of Treatment for Eating Disorders* (2nd edn) (pp. 50–63). New York: Guilford Press.

Garner, D. M., Vitousek, K., and Pike, K. M. (1997) Cognitive behavioral therapy for anorexia nervosa. In D. M. Garner and P. E. Garfinkel (eds), *Handbook of Treatment for Eating Disorders* (2nd edn) (pp. 91–144). New York: Guilford Press.

Geist, R., Heinmaa, M., Stephens, D., Davis, R., and Katzman, D. K. (2000) Comparison of family therapy and family group psychoeducation in adolescents with anorexia nervosa. *Canadian Journal of Psychiatry*, 45, 173–178.

Geller, J. (2002) What a motivational approach is and what a motivational approach isn't: reflections and responses. *European Eating Disorders Review*, 10, 155–160.

Gerlinghoff, M., Backmund, H., and Franzen, U. (1998) Evaluation of a day treatment programme for eating disorders. *European Eating Disorders Review*, 6, 96–106.

Golden, N. H., Lanzkowsky, L., Schebendach, J., Palestro, C. J., Jacobson, M. S., and Shenker, I. R. (2002) The effect of estrogen-progestin treatment on bone mineral density in anorexia nervosa. *Journal of Pediatric and Adolescent Gynecology*, 15, 135–143.

Goldner, E. M., Birmingham, C. L., and Smye, V. (1997) Addressing treatment refusal in anorexia nervosa: clinical, ethical, and legal considerations. In D. M. Garner and P. E. Garfinkel (eds), *Handbook of Treatment for Eating Disorders* (2nd edn) (pp. 450–461). New York: Guilford Press.

Goodsitt, A. (1985) Self psychology and the treatment of anorexia nervosa. In D. M. Garner and P. E. Garfinkel (eds), *Handbook of Psychotherapy for Anorexia Nervosa and Bulimia* (pp. 55–82). New York: Guilford Press.

Goodsitt, A. (1997) Eating disorders: a self-psychological perspective. In D. M. Garner and P. E. Garfinkel (eds), *Handbook of Treatment for Eating Disorders* (2nd edn) (pp. 205–228). New York: Guilford Press.

Gowers, S. G. and Smyth, B. (2004) The impact of motivational assessment interview on initial response to treatment in adolescent anorexia nervosa. *European Eating Disorders Review*, 12, 87–93.

Gowers, S. G., Weetman, J., Shore, A., Hossain, F., and Elvins, R. (2000) Impact of hospitalization on the outcome of adolescent anorexia nervosa. *British Journal of Psychiatry*, 176, 138–141.

Grigoriadis, S., Kaplan, A., Carter, J., and Woodside, B. (2001) What treatments patients seek after inpatient care: a follow-up of 24 patients with anorexia nervosa. *Eating and Weight Disorders*, 6, 115–120.

Hall, A. and Crisp, A. H. (1987) Brief psychotherapy in the treatment of anorexia nervosa: outcome at one year. *British Journal of Psychiatry*, 151, 185–191.

Halmi, K. A. (2000) Collaborative anorexia nervosa study: 6 months results. Paper presented at the meeting of the International Conference on Eating Disorders, New York.

Hay, P., Bacaltchuk, J., Claudino, A., Ben-Tovim, D., and Yong, P. Y. (2003) Individual psychotherapy in the outpatient treatment of adults with anorexia nervosa. *The Cochrane Database of Systematic Reviews*, Issue 4. Art. No. CD003909. DOI: 10.1002/14651858.CD003909.

Hornbacher, M. (1998) *Wasted*. New York: HarperCollins.

Howard, W. T., Evans, K. K., Quintero-Howard, C. V., Bowers, W. A. S., and Andersen, A. E. (1999) Predictors of success or failure of transition to day hospital treatment for inpatients with anorexia nervosa. *American Journal of Psychiatry*, 156, 1697–1702.

Johnson, W. G., Tsoh, J. Y., and Varnado, P. J. (1996) Eating disorders: efficacy of pharmacological and psychological interventions. *Clinical Psychology Review*, 16, 457–478.

Kaplan, A. S. and Olmsted, M. P. (1997) Partial hospitalization. In D. M. Garner and P. E. Garfinkel (eds), *Handbook of Treatment for Eating Disorders* (2nd edn) (pp. 354–360). New York: Guilford Press.

Kaye, W. H., Kaplan, A. S., and Zucker, M. L. (1996) Treating eating-disorder patients in a managed care environment: contemporary American issues and a Canadian response. *Psychiatric Clinics of North America*, 19, 793–810.

Kearney-Cooke, A. and Striegel-Moore, R. (1997) The etiology and treatment of body image disturbance. In D. M. Garner and P. E. Garfinkel (eds), *Handbook of Treatment for Eating Disorders* (2nd edn) (pp. 295–306). New York: Guilford Press.

Keesey, R. E. (1993) Physiological regulation of body energy: implications for obesity. In A. J. Stunkard and T. A. Wadden (eds), *Obesity: Theory and Therapy* (2nd edn) (pp. 77–96). New York: Raven Press.

Kennedy, S. H., Kaplan, A. S., and Garfinkel, P. E. (1992) Intensive hospital treatments for anorexia nervosa and bulimia nervosa. In P. J. Cooper and A. Stein (eds), *Feeding Problems and Eating Disorders in Children and Adolescents* (pp. 161–181). Chur, Switzerland: Harwood Academic Publishers.

Keys, A., Brozek, J., Henschel, A., Mickelson, O., and Taylor, H. L. (1950) *The Biology of Human Starvation* (2 vols). Minneapolis: University of Minnesota Press.

Lask, B. (1992) Management of pre-pubertal anorexia nervosa. In P. J. Cooper and A. Stein (eds), *Feeding Problems and Eating Disorders in Children and Adolescents* (pp. 113–122). Chur, Switzerland: Harwood Academic Publishers.

Lawrence, M. (1984) *The Anorexic Experience*. London: The Women's Press.

le Grange, D., Eisler, I., Dare, C., and Russell, G. F. M. (1992) Evaluation of family treatments in adolescent anorexia nervosa: a pilot study. *International Journal of Eating Disorders*, 12, 347–357.

Linehan, M. M. (1993) *Cognitive-behavioral Treatment of Borderline Personality Disorder*. New York: Guilford Press.

Litt, I. F. (1999) Managed care and adolescents with eating disorders. *Journal of Adolescent Health*, 24, 373.

Lock, J., le Grange, D., Agras, W. S., and Dare, C. (2001) *Treatment Manual for Anorexia Nervosa: A Family-based Approach*. New York: Guilford Press.

McIntosh, V. V., Bulik, C. M., McKenzie, J. M., Luty, S. E., and Jordan, J. (2000) Interpersonal psychotherapy for anorexia nervosa. *International Journal of Eating Disorders*, 27, 125–139.

McIntosh, V. V. W., Jordan, J., Carter, F. A., Luty, S. E., McKenzie, J. M., Bulik, C. M., Frampton, C. M. A., and Joyce, P. R. (2005) Three psychotherapies for anorexia nervosa: a randomized controlled trial. *American Journal of Psychiatry*, 162, 741–747.

McKenzie, J. M. and Joyce, P. R. (1992) Hospitalization for anorexia nervosa. *International Journal of Eating Disorders*, 11, 235–241.

MacLeod, S. (1982) *The Art of Starvation: A Story of Anorexia and Survival*. New York: Schocken Books.

Meads, C., Gold, L., and Burls, A. (2001) How effective is outpatient care compared to inpatient care for the treatment of anorexia nervosa? A systematic review. *European Eating Disorders Review*, 9, 229–241.

Miller, W. R. and Rollnick, S. (1991) *Motivational Interviewing: Preparing People to Change Addictive Behavior*. New York: Guilford Press.

Miller, W. R. and Rollnick, S. (2002) *Motivational Interviewing* (2nd edn). New York: Guilford Press.

Minuchin, S., Rosman, B. L., and Baker, L. (1978) *Psychosomatic Families: Anorexia Nervosa in Context*. Cambridge, MA: Harvard University Press.

Neumarker, K. J. (1997) Mortality and sudden death in anorexia nervosa. *International Journal of Eating Disorders*, 21, 205–212.

Orbach, S. (1985) Accepting the symptom: a feminist psychoanalytic treatment of anorexia nervosa. In D. M. Garner and P. E. Garfinkel (eds), *Handbook of Psychotherapy for Anorexia Nervosa and Bulimia* (pp. 83–104). New York: Guilford Press.

Orimoto, L. and Vitousek, K. (1992) Anorexia nervosa and bulimia nervosa. In P. W. Wilson (ed.), *Principles and Practices of Relapse Prevention* (pp. 85–127). New York: Guilford Press.

Palazzoli, M. S. (1978) *Self-starvation: From Individual to Family Therapy in the Treatment of Anorexia Nervosa*. New York: Jason Aronson.

Palmer, R. L. (2000) *Helping People with Eating Disorders: A Clinical Guide to Assessment and Treatment*. Chichester: Wiley.

Pike, K. M., Loeb, K., and Vitousek, K. (1996) Cognitive-behavioral therapy for anorexia nervosa and bulimia nervosa. In J. K. Thompson (ed.), *Body Image, Eating Disorders, and Obesity: An Integrative Guide for Assessment and Treatment* (pp. 253–302). Washington, DC: American Psychological Association.

Pike, K. M., Walsh, B. T., Vitousek, K., Wilson, G. T., and Bauer, J. (2003) Cognitive behavioral therapy in the posthospitalization treatment of anorexia nervosa. *American Journal of Psychiatry*, 160, 2046–2049.

Pinel, J. P. (2000) *Biopsychology* (4th edn). Boston: Allyn and Bacon.

Piran, N. and Kaplan, A. S. (eds) (1990) *A Day Hospital Group Treatment Program for Anorexia Nervosa and Bulimia Nervosa*. New York: Brunner/Mazel.

Pomeroy, C. and Mitchell, J. E. (2002) Medical complications of anorexia nervosa and bulimia nervosa. In C. G. Fairburn and K. D. Brownell (eds), *Eating*

Disorders and Obesity: A Comprehensive Handbook (pp. 278–285). New York: Guilford Press.

Powers, P. S. and Powers, H. P. (1984) Inpatient treatment of anorexia nervosa. *Psychosomatics*, 25, 512–527.

Rampling, D. (1978) Anorexia nervosa: reflections on theory and practice. *Psychiatry*, 41, 296–301.

Robin, A. L., Siegel, P. T., Koepke, T., Moye, A. W., and Tice, S. (1994) Family therapy versus individual therapy for adolescent females with anorexia nervosa. *Developmental and Behavioral Pediatrics*, 15, 111–116.

Robin, A. L., Bedway, M., Siegel, P. T., and Gilroy, M. (1996) Therapy for adolescent anorexia nervosa: addressing cognitions, feelings, and the family's role. In E. D. Hibbs and P. S. Jensen (eds), *Psychosocial Treatments for Child and Adolescent Disorders: Empirically Based Strategies for Clinical Practice* (pp. 239–259). Washington, DC: American Psychological Association.

Robinson, P. (1993) Treatment for eating disorders in the United Kingdom. Part I. A survey of specialist services. *Eating Disorders Review*, 1, 4–9.

Russell, G. F. M. (1977) General management of anorexia nervosa and difficulty in assessing the efficacy of treatment. In R. A. Vigersky (ed.), *Anorexia Nervosa*. New York: Raven Press, pp. 277–289.

Russell, G. F. M., Szmukler, G. I., Dare, C., and Eisler, I. (1987) An evaluation of family therapy in anorexia nervosa and bulimia nervosa. *Archives of General Psychiatry*, 44, 1047–1056.

Serfaty, M. A., Turkington, D., Heap, M., Ledsham, L., and Jolley, E. (1999) Cognitive therapy versus dietary counselling in the outpatient treatment of anorexia nervosa: effects of the treatment phase. *European Eating Disorders Review*, 7, 334–350.

Slade, P. (1982) Towards a functional analysis of anorexia nervosa and bulimia nervosa. *British Journal of Clinical Psychology*, 21, 167–179.

Smith, D. E., Heckemeyer, C. M., Kratt, P. P., and Mason, D. A. (1997) Motivational interviewing to improve adherence to a behavioral weight-control program for older obese women with NIDDM. *Diabetes Care*, 20, 52–54.

Steinhausen, H.-C. (1995) The course and outcome of anorexia nervosa. In K. D. Brownell and C. G. Fairburn (eds), *Eating Disorders and Obesity: A Comprehensive Handbook* (pp. 234–237). New York: Guilford Press.

Story, I. (1982) Anorexia nervosa and the psychotherapeutic hospital. *International Journal of Psychoanalytic Psychotherapy*, 9, 267–302.

Striegel-Moore, R. H., Leslie, D., Petrill, S. A., Garvin, V., and Rosenheck, R. A. (2000) One-year use and cost of inpatient and outpatient services among female and male patients with an eating disorder: evidence from a national database of health insurance claims. *International Journal of Eating Disorders*, 27, 381–389.

Strober, M. (2004) Managing the chronic, treatment-resistant patient with anorexia nervosa. *International Journal of Eating Disorders*, 36, 245–255.

Strober, M. and Yager, J. (1985) A developmental perspective on the treatment of anorexia nervosa in adolescents. In D. M. Garner and P. E. Garfinkel (eds), *Handbook of Psychotherapy for Anorexia Nervosa and Bulimia* (pp. 363–390). New York: Guilford Press.

Strober, M., Freeman, R., and Morrell, W. (1997) The long-term course of severe anorexia nervosa in adolescents: survival analysis of recovery, relapse, and outcome predictors over 10–15 years in a prospective study. *International Journal of Eating Disorders*, 22, 339–360.

Sullivan, P. F. (2002) Course and outcome of anorexia nervosa and bulimia nervosa. In C. G. Fairburn and K. D. Brownell (eds), *Eating Disorders and Obesity: A Comprehensive Handbook* (pp. 226–230). New York: Guilford Press.

Tanner, C. and Connan, F. (2003) Cognitive analytic therapy. In J. Treasure, U. Schmidt, and E. Van Furth (eds), *Handbook of Eating Disorders* (2nd edn) (pp. 279–290). Chichester: Wiley.

Touyz, S. W. and Beumont, P. J. V. (1997) Behavioral treatment to promote weight gain in anorexia nervosa. In D. M. Garner and P. E. Garfinkel (eds), *Handbook of Treatment for Eating Disorders* (2nd edn) (pp. 361–371). New York: Guilford Press.

Treasure, J. and Schmidt, U. (2001) Ready, willing, and able to change: motivational aspects of the assessment and treatment of eating disorders. *European Eating Disorders Review*, 9, 4–18.

Treasure, J. and Ward, A. (1997a) Cognitive analytical therapy in the treatment of anorexia nervosa. *Clinical Psychology and Psychotherapy*, 4, 62–71.

Treasure, J. and Ward, A. (1997b) A practical guide to the use of motivational interviewing in anorexia nervosa. *European Eating Disorders Review*, 5, 102–114.

Treasure, J., Todd, G., Brolly, J., Nehmed, A., and Denman, F. (1995a) A pilot study of a randomised trial of cognitive analytical therapy vs. educational behavioral therapy for adult anorexia nervosa. *Behaviour Research and Therapy*, 33, 363–367.

Treasure, J., Todd, G., and Szmukler, G. (1995b) The inpatient treatment of anorexia nervosa. In G. Szmukler, C. Dare, and J. Treasure (eds), *Handbook of Eating Disorders: Theory, Treatment, and Research*. Chichester: Wiley, pp. 275–291.

Vandereycken, W. (1987a) The constructive family approach to eating disorders: critical remarks on the use of family therapy in anorexia nervosa and bulimia. *International Journal of Eating Disorders*, 6, 455–467.

Vandereycken, W. (1987b) The management of patients with anorexia nervosa and bulimia – basic principles and general guidelines. In P. J. V. Beumont, G. D. Burrows, and R. C. Casper (eds), *Handbook of Eating Disorders: Part 1: Anorexia and Bulimia Nervosa* (pp. 235–253). New York: Elsevier.

Vandereycken, W. (2003) The place of inpatient care in the treatment of anorexia nervosa: questions to be answered. *International Journal of Eating Disorders*, 34, 409–422.

Vitousek, K. (1998) Procedures for in vivo therapy sessions. Unpublished manuscript, University of Hawaii.

Vitousek, K. (2002) Cognitive-behavioral therapy for anorexia nervosa. In C. G. Fairburn and K. D. Brownell (eds), *Eating Disorders and Obesity: A Comprehensive Handbook*. New York: Guilford Press, pp. 308–313.

Vitousek, K. and Gray, J. (2005) Eating disorders. In G. Gabbard, J. Beck, and J. Holmes (eds), *Concise Oxford Textbook of Psychotherapy*. Oxford: Oxford University Press, pp. 177–202.

Vitousek, K. and Hollon, S. D. (1990) The investigation of schematic content and processing in eating disorders. *Cognitive Therapy and Research*, 14, 191–214.

Vitousek, K. and Orimoto, L. (1993) Cognitive-behavioral models of anorexia nervosa, bulimia nervosa, and obesity. In K. S. Dobson and P. C. Kendall (eds), *Psychopathology and Cognition* (pp. 191–243). San Diego, CA: Academic Press.

Vitousek, K., Watson, S., and Wilson, G. T. (1998) Enhancing motivation for change in treatment-resistant eating disorders. *Clinical Psychology Review*, 18, 391–420.

Walsh, B. T. (2002) Pharmacological treatment of anorexia nervosa and bulimia nervosa. In C. G. Fairburn and K. D. Brownell (eds), *Eating Disorders and Obesity: A Comprehensive Handbook* (2nd edn) (pp. 325–329). New York: Guilford Press.

Wilfley, D., Stein, R., and Welch, R. (2003) Interpersonal psychotherapy. In J. Treasure, U. Schmidt, and E. Van Furth (eds), *Handbook of Eating Disorders* (2nd edn) (pp. 253–270). Chichester: Wiley.

Williamson, D. A., Thaw, J. M., and Varnado-Sullivan, P. J. (2001) Cost-effectiveness analysis of a hospital-based cognitive-behavioral treatment program for eating disorders. *Behavior Therapy*, 32, 459–477.

Wilson, G. T. and Agras, W. S. (2001) Practice guidelines for eating disorders. *Behavior Therapy*, 32, 219–234.

Wilson, G. T. and Vitousek, K. M. (1999) Self-monitoring in the assessment of eating disorders. *Psychological Assessment*, 11, 480–489.

Wilson, G. T., Fairburn, C. F., and Agras, W. S. (1997) Cognitive-behavioral therapy for bulimia nervosa. In D. M. Garner and P. E. Garfinkel (eds), *Handbook of Treatment for Eating Disorders* (2nd edn) (pp. 67–93). New York: Guilford Press.

Wilson, G. T., Vitousek, K. M., and Loeb, K. L. (2000) Stepped care treatment for eating disorders. *Journal of Consulting and Clinical Psychology*, 67, 451–459.

Wirtshafter, D. and Davis, D. J. (1977) Set points, settling points, and the control of body weight. *Physiology and Behavior*, 19, 75–78.

Wiseman, C. V., Sunday, S. R., Klapper, F., Harris, W. A., and Halmi, K. A. (2001) Changing patterns of hospitalization in eating disorder patients. *International Journal of Eating Disorders*, 30, 69–74.

Woodside, D. B., Carter, J. C., and Blackmore, E. (2004) Predictors of premature termination of inpatient treatment for anorexia nervosa. *American Journal of Psychiatry*, 161, 2277–2281.

Yager, J. (2002) Management of patients with intractable eating disorders. In C. G. Fairburn and K. D. Brownell (eds), *Eating Disorders and Obesity: A Comprehensive Handbook* (pp. 345–349). New York: Guilford Press.

Zastowny, T. R., O'Brien, C., Young, R., and Barclay, C. (1991) An outpatient eating disorders program in a CMHC. *Hospital and Community Psychiatry*, 42, 1256–1258.

Zerbe, K. J. (1996) Extending the frame: working with managed care to support treatment for a refractory patient. In J. Werne (ed.), *Treating Eating Disorders* (pp. 335–356). San Francisco: Jossey-Bass.

Zipfel, S., Reas, D. L., Thornton, C., Olmsted, M. P., Williamson, D. A., Gerlinghoff, M., Herzog, W., and Beumont, P. J. (2002) Day hospitalization program for eating disorders: a systematic review of the literature. *International Journal of Eating Disorders*, 31, 105–117.

Chapter 11

Outpatient treatment of bulimia nervosa

Peter J. Cooper

Introduction

The great majority of people with bulimia nervosa and related disorders do not seek treatment; and those who do present for treatment in specialist outpatient clinics therefore represent a highly selected group (Whitaker *et al.*, 1990; Fairburn *et al.*, 1996). The reason for this is at least partly because the shame people feel about having the disorder prevents them from being open about their difficulties. However, it is also the case that specialist services are not widely available and people will therefore not have access to the services they need. There are therefore two priorities for those concerned with providing therapeutic services to people with bulimia nervosa. The first is to be in a position to deliver evidence-based effective treatments to the cases that present for treatment. The second is to find an effective means of providing therapeutic help to those people who, for one reason or another, do not present to specialist clinics but nevertheless have the disorder and are distressed and disabled by it.

Over the past twenty-five years, there has been a considerable clinical and research effort into the development and evaluation of treatments for bulimia nervosa. Indeed, there have been over sixty randomised controlled trials evaluating such interventions. The picture to emerge from this body of work is a consistent one. Baldly stated, the evidence strongly supports the use of a specific cognitive behavioural treatment (CBT) for bulimia nervosa. This chapter will therefore concentrate on this form of intervention. However, there have been several studies of alternative therapeutic strategies, especially ones concerning the use of antidepressant medication, and antidepressant treatment will also therefore be briefly considered. In addition, since the studies of CBT have almost all been done in specialist clinics, attention will be paid to the question of how this form of intervention can be more widely delivered. In particular, the use of cognitive behavioural self-help manuals will be discussed and evidence for their utility will be presented.

The place of drug treatments

There have been more than twenty well-controlled trials of pharmacological treatments for bulimia nervosa. The great majority of these concern antidepressant medication, including tricyclic medication, monoamine oxidase inhibitors, selective serotonin uptake inhibitors, and other antidepressants. The original basis to these treatments was the supposition that bulimia nervosa was a form of affective disorder (Pope et al., 1983). Despite the fact that several lines of evidence run counter to this notion, and it is an hypothesis not now given credence, there is consistent evidence that antidepressants do have a positive impact on binge eating and purgative behaviour. Wilson and Fairburn (1998) summarised the results of fourteen controlled trials of antidepressants and reported a mean reduction in binge eating and purging frequency of 61 per cent and 59 per cent respectively. In twelve of these studies the therapeutic benefit was significantly superior to the placebo effect. However, these studies were all investigations of short-term outcome, and there is little convincing evidence that antidepressants have an impact on the long-term course of bulimia nervosa. One study (Romano et al., 2002) did find that, after one year, patients who had responded after eight weeks of treatment with fluoxetine did better if they were maintained on fluoxetine than those who were switched to placebo; but the main outcome variable was 'time to relapse', and the principal finding therefore was that those on placebo tended to relapse earlier than those on fluoxetine. Indeed, the findings of this study largely confirm those of earlier maintenance studies which indicated that the effectiveness of antidepressant medication was relatively short-lived. For example, two studies found that even amongst those patients with bulimia nervosa who had initially responded to the medication, the relapse rate was high for both those switched to placebo and those maintained on the original medication (Pyle et al., 1990; Walsh et al., 1991). It has been suggested that there could be benefit from switching from one antidepressant, which has been found in a given case to be relatively ineffective, to a second type of antidepressant; but this is a speculation without empirical support, and it remains doubtful whether this practice would improve the longer-term outcome of patients treated with these forms of medication.

Several studies have compared antidepressant medication with CBT for bulimia nervosa; and some studies have examined whether the addition of an antidepressant medication to CBT produces a superior outcome to CBT alone (for reviews see Bacaltchuk and Hay, 2005; NICE, 2004). Three major conclusions can be drawn from this work. First, in simple comparisons, CBT has been found to have a stronger therapeutic effect than antidepressant medication. Second, the combination of CBT with an antidepressant has not generally been found to produce a larger therapeutic effect than CBT alone. Third, no predictive factors have emerged suggestive of a subgroup for whom antidepressant medication would be appropriate.

A problem with the use of antidepressant medication in this patient group is that it is not generally well tolerated by people with bulimia nervosa, with many refusing this form of treatment and many dropping out of treatment. The NICE recommendations state that, despite the lack of firm evidence for a long-term benefit of antidepressant medication, this form of treatment can be considered in adult patients (SSRIs being the first choice) as an alternative or addition to an evidence-based first step. Unfortunately, the clinical basis on which the decision to prescribe an antidepressant should be made has not been specified. Significant comorbid depressive symptomatology, or a history of depressive disorder, do not reliably identify those who will respond to the medication (and neither do they, incidentally, predict a poor response to psychological treatment). In reality the decision whether to prescribe an anti-depressant is likely to come down to the question of whether a patient has failed to respond to the first line treatment (see below) and what further options are available within a particular clinical service.

The place of psychological treatments

Several forms of psychological treatment have been developed for the treat-ment of bulimia nervosa and many have been subjected to rigorous empirical testing. These include purely behavioural forms of treatment, notably some involving specific exposure and response prevention techniques (Leitenberg and Rosen, 1985; Leitenberg et al., 1988), psychoeducational treatment (Olmsted et al., 1991), and interpersonal psychotherapy (Fairburn et al., 1993a; Fairburn, 1997). However, the treatment which has been most well developed and most extensively researched is a form of cognitive behaviour therapy (CBT), developed specifically for this patient group, first described by Fairburn (1981). Since the evidence most strongly supports the use of this form of treatment in the management of bulimia nervosa, it is the only form of psychological intervention that will be considered within this chapter.

The nature of CBT for bulimia nervosa

CBT for bulimia nervosa derives from a cognitive behavioural model of the maintenance of the disorder (Fairburn, 1981). This sees the behavioural dis-turbances characteristic of the disorder – the loss of control over eating and the extreme compensatory measures – as emanating from both a general poor regard of self and, more specifically, from overvalued ideas about body weight and shape. The link between these ideas and behaviours is the dietary restraint provoked by the extreme concerns about weight and shape. Thus, there is a wealth of both experimental evidence (see Polivy and Herman, 1993) and clinical experience which points to dietary restraint being causally linked to episodes of overeating. Binge eating, in turn, encourages further efforts at dietary restraint. People with bulimia nervosa are therefore trapped in a vicious cycle where their concerns about weight and shape lead them to diet; dieting leads them to lose control of their eating and binge; and to compensate for having overeaten, they induce vomiting, abuse laxatives, and renew their efforts to diet. It is a basic tenet of the cognitive behavioural approach to the treatment of bulimia nervosa that both the cognitive and the behavioural features which maintain the disorder must be directly addressed in treatment.

CBT for bulimia nervosa has been fully described in a comprehensive treatment manual (Fairburn *et al.*, 1993b). (Only a brief summary of this treatment will be provided here. For a full appreciation of all the components of the treatment, the original manual must be consulted.) Within this manual the treatment is described in considerable detail. The treatment involves approximately nineteen sessions of individual therapy over about twenty weeks. It is problem-oriented and principally focused on present problems and future potential difficulties, rather than on the past circumstances which may have contributed to the development of the eating disorder. The style of therapy described is essentially a collaborative one in which patient and therapist work together, with the therapist providing guidance and encouragement, but the main therapeutic work being done by the patient between sessions. Fairburn *et al.* (1993b) emphasise that mutual trust and respect are essential for the therapeutic relationship to work effectively. An understanding by the therapist of the psychological and physiological factors involved in bulimia nervosa is essential, both because the therapist must re-educate patients in certain areas (such as body weight regulation), and because patients are at risk of a variety of physical complications which need to be closely monitored. Initially, the cognitive model of the maintenance of the disorder is presented as the theoretic basis underpinning the treatment programme, and the importance of both behavioural and cognitive change is emphasised. Throughout the course of treatment aspects of the patient's experience are discussed in terms of this model, as a means of providing the patient with an explanatory framework for their difficulties and thereby enhancing their sense of control over their thoughts, feelings and behaviour.

The treatment is divided into three distinct stages. In stage one, where therapy sessions are held twice weekly over a four-week period, the focus is on behavioural change. The aim is to displace the chaotic pattern of binge eating, vomiting, laxative abuse and dietary restriction, by the establishment of a pattern of regular eating. During this phase of treatment, patients should be provided with information about body weight regulation (such as the normal body mass index range, and the medical implications of being too thin), the physical consequences of binge eating, self-induced vomiting and laxative abuse, and the ineffectiveness of vomiting and laxative abuse as weight control measures. They should also be informed of the adverse effects of dieting. Patients with bulimia nervosa typically restrict the amount they eat, avoid eating particular sorts of food, and avoid eating at all for long periods of time. Commonly it becomes apparent early in the treatment that perceived transgressions of rigidly held dietary rules lead to feelings of failure and despair which in turn lead to a breakdown of dietary control and binges. It is important that patients become aware that the fault here lies not in their own poor self-control, but in the dietary rules themselves, and that it is these rules that promote overeating.

A crucial aspect of stage one of treatment is that patients are instructed to record their eating on monitoring sheets throughout the day. This monitoring includes recording of the time of day, exactly what was eaten (nature and amount), and whether it was a meal, a snack or a binge. Patients are also encouraged to record any notable thoughts and emotions that might have been present before, during or after the episodes of eating. Patients are instructed to keep this diary of their eating by making entries throughout the day as events occur, rather than by trying to recall the information at the end of the day. Since review of these records largely forms the substance of the therapy sessions, the importance of accurate and comprehensive monitoring is strongly emphasised. In addition to providing the material of therapy sessions, monitoring serves to heighten patients' awareness of patterns in their eating habits, which helps in the process of regaining control. For example, commonly patterns become apparent of binge eating episodes following episodes of marked dietary restraint, minor trangressions of dietary rules, and negative emotional states. Awareness of these patterns is used as evidence supporting the case for the patients attempting to make particular changes in their life. One of these concerns the tendency, common in these patients, to monitor body weight excessively by frequent weighing (although some patients deal with the heightened concern over body weight by avoiding weighing altogether). Patients are advised to weigh themselves once a week. This suggestion is commonly met with resistance, but patients can be reassured that people rarely gain any weight during the course of this treatment. They should also, where possible, be alerted, through reference to their monitoring sheets, to the way in which minor temporary fluctuations in weight adversely affect their mood and behaviour.

A major component of the first phase of treatment is the generation, with the patient, of a meal plan. The purpose here is to impose a regular pattern of eating to displace the episodes of loss of control. So patients are asked to plan to eat, at set times of the day, three 'meals' and two or three 'snacks'. Patients commonly resist this step as they fear it will lead to weight gain. However, it is not difficult to demonstrate that if the adoption of planned episodes of eating does displace episodes of loss of control and binges, overall calorie consumption will not be increased. The content of these meals and snacks is left at this stage to the discretion of the patient, although they should be told only to include a quantity and type of food that will not provoke compensatory behaviour (such as vomiting). These meals and snacks therefore invariably comprise small amounts of low-calorie foods; however, this is not an issue of concern at this point in treatment, as what matters is when patients eat. One problem patients commonly experience with this aspect of treatment is discomfort following eating because of a sense of 'fullness'. This is an opportunity to highlight the links between the patient's concerns about becoming fat and their feelings and behavioural urges (i.e. the urge to vomit). Patients are strongly encouraged to resist the urge to purge and encouraged to attempt to console themselves with the thought that planned meals and snacks are the means to regain self-control over their eating. Patients also need to be helped to develop self-control strategies which they can deploy to refrain from binge eating and purging. For example, patients can be asked to generate a list of activities that are pleasurable and incompatible with binge eating. They might come up with having a bath or speaking to a friend or relative on the telephone. They are then advised to consult their list whenever they have an urge to binge, and to work their way through their list until the urge has passed (or it is time for the next planned meal or snack). Patients should also be advised to avoid 'dangerous' activities, such as exposing themselves to food when they feel especially vulnerable. Other stimulus control strategies can also be helpful, such as restricting eating to one place in the house.

In the great majority of cases, by the end of stage one of treatment the frequency of episodes of loss of control over eating has decreased substantially, as have episodes of self-induced vomiting and laxative abuse. General mood has also usually improved and patients feel more in control of their lives. Fairburn and colleagues (1993b) note that patients who have not improved at all by this stage of treatment rarely benefit from continuing in this therapy. Instead, if, for example, depressive symptoms remain prominent, a course of antidepressants could be considered. Day patient (see Chapter 12) or inpatient treatment might also be indicated.

In the second stage of the treatment, during which therapy sessions are held weekly over a two-month period, the self-control strategies established in stage one are supplemented with a variety of procedures designed to reduce dietary restraint, to increase coping skills for resisting binge eating, and to introduce the patient to cognitive techniques to address their extreme concerns about shape and weight. By the end of the first stage of the treatment programme the link between dietary restraint and episodes of loss of control over eating will have become clear to the patient. A regular pattern of eating will have been established. Patients must now be encouraged to make changes to both the quantity of their meals and snacks and their composition. Initially, patients are asked to generate a list of foods they would normally avoid – either because they are perceived as fattening or because they are seen as foods which trigger binge eating – and to rank these in terms of how threatening they are regarded. They are then instructed to introduce these foods gradually, beginning with the least threatening, in their planned meals and snacks at times when they feel they are reasonably in control of their eating. By the end of the eight weeks of the second phase of treatment they should aim to have worked their way through their list such that no foods are avoided because of the threat they might carry. At this point the patient is able to make a free choice about which of these foods they actually enjoy eating and would therefore wish to retain in their diet and which they might wish to exclude. During this process of gradual exposure to previously avoided foods, the question of the quantity being eaten should be addressed. Commonly, remaining episodes of loss of control over eating can be seen to have occurred at times when rather little has been eaten; and this evidence can be used as the basis for the patient increasing the quantity consumed in planned meals. Finally, in an effort to establish normalised eating habits, patients should be encouraged to organise opportunities for eating in a wide range of circumstances, such as restaurants, dinner parties and situations where food quantity is difficult to control (such as a cocktail party or buffet meal).

As with many cognitive behaviourally oriented treatments, this treatment programme explicitly introduces formal problem-solving techniques as a means of enhancing patients' sense of control over their eating. In stage two it commonly becomes apparent that the remaining intermittent episodes of loss of control over eating are precipitated by external problems in patients' lives, commonly of an interpersonal nature. By developing the skills to deal with these problems, patients have the capacity to address such problems without them disrupting their eating. There are several steps to be followed in this process: identifying and specifying the problem; generating alternative ways of dealing with the problem; evaluating the feasibility and potential effectiveness of each of these alternatives; choosing the best alternative to follow; specifying how this alternative is to be effected; carrying out this alternative; and evaluating the outcome and the problem-solving process. Many patients find this process enormously helpful and utilise it widely to help them deal with difficulties not just concerning food and eating but many other aspects of their lives.

The final aspect of the second phase of this treatment programme is cognitive in nature and involves addressing patients' concerns about their shape and weight and dealing with their associated dysfunctional cognitions. Cognitive restructuring techniques are used, adapted from Beck's cognitive restructuring for depression (Beck et al., 1979). Briefly, patients are helped to identify and specify problematic thoughts (e.g. 'only by being thin can I possibly be happy') and the context in which these occurred. They are encouraged to question the validity of the thought and rationally to evaluate the evidence in favour of and against the thought. The aim is to help the patient reach a reasoned conclusion which itself can enable a change in behaviour. The general technique of cognitive restructuring is implemented in somewhat different ways in different treatment programmes. Fairburn and colleagues (1993b) stipulate that patients should record their efforts at cognitive restructuring on the back of their monitoring sheets, so that they can be reviewed with the therapist.

Extreme concerns about weight and shape are not always easy to specify in terms of clearly articulated problematic thoughts; however, they can be elicited by certain behavioural techniques. These involve planning episodes of exposure to feared or avoided stimuli, such as situations where the quantity of food being served is not under the direct control of the patient, or where body shape is revealed (by, for example, wearing tight clothing). These challenges commonly provoke anxiety and thoughts which themselves can then be subjected to cognitive appraisal and, where appropriate, restructuring.

The third and final stage of the treatment, during which therapy sessions are held fortnightly over six weeks, is concerned with relapse prevention strategies to ensure the maintenance of therapeutic gains. The major goal is for patients to be in a position to anticipate difficulties which might arise in the future, and to have prearranged strategies to deal with these. This last phase of treatment should therefore be used to devise and rehearse strategies for coping with situations which could in the future cause problems. These situations commonly involve occasions where there are large amounts of unregulated food (e.g. attending a buffet), or where exposure of body shape is involved (e.g. a swimming pool party). By rehearsing the feelings which are likely to arise and the behaviours these feelings are likely to provoke, patients can come to devise benign solutions. However 'cured' a patient may feel, it is prudent for someone who has successfully come through a treatment for bulimia nervosa to regard themselves as always potentially vulnerable to the recurrence of problems with their eating. It is also important that they do not regard occasional minor setbacks as catastrophic. Indeed, in so far as they are able successfully to respond to such setbacks by reinstating previously effective therapeutic strategies, these recurrences can be seen as evidence of the fact that self-control has been successfully achieved. Fairburn and colleagues (1993b) advise that each patient devise their own written 'maintenance plan', which the therapist reviews, to be used as a guide following the termination of treatment and, in particular, to be consulted and adhered to at times when difficulty is being experienced.

The evidence for CBT for bulimia nervosa

Wilson and Fairburn (1998), in their review of the effectiveness of CBT for bulimia nervosa, reported, on the basis of ten of the best-controlled treatment trials of CBT, that the mean percentage reduction in binge eating ranged from 73 per cent to 93 per cent; and for purging, the mean reduction ranged from 77 per cent to 94 per cent. Rates of remission from binge eating in these studies ranged from 51 per cent to 71 per cent, and for purging from 36 per cent to 56 per cent (e.g. Agras *et al.*, 1989, 1992; Fairburn *et al.*, 1991; Garner *et al.*, 1993). In addition, these studies consistently showed marked improvements in terms of dietary restraint and attitudes to body shape and weight (e.g. Fairburn *et al.*, 1991; Garner *et al.*, 1993; Wilson *et al.*, 1991). These studies have also consistently revealed improvements in the general psychopathology of the disorder, with benefits found in terms of depressed mood, self-esteem and social functioning (e.g. Fairburn *et al.*, 1986, 1992; Garner *et al.*, 1993). Maintenance of change has, when assessed, generally been shown to be impressive. The longest follow-up has been reported by Fairburn and colleagues (1993a): five and a half years after the end of CBT, improvements in all major aspects of post-treatment outcome had been maintained, with total abstinence from binge eating and purging evident in just under half the patients.

CBT has been systematically compared to other forms of treatment for bulimia nervosa, such as antidepressant medication (discussed above) and other forms of psychotherapy. In comparison with other forms of psychological treatment it has, in all cases, either proved as effective or more effective. For example, Agras *et al.* (1989) found CBT to be more effective than supportive psychotherapy both at the end of treatment and at a one-year follow-up. Garner *et al.* (1993) found CBT and supportive-expressive psychotherapy to be comparable in terms of some outcomes, but CBT to be superior in terms of reducing levels of dietary restraint, normalising dysfunctional attitudes to weight and shape, and improving general mood and self-esteem. Fairburn *et al.* (1991, 1993a) found CBT to be far superior to a behavioural treatment but comparable on a wide range of specific and non-specific outcomes to interpersonal psychotherapy (IPT); however, the positive benefits of CBT were evident far sooner than they were for IPT.

It will be apparent from the figures cited above that, impressive though the results from CBT might be, this treatment does not invariably produce a favourable clinical outcome. Wilson and Fairburn (1998) list the contraindications for this treatment as psychotic states, severe depression or the risk of suicide, and substance use disorders that effectively prevent patients from fully engaging in the cognitive behavioural treatment programme.

The place of CBT self-help

CBT for bulimia nervosa was developed as a specialist form of therapy for use within specialist centres. As such, its availability is highly restricted. Once the effectiveness of the CBT approach had been demonstrated, there was recognition of a need for there to be brief or simple forms of this treatment which could be made more widely available. One approach was to produce a self-help manual based on the principles of full CBT for bulimia nervosa. About a decade ago, two such manuals became available (Cooper, 1993, 1995; Fairburn, 1995). Both provide an overview of the disorder followed by a structured cognitive behavioural manual, based on the account of full CBT for bulimia nervosa described by Fairburn and his colleagues (Fairburn,

1985; Fairburn and Cooper, 1989; Fairburn et al., 1993b), but designed to be used by people on their own or under the guidance of a clinician. Figure 11.1 shows a page taken from one of these manuals which specifies the stepped structure of the self-help programme.

The effectiveness of the cognitive behavioural self-help approach as a purely self-help form of treatment (i.e. where the manual is followed by patients without any support or supervision) has been shown to be rather modest (Palmer et al., 2002; Carter et al., 2003). However, far more promising results have been produced in studies of the effectiveness of 'guided self-help'. Here the patient works through the self-help manual guided and encouraged in brief sessions by a specialist or non-specialist health professional. The early findings using this guided CB self-help approach were encouraging. Thus, in an open series of eighteen patients referred to a specialist eating disorder clinic, Cooper et al. (1994) reported that CB self-help, with guidance provided by a social worker over eight twenty- to thirty-minute sessions, led to substantial reductions in both binge eating and vomiting. In a subsequent report of eighty-two patients treated using the same guided self-help format, these promising findings were confirmed and extended, with evidence of lasting benefit in terms of both behavioural change and improvement in dietary

Step 1. Monitoring
(keeping a systematic written record of your eating so that you can know precisely what has been happening)

↓

Step 2. Establishing a meal plan
(deciding on what pattern of eating is sensible and attempting to adhere to it)

↓

Step 3. Learning to intervene
(learning what sort of circumstances cause you to binge and what sort of things you can do to prevent this happening)

↓

Step 4. Problem solving
(learning how to define problems which cause you difficulty with your eating, and learning to deal with them)

↓

Step 5. Eliminating dieting
(systematically widening the range of foods you eat)

↓

Step 6. Changing your mind
(identifying some of the beliefs which underlie your difficulties with eating and attempting to modify them)

Figure 11.1.

Source: Cooper, 1995.

restraint and concerns about body shape and weight (Cooper *et al.*, 1996). Several controlled trials, conducted in eating disorder clinics, have evaluated guided self-help. For example, Palmer *et al.* (2002) compared the efficacy of three treatment conditions: self-help alone, self-help with face-to-face guidance, and self-help with telephone guidance. Half the sample was on antidepressant medication. At the end of treatment, patients in the face-to-face guided self-help condition showed significantly greater improvement on key behavioural variables (i.e. binge eating, vomiting) than those in the other conditions, although the recovery rate (i.e. cessation of binge eating and vomiting) was only 10 per cent.

While guided self-help could well constitute a useful first line treatment in specialist clinics, this would still mean that CBT principles were only reaching the minority of those with bulimia nervosa who gained referral to specialist services. Dissemination would be better served if self-help could be managed within primary care facilities. Three recent studies, conducted in three different countries, have examined the utility of guided CB self-help for bulimia nervosa delivered within primary care. The first of these was conducted in London (Durand and King, 2003) and involved a comparison between CB self-help, with guidance provided by the general practitioner, and specialist outpatient treatment (combined CBT and interpersonal psychotherapy). Both groups experienced significant and similar degrees of benefit, in terms of both primary symptoms (i.e. binge eating and vomiting) and secondary ones (i.e. depression and social adjustment). The remission rates were very similar for the two groups: 29 per cent for the self-help group and 27 per cent for the participants in the specialist treatment group – rates similar to those reported by other CBT trials (e.g. Agras *et al.*, 2000). These promising results have not been supported by a recent study, of similar design, from the United States (Walsh *et al.*, 2004). Four groups of patients with bulimia nervosa (or a bulimic form of the DSM category EDNOS ('eating disorders not otherwise specified')) were compared: placebo; fluoxetine; placebo plus guided CB self-help; and fluoxetine plus CB self-help. Fluoxetine was found to be superior to placebo in reducing binge eating and improving other psychological symptoms, but there were no important clinical differences in outcome between the guided CB self-help group and those receiving pills. Overall recovery rates were modest at around 10 per cent for both the self-help and the medication groups. The significance of this study is, however, somewhat difficult to discern, since over two-thirds of the patients failed to complete treatment.

Finally, the most recent study of guided CB self-help in primary care (Banasiak *et al.*, 2005), carried out in Australia, produced findings much more in line with those of the London study than those of the US study. Patients fulfilling similar diagnostic criteria to those employed by Walsh *et al.* (2004), recruited in general practice or via advertisement, were randomly allocated to a delayed treatment condition (effectively a waiting list control) or CB self-help with guidance provided by general practitioners who had attended a half-day workshop on guided self-help. After a seventeen-week intervention period, the frequency of binge eating in the guided self-help group had reduced by 60 per cent, compared with a 6 per cent reduction in the control group. Remission rates (from binge eating and compensatory behaviours) were 28 per cent and 11 per cent respectively. These treatment gains, along with secondary improvements in depression, anxiety, life satisfaction and occupational functioning, were maintained at a six-month follow-up.

It is unclear why the findings of the US study are in such contrast to those of the British and the Australian studies. The unusually high drop-out rate points to a mismatch between the treatment delivery and the patients' expectations, although there are several other possible reasons for the relative ineffectiveness of the self-help approach (Banasiak *et al.*, 2005). Whatever the reason, the question remains open whether this mode of treatment delivery is appropriate for the US primary care system and, if so, under what conditions its efficacy can be optimised. The conclusions are far more optimistic for delivery within British and Australian primary care services.

In summary, the evidence to date, from well-controlled clinical trials, suggests that guided CB self-help, delivered both in a specialist clinic setting and in primary care, offers considerable benefit to a significant proportion of patients with bulimia nervosa and its variants. Although some form of informed guidance appears essential, no specialist therapist expertise seems to be necessary. This form of treatment could, therefore, readily be incorporated within primary care services, thereby making at least a simplified form of CBT available for those with bulimia nervosa and related binge eating problems. This is the conclusion reached by the NICE committee which stated that 'as a possible first step, patients with bulimia nervosa should be encouraged to follow an evidence-based self-help programme'; and that 'health care professionals should consider providing direct encouragement and support to patients undertaking an evidence-based self-help programme'.

Conclusion

Where there are several different treatments available for a disorder, the ideal is to be able to match particular sorts of patients to particular treatments, on the basis of empirically grounded criteria which optimise treatment response. However, no such grounds currently exist for bulimia nervosa (Wilson and Fairburn, 1998). Accordingly, a stepped care approach has been recommended (Fairburn *et al.*, 1992; Wilson and Fairburn, 1998), in which treatments are provided sequentially. Initially all patients receive the simplest, least expensive form of treatment; only those who do not respond adequately to the first level of treatment are offered the next level of treatment; and so on, moving progressively, on the basis of need, to increasingly more complex (or more expensive) forms of treatment. While in practice the structure of the particular stepped care programme adopted will depend on the expertise and resources available, the evidence currently supports a first step of guided self-help followed, where necessary, by a full course of CBT. The place of other forms of intervention, such as antidepressant medication, interpersonal psychotherapy, psycho-educational groups, or day patient and inpatient treatment, is uncertain.

References

Agras, W.S. Schneider, J.A., Arnow, B., Raeburn, S.D. and Telch, C.F. (1989) Cognitive-behavioural and response-prevention treatments for bulimia nervosa. *Journal of Consulting and Clinical Psychology*, 57, 215–221.

Agras, W.S., Rossiter, E.M., Arnow, B., Schneider, J.A., Telch, C.F., Raeburn, S.D., Bruce, B., Perl, M. and Koran, L.M. (1992) Pharmacologic and cognitive-behavioural treatment for bulimia nervosa: a controlled comparision. *American Journal of Psychiatry*, 149, 82–87.

Agras, W.S., Walsh, B.T., Fairburn, C.G., Wilson, G.T. and Kraemer, H.C. (2000) A multicenter comparison of cognitive behavioural therapy and interpersonal psychotherapy for bulimia nervosa. *Archives of General Psychiatry*, 57, 459–466.

Bacaltchuk, J. and Hay, P. (2005) Antidepressants versus placebo for people with bulimia nervosa. The Cochrane Library, issue 2, Chichester: Wiley.

Banasiak, S.J., Paxton, S.J. and Hay, P. (2005) Guided self-help for bulimia nervosa in primary care: a randomised controlled trial. *Psychological Medicine*, 35, 1283–1294.

Beck, A.T., Rush, A.J., Shaw, B.F. and Emory, G. (1979) *Cognitive Therapy of Depression*. New York: Guilford Press.

Carter, J.C., Olmsted, M.P., Kaplan, A.S., McCabe, R.E., Mills, J.S. and Aime, A. (2003) Self-help for bulimia nervosa: a randomised controlled trial. *American Journal of Psychiatry*, 160, 973–978.

Cooper, P.J. (1993) *Bulimia Nervosa: A Guide to Recovery*. London: Robinson.

Cooper, P.J. (1995) *Bulimia Nervosa and Binge Eating: A Guide to Recovery*. London: Robinson.

Cooper, P.J., Coker, S. and Fleming, C. (1994) Self-help for bulimia nervosa: a preliminary report. *International Journal of Eating Disorders*, 16, 401–404.

Cooper, P.J., Coker, S. and Fleming, C. (1995) An evaluation of the efficacy of supervised cognitive behavioural self-help for bulimia nervosa. *Journal of Psychosomatic Research*, 40, 281–287.

Cooper, P.J., Coker, S. and Fleming, C. (1996) An evaluation of the efficacy of supervised cognitive behavioral self-help bulimia nervosa. *Journal of Psychosomatic Research*, 40, 281–287.

Durand, M.A. and King, M. (2003) Specialist treatment versus self-help for bulimia nervosa: a randomised controlled trial in general practice. *British Journal of General Practice*, 53, 371–377.

Fairburn, C.G. (1981) A cognitive behavioural approach to the management of bulimia. *Psychological Medicine*, 11, 707–711.

Fairburn, C.G. (1985) Cognitive-behavioral treatment for bulimia. In D.M. Garner and P.E. Garfinkel (eds) *Handbook of Psychotherapy for Anorexia Nervosa and Bulimia*. New York: Guilford Press.

Fairburn, C.G. (1995) *Overcoming Binge Eating*. New York: Guilford Press.

Fairburn, C.G. (1997) Interpersonal psychotherapy for bulimia nervosa. In D.M. Garner and P.E. Garfinkel (eds) *Handbook of Treatment for Eating Disorders*. New York: Guilford Press.

Fairburn, C.G. and Carter, J.C. (1997) Self-help and guided self-help for binge-eating problems. In D.M. Garner and P.E. Garfinkel (eds) *Handbook of Treatment for Eating Disorders*. New York: Guilford Press.

Fairburn, C.G. and Cooper, P.J. ((1989) Eating disorder. In K. Hawton, P. Salkovskis, J. Kirk and D.M. Clark (eds) *Cognitive-behaviour Therapy for Psychiatric Problems: A Practical Guide*. Oxford: Oxford University Press.

Fairburn, C.G., Kirk, J., O'Connor, M. and Cooper, P.J. (1986) A comparison of two psychological treatments for bulimia nervosa. *Behaviour Research and Therapy*, 24, 629–643.

Fairburn, C.G., Jones, R., Pevler, R.A., Carr, S.J., Solomon, R.A., O'Connor, M.E., Burton, J. and Hope, R.A. (1991) Three psychological treatments for bulimia nervosa. *Archives of General Psychiatry*, 48, 463–469.

Fairburn, C.G., Stein, A. and Jones, R. (1992) Eating habits and eating disorders during pregnancy. *Psychosomatic Medicine*, 54, 6, 665–672.

Fairburn, C.G., Jones, R., Pevler, R.A. and O'Connor, M. (1993a) Psychotherapy and bulimia nervosa: the longer-term effects of interpersonal psychotherapy, behavior therapy and cognitive therapy. *Archives of General Psychiatry*, 50, 419–428.

Fairburn, C.G., Marcus, M.D.M. and Wilson, G.T. (1993b) Cognitive-behavioral therapy for binge eating and bulimia nervosa: a comprehensive treatment manual. In C.G. Fairburn and G.T. Wilson (eds) *Binge Eating: Nature, Assessment, and Treatment*. New York: Guilford Press.

Fairburn, C.G., Jones, R., Peveler, R., Hope, T. and O'Connor, T. (1993c) Predictors of 12 month outcome in bulimia nervosa and the influence of attitudes to shape and weight. *Journal of Consulting and Clinical Psychology*, 61, 696–698.

Fairburn, C.G., Welsh, S.L., Norman, P.A., O'Connor, M.E. and Doll, H.A. (1996) Bias and bulimia nervosa: how typical are clinic cases? *American Journal of Psychiatry*, 153, 386–391.

Leitenberg, H. and Rosen, J.C. (1985) Exposure plus response prevention treatment of bulimia. In D.M. Garner and P.E. Garfinkel (eds) *Handbook of Treatment for Eating Disorders*. New York: Guilford Press.

Garner, D.M., Rockert, W., Davis, R., Garner, M.V., Olmsted, M. and Eagle, M. (1993) Comparison of cognitive-behavioural and supportive-expressive therapy for bulimia nervosa. *American Journal of Psychiatry*, 150, 37–46.

Leitenberg, H., Rosen, J.C., Gross, J., Nudelman, S. and Vara, L.S. (1988) Exposure plus response prevention treatment of bulimia nervosa. *Journal of Consulting and Clinical Psychology*, 56, 535–541.

National Institute for Clinical Excellence (2004) Eating Disorders: core interventions in the treatment and management of anorexia nervosa, bulimia nervosa and related disorders. www.nice.org.uk

Olmsted, M.P., Davis, R., Garener, D.M., Eagle, M., Rockert, W. and Irvine, M.J. (1991) Efficacy of a brief psychoeducational intervention for bulimia nervosa. *Behaviour Research and Therapy*, 29, 71–84.

Palmer, R.L., Birchall, H., McGrain, L. and Sullivan, V. (2002) Self-help for bulimic disorders: a randomised controlled trial comparing minimal guidance with face-to-face or telephone guidance. *British Journal of Psychiatry*, 181, 230–235.

Polivy, J. and Herman, C.P. (1993) Etiology of binge eating: psychological mechanisms. In C.G. Fairburn and G.T. Wilson (eds) *Binge-eating: Nature, Assessment and Treatment*. New York: Guilford Press.

Pope, H.G., Hudson, J.I., Jonas, J.M. and Yurgelum-Todd, D. (1983) Bulimia treated with imipramine: a placebo-controlled, double-blind study. *American Journal of Psychiatry*, 140, 554–558.

Pyle, R.L., Mitchell, J.E., Eckert, E.D., Hatsukami, D., Pomeroy, C. and Zimmerman, R. (1990) Maintenance treatment and six month outcome for bulimic patients who respond to initial treatment. *American Journal of Psychiatry*, 147, 871–875.

Romano, S.J., Halmi, K., Sarkar, N.P., Koko, S.C. and Lee, J.S. (2002) A placebo-controlled study of fluoxetine in continued treatment of bulimia nervosa after successful acute fluoxetine treatment. *American Journal of Psychiatry*, 159, 96–102.

Walsh, B.T., Haddigan, C.M., Devlin, M.J., Gladis, M. and Roose, S.P. (1991) Long term outcome of antidepressant treatment for bulimia nervosa. *Journal of Psychiatry*, 148, 1206–1212.

Walsh, B.T., Fairburn, C.G., Mickley, D., Sysko, R. and Parides, M.K. (2004) Treatment of bulimia nervosa in a primary care setting. *American Journal of Psychiatry*, 161, 556–561.

Whitaker, A., Johnson, J., Shaffer, D., Rapoport, J.L., Kalikow, K., Walsh, B.T., Davies, M., Braiman, S. and Dolinsky, A. (1990) Uncommon troubles in young people: prevalence estimates of selected psychiatric disorders in a nonreferred adolescent population. *Archives of General Psychiatry*, 47, 487–496.

Wilson, G.T. and Fairburn, C.G. (1998) Treatments for eating disorders. In P.E. Nathan and J.M. Gorman (eds) *A Guide to Treatments that Work*. New York: Oxford University Press.

Wilson, G.T., Eldredge, K.L., Smith, D. *et al.* (1991) Cognitive-behavioral treatment with and without response prevention for bulimia. *Behaviour, Research and Therapy*, 29, 6, 575–583.

Chapter 12

Day hospital treatment for eating disorders

Marion Olmsted, Traci McFarlane, Lynda Molleken and Allan Kaplan

Introduction

The day hospital program at Toronto General Hospital is an intensive group therapy program for patients with moderate to severe eating disorders. The day hospital is part of an integrated ambulatory care program for eating disorders staffed by an experienced multi-disciplinary team of professionals from the fields of social work, psychology, psychiatry, nursing, and nutrition. Other components of this program include a transition program available to both day hospital patients and inpatients, and a variety of outpatient groups. This chapter will discuss the evolution of the program, advantages and disadvantages of day hospital treatment, the current day hospital program and the transition program, and will conclude with a section on future directions for the program.

Evolution of the day hospital

The day hospital program at Toronto General Hospital opened its doors in 1985. The program was modeled on the structure of an inpatient unit, and was designed to provide more cost-effective treatment for patients who would otherwise need hospitalization (Piran and Kaplan, 1990). At this time the program ran five days weekly, and did not offer on-site follow-up treatment or a vegetarian meal plan. In 1990 one follow-up group was introduced that was held on a weekly basis for ninety minutes. In 1994 the day hospital was reduced to a four-day program and resources were re-allocated for a more extensive follow-up program. From 1994 to the present the follow-up treatment (i.e. the transition program) has included three or four groups per week. The degree of structure in the follow-up program has progressively increased over time.

In 1995 a vegetarian option was introduced in the day hospital. This option is available to all patients, including those who avoid meat because of its fat or calorie content. Patients who avoid meat for eating disordered reasons are encouraged (but not required) to eat it, similar to our approach with other specific phobic foods. This is consistent with our philosophy of supporting full recovery while being responsive to patients' goals and preferences.

Advantages of day hospital treatment

The day hospital treatment of eating disorders has both financial and clinical advantages over inpatient treatment. The day hospital removes the need for hospital beds and nursing care, and allows resources to be directed at providing treatment rather than housing patients (Kaplan and Olmsted, 1997). In comparison to inpatient treatment, day hospital treatment is a highly cost-effective method for treating patients who do not require full hospitalization.

There are also clinical advantages to day hospital over inpatient treatment. Day treatment is less disruptive than inpatient care, as patients are able to maintain regular contact in relationships outside of the program. For some, these relationships may be supportive and facilitate the process of recovery. For others these relationships may serve as stressors or factors that have historically maintained the eating disorder and can now be explored in treatment. Patients have daily opportunities to apply the skills of normalized eating and symptom control that they learn in the program to their lives outside of the program. This increases the probability that the new skills will be internalized and generalized beyond the confines of the program.

Many patients who suffer from eating disorders have underlying personality deficits including maturity fears, interpersonal distrust, and an overwhelming sense of ineffectiveness (Bruch, 1982, Garner *et al.*, 1984). Such patients often perceive external control as punitive and are compelled to oppose treatment. This may manifest itself during hospitalization through the development of regression, dependence, unstable mood and impulsive behavior. Alternatively, patients may comply superficially with treatment, but secretly continue to engage in eating disordered behavior. In the day hospital setting these responses are attenuated by the limited control exerted by the program and the requirement that patients maintain themselves in a functioning state outside the hospital each day.

Disadvantages of day hospital treatment

Treating severely ill patients in an intensive day hospital setting provides challenges for both patients and staff. For some patients this model does not provide enough containment and inpatient hospitalization is required. The containment in a day hospital setting comes largely from interaction with other group members and staff. For those patients who are not equipped to engage in this interpersonal process or who cannot tolerate extreme affect, the intensity of this experience can be overwhelming and can lead to psychological deterioration. The risk of this occurring in vulnerable patients increases as eating and weight improve because the intense affect that was managed through starvation or bingeing and purging begins to surface and may feel intolerable or beyond control. At times some patients resort to maladaptive coping methods such as self-harm or substance abuse.

For staff, working in such an intensive setting can be extremely stressful, and requires considerable clinical skill and self-care. The need for continuous monitoring of patients' mental status, the constant staff–patient interaction required to maintain an empathically controlling environment, and the high degree of vigilance needed, especially around meals, can contribute to staff burn-out. Staff work closely together, providing ample opportunity for inter-personal tensions and/or mutual support and enrichment. Frequent com-munication and careful attention to team and countertransference issues are important (Kaplan *et al.*, 1997).

The day hospital programme

Structure

The day hospital program treats a maximum of twelve patients at any one time. The average length of stay is six to eight weeks for patients with bulimia nervosa, and ten to twelve weeks for patients with anorexia nervosa, depend-ing on their weight gain requirements. Currently the day hospital runs from Tuesday to Friday from 10:00 or 11:30 a.m. to 6:15 p.m. (see schedule in Figure 12.1). Patients are expected to attend each program day, and to remain on the unit unless supervised by a staff member. Program days are very structured with limited free time for patients. The time is divided into meals and therapy groups. Both staff and patients are expected to adhere closely to the schedule, starting and ending each activity on time. Purging is not permit-ted on the unit, and bathrooms are locked except for brief periods before meals and snacks.

Patients

To enter the day hospital program patients must meet the diagnostic criteria for an eating disorder (American Psychiatric Association, 1994). As part of a stepped care model, many patients have attended an outpatient group such as a six-session psychoeducation group or a ten-session outpatient symptom interruption group before admission to the day hospital. Some patients use the less intense outpatient groups to decide if a day hospital stay is necessary for their recovery or to prepare for their day hospital stay. Patients who are suffering from a severe eating disorder, or are from out of town, may be admitted directly into the day hospital program.

Patients must be motivated to change their eating disordered behavior, and are selected based on their willingness to work toward the program goals.

🕖	Tuesday	Wednesday	Thursday	Friday
9:15		GROCERY SHOPPING (4 patients)		
10:00				
10:15	WEEKEND SUMMARY	WEEK-IN-REVIEW		
11:30	COMMUNITY MEETING		CHECK-IN GROUP OR COOKING (2 patients)	CHECK-IN GROUP OR COOKING (2 patients)
12:00	LUNCH OR LUNCH OUTING (3 patients)	LUNCH	LUNCH	LUNCH
1:00	FREE TIME	COMMUNITY MEETING	COMMUNITY MEETING	COMMUNITY MEETING
1:30	EDUCATION GROUP	FREE TIME	MEAL PLAN CHANGES	FREE TIME
1:45 / 2:30	FREE TIME	GYM	GROUP'S CHOICE	BODY IMAGE
2:45	SNACK OUTING (4 patients)			
3:00	SNACK	SNACK	SNACK	SNACK
3:30	RELATIONSHIP GROUP	BODY IMAGE	MENUS/ NUTRITION	WEEKEND PLANNING
5:00–6:15	DINNER and EVENING PLANS	DINNER and EVENING PLANS	DINNER and EVENING PLANS	DINNER and EVENING PLANS

Figure 12.1 Day hospital schedule.

They must also demonstrate a capacity to tolerate a group setting. Patients are required to interrupt their daily activities in order to attend the program (e.g. take a leave of absence from work, defer school, or delay a vacation). Ninety per cent of patients admitted to the day hospital are female; their ages range from 17 to 60 years with an average age of 26 years. Comorbidity is high and includes affective disorders, anxiety disorders, personality disorders and substance abuse.

Contraindications for admission to the day hospital are few but include: (1) acute medical risk such as severe emaciation or cardiovascular complications requiring inpatient care; (2) severe substance abuse or dependence interfering with the ability to normalize eating or participate in groups; and (3) acute suicide risk (Kaplan and Olmsted, 1997).

Goals

The primary goals of the day hospital program are discussed with patients before their admission is planned. These goals include: (1) the normalization of eating behavior through the prescription of a balanced meal plan; (2) the cessation of bingeing, purging (i.e. vomiting, laxatives, exercise), and other behaviors used to control weight; (3) weight gain for patients who are below the average weight range (i.e. BMI less than 20); and (4) the identification and exploration of current stressors and underlying issues that serve to maintain the eating disorder.

(1) Normalized eating: an individualized balanced meal plan including three meals and two snacks per day is prescribed. Patients who are at or above a BMI of 20 start on 1500 to 1800 calories per day, and this is gradually increased until they reach the maintenance calorie level for their age and height (usually between 1800 and 2300 calories per day). The program advocates healthy non-dieting. From the first day all food groups (including fats and desserts) are included in the patient's meal plan. Over time patients are encouraged to increase their exposure to progressively more phobic foods. Through repeated exposure they learn that the anxiety triggered by eating phobic foods eventually subsides without the use of symptoms.

Meals within the program are an important feature of the day hospital treatment. Each program day includes lunch, afternoon snack, and dinner. Patients eat their meals together and are supervised by two therapists. The therapists coach patients in normal eating and guide conversation away from food, weight, and upsetting events. Patients are expected to complete their entire meal within a time frame of forty minutes for lunch or dinner and twenty minutes for snacks. Patients are expected to eat breakfast, evening snacks, and all meals on Saturdays, Sundays, and Mondays on their own. This provides them with the opportunity to incorporate normalized eating into their natural environment. Grocery shopping, cooking, and restaurant outings with staff occur regularly to expose patients to situations they may find difficult to manage on their own. During lunch and snack outings the staff eat with the patients to model normalized eating behavior.

(2) Symptom control: the containment of the day hospital provides a safe environment where symptoms are not an option during program hours. Patients are not allowed to bring food onto the unit, they must complete the meals provided by the program, and the washrooms are locked after all meals to prevent purging. In addition, there is a strong focus on cognitive-behavioral strategies to control symptoms outside of program hours (e.g. delay, distraction, stimulus control, and coping self-statements).

(3) Weight gain: patients who need to gain weight as part of their recovery start on 1500 to 1800 calories per day. This amount is gradually increased to support a weight gain of 1 to 2 kilograms per week. The maximum daily intake is 3600 calories. Patients follow a maintenance meal plan (1800–2300 calories per day) in order to learn normal food portions, with additional calories in the form of supplements. Activity levels may need to be kept to a minimum to promote weight gain.

(4) Underlying therapeutic issues: underlying issues and stressors that are maintaining the eating disorder are identified and processed in group and family therapy.

Groups

Many groups use cognitive-behavioral principles to focus on normalized eating and symptom control. These groups include nutrition, weekend planning, weekend summary, check-in, and week-in-review. During these groups, meals and activities are carefully planned, high risk situations are discussed and prepared for, strategies are formulated, and symptoms are examined in detail with the goal of identifying triggers and treating any symptom occurrence as a learning experience. Other groups such as 'group's choice' and 'relationship group' are more psychodynamic and focus on psychological issues underlying the eating disorder. These issues may include, but are not limited to, the function of the eating disorder, interpersonal relationships, autonomy, and past abuse. The body image groups explore the meaning of weight and shape specific to each individual (see Jarry, 1998). One body image group includes imagery and relaxation exercises, which help patients to explore the way they perceive their bodies, and learn ways to become more comfortable with their bodies. The other body image group is based on a more cognitive-behavioral model.

In the education group, staff teach patients about various topics related to eating disorders such as medical complications, cultural influences, exercise, setpoint, and metabolism. Patients also attend gym once weekly and play badminton, volleyball or frisbee as a group. The goal of the gym time is to model activity that is fun and social, in contrast to exercise that is solitary and focused on burning calories or changing weight and shape. Gym occurs early Wednesday afternoon (see Figure 12.1) after the patients have been weighed in the morning and before a body image group later in the afternoon; the gym time provides an outlet on this stressful day.

The community meeting, which takes place daily, includes all staff and patients and has an open agenda which provides an opportunity to address therapeutic issues, share feedback from staff, or discuss practical aspects of treatment such as planned absences from the program or the rationale for any program rule or requirement.

Weighing

All patients are weighed on a weekly basis. For many patients this can be an extremely distressful event because weight is tied to self-worth (Fairburn and Garner, 1988; Vitousek and Hollon, 1990). Patients are weighed individually and then come together in a week-in-review group to process changes in weight, express affect and start the process of separating weight and shape from self-esteem.

Self-monitoring

Patients keep a detailed record of their meals, eating disorder symptoms, urges, risks, strategies, and feelings in a weekly eating diary. This encourages patients to make connections between emotions and eating disorder symptoms, learn from symptoms, and become aware of progress toward recovery. These diaries are reviewed by staff, and patients are given feedback and recommendations each week.

Family therapy

Family therapy is available to all patients in the ambulatory care program for eating disorders. Patients in the day hospital are strongly encouraged to invite their close friends and family members in to address issues connected to the eating disorder and/or to help family members cope with the situation.

Psychiatric and medical treatment

Patients meet with the psychiatrist on admission for a medical and psychiatric assessment. At that time laboratory investigations are ordered which include an electrocardiogram, complete blood count, electrolytes, creatinine, and urea, with more specialized tests as needed. During the admission the psychiatrist follows up on routine medication and medical issues in the community meeting. More detailed or complicated psychiatric or medical issues are addressed in individual meetings with the patient, but care is taken not to drift on to therapeutic issues in these meetings. SSRI antidepressants are commonly prescribed, especially for patients with bulimia. Hypnotics and anxiolytics are prescribed as necessary. Common medical concerns requiring attention include gastrointestinal problems, cardiac symptoms, and osteoporosis.

Therapeutic milieu

While patients are encouraged to express their emotions, staff also monitor the patients closely and provide containment by coaching and educating patients about the need to explore painful issues at a pace that is tolerable for them. Patients need to work on issues at a pace that does not prohibit eating or efforts to control symptoms. The containment of the day hospital can trigger issues related to autonomy, control, anger, and perfectionism in some patients. When this occurs, patients are encouraged to explore the underlying psychological issues rather than focus on the details of the day hospital program.

Patients are allowed some control by the emphasis on the voluntary nature of the program, and the ability to choose from a menu of foods to fulfill their prescribed meal plan. The staff make every effort to establish a trusting relationship with the patients and a good rapport is the norm. Staff try to maintain the delicate balance between the containment required for normalized eating and symptom control, and the promotion of autonomy and self-responsibility necessary for recovery.

Advantages and disadvantages of group treatment

Group treatment provides an atmosphere of safety and mutual support for patients because all group members are struggling with similar issues. The isolation that often develops as a result of the shame connected to the eating disorder is alleviated by the mutual sharing of these feelings in the group (Kaplan *et al.*, 1997). Many emotional and behavioral responses are normalized by other group members. The open group format of the day hospital allows senior members who have been through the initial stages of weight gain, normalized eating, and symptom control to guide and support junior members who are unclear about what to expect during treatment and recovery. Finally, group pressure and confrontation is a powerful therapeutic tool, especially during mealtimes.

The day hospital does not provide individual therapy. Many patients require intense individual therapy to work on core issues, and are therefore encouraged to work with an individual therapist on these issues after completion of their day hospital stay. Patients who already have an individual therapist when they start the program are asked to limit their contact to weekly meetings focused on maintaining the patient's connection to the therapist and on keeping the therapist informed. The day hospital currently offers a standardized approach to all participants. Although this consistency plays an important role in fostering containment, the lack of flexibility keeps some patients out of the program and makes it stressful for others.

The transition program

An important component of day hospital treatment is the transition program, which provides follow-up care for patients. Upon completion of the day hospital program or the inpatient program patients are strongly encouraged to attend the transition program. The goal of the transition program is to maintain the progress that has been achieved during day hospital or inpatient treatment when patients return to the challenges of life outside the program. At this time, patients can begin to reintegrate work, school, and leisure activities back into their daily schedules.

The transition program consists of four weekly groups each structured around a specific therapeutic task. Each group lasts ninety minutes to two hours, and groups are co-led by day hospital and inpatient staff. On Mondays patients are weighed, and given an opportunity to have their nutrition questions answered by the dietician. This group involves bringing a lunch consistent with the patient's meal plan and eating together as a group. Patients are encouraged to bring risky foods to consume at this time. After lunch a therapy group allows patients to process any changes in their weight and review how their week went in terms of their meal plan, risks, urges, symptoms, and other significant events and issues.

Patients in the transition program are required to monitor their eating behavior in a weekly food diary. Staff review this food diary and provide feedback to patients in a feedback group. The remainder of this group focuses on strategies and/or relevant psychological issues. The third group focuses on body image work and the fourth group is an open agenda group focused on psychological issues. Depending on their progress, patients can remain in the transition program for up to twelve weeks.

Relapse prevention group

Patients who are able to normalize their eating and remain almost symptom-free for a minimum of four weeks are invited to attend the relapse prevention group. This group meets every Monday evening, so that patients can fully reintegrate back into their normal lifestyle and begin to develop regular daily activities while attending. This group focuses on factors such as identification and expression of emotions, building self-esteem in areas other than weight and shape, challenging maladaptive thoughts, and assertiveness training. Patients who remain well can attend this group for up to twenty weeks.

Future directions

Our thoughts for the future include making the day hospital program more flexible. We have been experimenting with 'pieces' of treatment, such as having patients attend the day hospital to accomplish part of their weight gain or for a limited stay tied to their ability to tolerate the program. In addition, we are considering the idea of encouraging patients to negotiate their own treatment goals in order to enhance their control and autonomy in the context of working toward recovery. Ideally, we will find a way to respect and support patients' personal goals, while sharing our hope and belief in a full recovery for each of them.

References

American Psychiatric Association (1994) *Diagnostic and Statistical Manual of Mental Disorders* (4th ed). Washington, DC: APA.

Bruch, H. (1982) Psychotherapy in anorexia nervosa. *International Journal of Eating Disorders*, 2, 3–14.

Fairburn, C.G. and Garner, D.M. (1988) Diagnostic criteria for anorexia nervosa and bulimia nervosa: the importance of attitudes to shape and weight. In D.M. Garner and P.E. Garfinkel (eds), *Diagnostic Issues in Anorexia Nervosa and Bulimia Nervosa*. New York: Brunner/Mazel.

Garner, D.M., Olmsted, M.P., Polivy, J., and Garfinkel, P.E. (1984) Comparison between weight-preoccupied women and anorexia nervosa. *Psychosomatic Medicine*, 46, 255–266.

Jarry, J. (1998) The meaning of body image for women with eating disorders. *Psychosomatic Medicine*, 43, 367–374.

Kaplan, A. and Olmsted, M.P. (1997) Partial hospitalization. In D.M. Garner and P.E. Garfinkel (eds) *Handbook of Treatment for Eating Disorders*. New York: Guilford Press.

Kaplan, A.S., Olmsted, M.P., and Molleken, L. (1997) Day treatment of eating disorders. *Bailliere's Clinical Psychiatry*, 3, 275–289.

Piran, N. and Kaplan, A. (eds) (1990) *A Day Hospital Group Treatment Program for Anorexia Nervosa and Bulimia Nervosa*. New York: Brunner/Mazel.

Vitousek, K.B. and Hollon, S.D. (1990) The investigation of schematic content and processing in eating disorders. *Cognitive Therapy and Research*, 14, 191–214.

Chapter 13

Inpatient treatment of anorexia nervosa

The Toronto General Hospital program

D. Blake Woodside, Sandy Sonnenberg, Kelli Young, Debbi Jonas, Jacqueline Carter, Allan Kaplan, Rochelle Martin, Regina Cowan and Sophie Grigoriadis

Introduction

The inpatient treatment of anorexia nervosa has been a neglected topic in the academic literature over the last two decades. This has partly been due to the explosion of interest in the assessment and treatment of bulimia nervosa. In North America, there has been some decrease in interest in inpatient treatment because of the very difficult situations that have been encountered as a result of marked constraints in the funding of inpatient treatments.

As a result, the majority of inpatient treatment programs appear to have remained relatively unchanged for the last two decades. Emphasis continues to be placed on the use of behavioral techniques to generate weight gain, usually as quickly as possible, with little attention paid to the psychological and cognitive aspects of treatment, at least during the inpatient phase. And while a number of authors have commented on the relatively disappointing results of inpatient treatments (Eckert *et al.*, 1995; Norring and Sohlberg, 1993; Kreipe *et al.*, 1995; Herzog *et al.*, 1993), these commentaries have not generated much interest in how the outcome of these treatments might be improved. Given the very large expense involved in the provision of inpatient treatment, and the recognized mortality and morbidity that occur in patients who are sick enough to require inpatient treatment, the lack of attention to this area in eating disorders is unfortunate.

Literature describing inpatient treatments in the last decade

Although there has been little written on comprehensive inpatient treatment for anorexia nervosa, the first practice guidelines for a set of psychiatric disorders were developed for the eating disorders (APA, 1993). Inpatient hospitalization is recommended for patients whose weight is below 70 per cent of average weight for height, those with rapidly falling weight, or those who show physiological instability for medical management and comprehensive treatment for support of weight gain. Bowers and Andersen (1994) described additional indications for hospitalization: patients with serious comorbid psychiatric symptoms or relentless binge or purge related behaviors (such as vomiting, laxative and diuretic abuse, and compulsive over-exercise); patients with untreated ongoing anorexia for over a year; patients who fail twelve to sixteen weeks' outpatient management and those in a destructive family relationship should also be admitted for inpatient treatment. Aims of inpatient treatment are diverse and include the restoration to a healthy weight, restoration of healthy eating patterns, management of medical complications, addressing dysfunctional thoughts, feelings and beliefs, correcting defects in affect and behavioral regulation, improvement of psychological difficulties, enlisting family support when necessary, and lastly preventing relapse (APA, 1993). It has been noted that chronic patients who have had a number of admissions may need alternative approaches to inpatient hospitalization (Hsu, 1986).

Following from the diverse goals of impatient admission, programs need to be multidimensional and multidisciplinary in their approach. Integrated programs generally include a nutritional regimen, target weights with a specific speed of weight restoration, psychoeducation, psychotherapy with the incorporation of individual, group or family approaches, occupational or activities therapy, and informational feedback. Unfortunately, the literature on comprehensive inpatient management for anorexia nervosa remains sparse and few controlled studies have been done to address their effectiveness. One of the central aims of hospitalization is the restoration of weight and there is a body of literature on how that can be achieved effectively.

The APA (1993) guidelines recommended 1–3 lbs./week as a rate of weight gain with a usual starting intake of 30–40 kcal/kg per day. An individual patient should achieve a weight that allows return to normal reproductive function and reversal of bone demineralization. There are a variety of successful interventions to restore weight. A detailed review is beyond the scope of this chapter but methods shown to be efficacious include a supportive nursing management with emphasis on encouragement of eating and bed rest with a high-calorie diet (Russell, 1977). Tube feeding and hyperalimentation (enterally or parenterally (Silverman, 1974; Maloney and Farrell, 1980)) can also induce weight gain. However, as these approaches have not been found to effect long-term maintenance of weight gain and are associated with many complications (Garfinkel and Garner, 1982), it is suggested that they be used only in 'life threatening or very unusual circumstances' and only for brief periods of time while normal eating is developed (APA, 1993). Electroconvulsive therapy (ECT), psychosurgery and pharmacotherapies have not been as successful in inducing weight gain (Ferguson, 1993; Crisp and Kalucy, 1973; Goldbloom *et al.*, 1989). Bowers and Andersen (1994) report that the most 'prudent' programs combine several interventions and emphasize the restoration of a normal pattern of eating behavior in addition to a healthy weight. Regardless, however, nutritional assessment, education and continued support are essential.

Inpatient admission also allows for the treatment of medical complications associated with starvation. Dehydration, electrolyte imbalances, leukopenia and delayed gastric emptying are usually the first to require treatment. More complicated issues such as generalized brain atrophy and decreased cardiac diameter may also need to be addressed (Kaplan and Garfinkel, 1993). There is no doubt that hospitalization within a well-structured program is the most rapid and efficient way to deal with weight and medical issues (Eckert and Mitchell, 1989). Typically patients remain in hospital from two to four months. Bowers and Andersen (1994) consider that another vital task of inpatient admission is to initiate psychotherapy and behavioral relearning within a safe holding environment.

Various forms of psychotherapy have also proven helpful in the induction of weight gain. The reader is directed to Hsu (1986) and Eckert and Mitchell (1989) for a comprehensive review. Briefly, behavioral programs with both positive and negative reinforcers in addition to feedback regarding weight gain, caloric intake and large meals have been shown to influence weight gain at least in the short term (Agras, 1987). Moreover, 'strict' behavioral programs associating caloric intake or weight gain with a schedule of privileges have not been found to be more effective than 'lenient' ones (Touyz et al., 1984) Behavioral programs have produced the most consistent results in terms of promoting weight restoration but not in terms of changing body image or alleviating interpersonal problems. Other forms of psychotherapy are used in inpatient settings to address core psychological issues and include individual, group and family therapy but controlled trials utilizing only inpatients have yet to be reported. As a result, little is known about the efficacy of any single psychotherapy during inpatient hospitalization. The APA guidelines (1993) state that the exact role of psychotherapy in the hospitalized severely malnourished patient remains unclear. This seems paradoxical in light of the many psychological issues and associated psychiatric symptoms that these patients face.

The most comprehensive treatment program described in the literature is that of Andersen et al. (1997), with an earlier version found in Andersen et al., (1985). Given its depth and breadth it will be reviewed in detail. Achievable goals include: re-establishing a healthy weight, improvement in eating patterns, the learning of healthy social behavior, decrease in core psychopathology, the promotion of healthy age-appropriate patterns of conflict resolution in addition to the promotion of healthy living, the treatment of comorbid disorders and medical complications, aftercare and relapse prevention plans. The program is a structured multidisciplinary one that integrates nutritional rehabilitation, psychotherapy and behavioral relearning. Following medical stabilization, patients enter a 'therapeutic milieu' which emphasizes consistency in goals and methods by a protocol designed to deal with issues related to weight restoration, exercise, level of observation and privileges. Psychological principles of treatment are derived from cognitive behavioral therapy, although psychoeducation and psychodynamic treatment are also incorporated. Treatment modalities include individual, group and family methods and patients are involved in treatment much of the day.

This program strives for a healthy weight based on a number of criteria with an average weight restoration of 9–12 kg. The goal weight range is kept from the patient until she is within the range. Food is prescribed as medicine and is eaten in formal conditions. Nursing staff remain with the patient and provide twenty-four-hour support and supervision until a normal eating pattern is established. A graduated exercise program is permitted. Medications to stimulate appetite are not used although prokinetic agents are. Selective serotonin reuptake inhibitors (SSRIs) are used for the treatment of the binge-eating/purging subtype of anorexia. Comorbid psychiatric illnesses can be treated pharmacologically. Although this program is ambitious it is appealing because it tries to address the multifactorial nature of the disorder. Unfortunately, data on its effectiveness are lacking.

Vandereycken (1985) describes a multifaceted group approach to inpatient treatment. The group operates on a standardized behavioral contract system with regard to short-term weight restoration. Group dynamics are used as well as the family in the treatment process. This program seems intuitively appealing given the increased awareness of health care spending; however, data on the effectiveness of this program also are not presented.

Engel and Wilfarth (1988) and Engel *et al.* (1989) describe a program for eating disorders which spans inpatient and outpatient treatment. The inpatient component includes a strict regimen component comprising bed rest, phenothiazines and tube feeding. Psychotherapeutic measures within the strict regimen incorporate behavioral contingencies, a confrontational technique and separation of the patient from their regular environment with no visitors, telephone or mail. Supportive and conflict-oriented psychotherapy are also incorporated. The authors quote a 53 per cent success rate following treatment, which falls to 51 per cent at two-year follow-up. At approximately nine-year follow-up, 53 per cent of patients are still able to maintain a job and relationship. The authors note that the addition of an outpatient psychotherapeutic component does not result in optimization of their earlier model which included only the strict regimen associated with medical treatment. The methods used in the inpatient component are not routinely recommended by the guidelines for eating disorders and indeed are not conventional by today's standards. Although not reviewed here, over 50 per cent of patients with anorexia ultimately recover (see Bowers and Andersen, 1994).

Research on comprehensive inpatient treatment of anorexia nervosa remains limited. Most of the work has been done in the area of weight restoration. Less is known on how to achieve psychological change during admission and how to maintain weight gain after discharge. The current status of the literature may reflect the complexity of inpatient treatment that is needed to treat this disorder. Given the multifaceted etiology and the compounding effects of starvation, several therapeutic approaches are often necessary simultaneously. Controlled research is necessary, addressing the effectiveness of a comprehensive approach.

Development of the Toronto General Hospital program

With the above in mind, we set about to reorganize our approach to the treatment of adults in Toronto in 1993. The treatment of children and adolescents is totally separate from that of adults in our province. At that time, we had four to six beds available for a population base of approximately 10 million individuals, and we were the only significant source of treatment for this population. While our day hospital program was able to treat less severely ill patients, the most ill patients continued to require inpatient treatment. At the time, our waiting list was routinely six months for inpatient treatment, and a previous version of the treatment, an individually based behavioral program, had largely become non-operational because of administrative reorganizations and budget reductions.

Assessing the situation, it was clear that no additional resources were likely to be available in the immediate future. A review of the types of patients referred suggested that they could be broken down into two main groups: those being referred for definitive treatment, and those being referred for emergency management and stabilization.

We needed to make a decision about how to apply a very limited resource – either to those who at least appeared to be interested in making a significant change in their condition, or to those who were in the worst shape physically and nutritionally, most of whom were involuntary patients who did not wish to receive active treatment.

Our decision to focus on the former group was affected by a number of factors. First, we had not had a good experience in the previous years with involuntary treatment: many of those to whom we had provided involuntary re-feeding had subsequently died and there seemed little to be gained from putting all of our resources into what amounted to management rather than treatment. In addition, we had been able to develop some ability to arrange for emergency management, such as short-term re-feeding and medical interventions, in settings other than our inpatient eating disorders program. We had observed fairly good results in treating less ill patients in the day hospital program, where we had made some attempts to assess motivation for change, and all treatment was voluntary.

Our final decision was to focus our resources on the group we felt was most likely to have a good response – those patients with severe anorexia nervosa who were prepared to come into treatment voluntarily, and who were willing to make a commitment to attempt to fully eradicate all traces of the illness. This decision went hand-in-hand with an ongoing commitment to assist in arranging emergency medical interventions, including re-feeding when necessary, in other settings, be they psychiatric or medical.

Once this decision had been made, it was then possible to develop some other basic elements of the program. Since the program was to be voluntary, we felt that we could offer a greater amount of freedom and a relatively lesser amount of constraint to the patients, who could, after all, leave the program at any time. In this regard, we were influenced not only by our experience in treating anorexic patients in the day hospital, but also by the writings of Touyz *et al.* (1984), and Vandereycken in Belgium (1985), who were advocating a more 'lenient' approach to the treatment of such patients. A growing familiarity with feminist thinking in this area (Sesan, 1994) also suggested to us that there were less coercive measures that could be at least equally effective in the medium term, and perhaps more effective in the long term, than traditional involuntary behavioral approaches. We were aware at the time that our short-term results were likely to be less successful compared to involuntary treatments, where patients simply were not permitted to leave the program.

What this approach has produced is an environment that is relatively free of external coercion. All those attending have made a positive decision to be in the program, and a given patient's ongoing participation in the program is contingent on her continuing to make changes that are in the direction of recovery. Rather than fighting to exit our treatment (as is often the case in more coercive environments), our patients fight to remain in the treatment. This profoundly alters the relationship between the patient group and staff – from one that is primarily focused on policing to one that is much more about assisting in the process of change.

We were fortunate to receive some additional funds to expand the program in 1997, and we were able to increase the size of the program to ten beds, and develop a complete specialty team. At that time we made a large number of changes to the content of the program, without altering the basic approach that we have described above. It is the later, expanded version of the program that is described below.

Goals and objectives for inpatient treatment in Toronto

As described above, we have made a decision to apply our limited resources to those severely ill patients who appear to be the most likely to respond to treatment. At the present time, the assessment of such a likelihood is completely clinical, there being essentially no empirical research available to act as a guide.

Because our goal is to begin the process of complete recovery, and because we are still not externally constrained as to such factors as length of stay, we have set complete weight restoration as part of our goal. This is related to our reading of the very limited literature on this topic (Commerford *et al.*, 1997; Baran *et al.*, 1995) which suggests that exiting inpatient treatment at a lower than normal weight is associated with worse outcome. So, for example, we do not contract for partial weight restoration, although patients may covertly have this in mind as they may leave the program at any time.

This goal rests alongside a goal to allow our patients the maximal chance to normalize their eating, both inside and outside of the hospital setting. We hope that patients by the time they complete our program will be able to eat reliably inside and outside the hospital, although possibly in a mechanical fashion.

With regard to cognitive and psychological goals, we hope that over the course of treatment patients will at least be able to identify the main issues that are pertinent to their own situation, and have a plan in place to effect a positive resolution to these difficulties. This plan could include further therapy or counseling, or perhaps a return to school or a course of vocational rehabilitation. The extent to which resolution is achieved is highly variable, and cannot be prescribed.

While these goals are ambitious, they are framed to the patients as part of a longer process, one which will take some time to complete. The individual-specific nature of the process of recovery is emphasized to all patients.

Current program description

General description

The program is an intensive, primarily group-therapy program. The majority of the programming is provided from Monday to Friday, from about 8:00 a.m. until 9:00 p.m. (see Figure 13.1). A limited amount of individual therapy is provided, along with family and couple therapy as required. Pharmacotherapy and medical interventions are provided as needed. All meals are supervised by staff. Patients also record their eating and other symptoms in a self-report booklet, called a weekly eating behavior book, or WEB.

The program is voluntary and the group is open – that is, new patients are admitted continuously as more senior patients either complete their stay or exit the program for one reason or another.

The program is staffed by a multidisciplinary team that includes a psychiatrist, psychologist, social worker, dietician, occupational therapist, an integrative and expressive arts therapist, and five specialty nurses. Program staff provide coverage Monday through Friday, 7:30 a.m. until 7:30 p.m.

The program is housed on a general psychiatry unit. All program treatment is provided separately from that provided to general psychiatry patients. The

	Monday	Tuesday	Wednesday	Thursday	Friday
8:00	Breakfast	Breakfast	Breakfast	Breakfast	Breakfast
8:30					
9:00	Expressive Arts		Menu Marking Group	Ward meeting	Research Group
9:30	Therapies				
10:00				Sexuality Group	Ward meeting
10:30			Shopping		
11:00					Weekend Activities
11:30	Weighing		Lunch prep		
12:00	Lunch	Lunch	Lunch	Lunch/ Lunch	Lunch
12:30				Outing	
1:00	Weekend Review	Ward Meeting/	Ward meeting		Weekend
1:30		Feedback		Relationship Group	Menus
2:00			Relaxation/ Spirituality		Reconnection Group/
2:30			Group		Nutrition Group
3:00	Snack	Snack/ Snack Outing	Snack	Snack	Snack
3:30	Family Relations	Self Image	Rethinking Group	Dinner prep	
4:00	Group	Group			Education Group
4:30					
5:00	Dinner/After dinner	Dinner/After dinner	Dinner/After dinner	Dinner/After dinner	Dinner/After dinner
5:30	discussion	discussion	discussion	discussion	discussion
6:15	Visiting hours	Visiting hours	Visiting hours	Visiting hours	Visiting hours
9:00	Snack	Snack	Snack	Snack	Snack

Figure 13.1 Inpatient eating disorders program.

program has a separate dining room and a group therapy room that is usually reserved for the program. Patients are usually housed in a double room, with another program patient or not, according to their preference.

There is no external limit placed on the length of admission. As will be reviewed below, length of stay ranges from a few hours to nearly thirty weeks, with a mean of about sixteen weeks. Patients who complete the program are then transferred to a follow-up program which runs three to four days per week for one to two hours per day. This program lasts four to twelve weeks, and is followed by further less intensive outpatient treatment.

Patients progress through a sequence of gradual reductions in containment that generally occur independent of weight or other symptoms. Patients are restricted to the ward for the first week and, if there is a history of bingeing or purging, have their bathroom locked. In the second week of treatment, patients are allowed to leave the ward, but must stay on hospital grounds. The bathroom remains locked during this week. In the third week, patients may leave the hospital grounds when not engaged in program activities, and are sent home for the weekend. Patients then continue on this program until they are roughly half-way through the process of weight gain. If their eating on the weekends is fairly stable, they will then be shifted to attending the inpatient program as a day attendee. That is, they will leave the hospital at the end of each day, spend the night at home, and return to the hospital the next morning to continue the program. Patients then complete their treatment as day attendees until they are ready for transfer to our follow-up program, which usually occurs a few weeks after they have reached a body mass index (BMI) of 20.

There are some significant program norms that all patients are expected to observe; patients who are consistently unable to do so may be asked to leave the program. Patients must agree to complete all of their supervised meals. Patients are further asked to refrain from self-harm, the use of alcohol and street drugs while in the program.

There is no bed rest in the program, and the program is devoid of behavioral contingencies, except that calories will be raised if the rate of weight gain does not reach our goal of 1–2 kg/week.

Health care in Ontario is a publicly funded service, with all medically necessary treatments provided by physicians and in hospitals covered at no direct cost to the patient. Resource constraints are global, rather than specific. It is illegal for a physician to provide an insured service at a cost to the patient in excess of that allowed by the provincial schedule of fees. Private hospitals are not allowed to provide insured services at cost to the patient, and thus they do not generally exist.

Assessments and entry into the program

Patients are referred to the program from the consultation service. These referrals are reviewed by the attending psychiatrist and triaged if necessary. Referred patients are then scheduled for a team assessment, where the relevant parts of their history are reviewed and their motivation to enter the treatment and their understanding of the treatment are assessed. Patients who are accepted into the program are then placed on a waiting list for a bed. The entire process, from referral to the inpatient program to admission, typically takes four to eight weeks, but can be as short as two weeks, depending on the demands on the program and the availability of beds.

Specific treatments in the program

Nutritional treatments

Nutrition therapy is essential and integral to the treatment of individuals suffering from anorexia nervosa or bulimia nervosa. Broadly speaking, the goals of nutrition intervention are twofold: (1) to improve and normalize physical nutrition parameters; (2) to normalize food intake patterns while eliminating eating disorder symptoms. The techniques and tools used must be science-based, and delivered with a unique combination of empathy and firmness (Rock and Curran-Celentano, 1996; Reiff and Reiff, 1992).

Nutritional assessment

A detailed nutrition history is key to developing an appropriate nutrition care plan. It is crucial to obtain a good understanding of each individual's food intake patterns in order to challenge the cognitive and perceptual distortions that determine her/his food choices and eating pattern. Food intake patterns usually vary with stage of illness, as increasing restriction is necessary to maintain weight loss. Patients often follow idiosyncratic, highly individual-ized rituals: eating only certain foods on certain days, eliminating entire food groups, allowing only a certain number of calories per food group, etc. Foods are also frequently dichotomized as 'good' or 'bad'. Diet products (i.e. foods labeled 'light', 'low fat', etc.) are commonly used, as are diet aids (diet pills, slimming teas, laxatives, diuretics, etc.). Many strategies are used to reduce energy intake and deny hunger cues, such as the overuse of chewing gum and caffeinated beverages. It is important to explore the meaning attached to the use of these foods and diet products, and then to progressively challenge this throughout treatment.

Common food-related behaviors include controlling the household food budget by shopping and cooking for the entire family. Usually little or no food is consumed with the family. As well, patients often have a strong aver-sion to spending money on food for their own consumption. They may spend hours reading cookbooks, fliers, calorie-counters, etc. By identifying these behaviors as part of the eating disorder, the individual can begin to make changes and incorporate healthier, normal food patterns.

Eating disorder patients often suffer from numerous gastrointestinal com-plaints, such as heartburn, reflux, bloating, cramps, diarrhea, constipation, sore mouth and poor dental health. It is important to acknowledge the dis-comfort of these symptoms, to normalize their presence in the context of an eating disorder, and if possible to treat them. However, it is just as important to identify that these kinds of complaints often serve to legitimize the patient's desire to restrict or omit certain foods.

Weight and body mass index (BMI: an indicator of weight relative to height (Ontario Ministry of Health, 1991)) upon admission generally reflect the severity of starvation; however, fluid status often influences true weight. Patients who binge/purge or abuse laxatives will often have fairly large fluctuations in weight gain early on, due to rehydration and stabilization of electrolytes. Similarly, the extremely underweight restricting anorexic may experience re-feeding edema, and initially gain significant weight as fluid. Preparing patients for expected fluid shifts and the resulting weight changes can help reduce their initial anxiety. It is also valuable to assess patterns of weight gain/loss (maximum weight, minimum weight, weight changes in the past six months, phobic weights), particularly when developing strategies to tolerate weight change.

Typically patients are extremely anxious regarding their so-called 'target' weight. We have eliminated the use of this term, using instead 'low end' weight, referring to the 'low end of a healthy weight'. This is set at a BMI of 20; however, patients are constantly encouraged not to focus on the particular number, but to understand that there is a range of healthy weights, i.e. BMI 20–25.

Finally, it is important to assess and monitor laboratory values, including electrolytes, magnesium, calcium, phosphate, albumin, total protein, and hemoglobin. Starvation and eating disorder symptoms influence the interpretation of these nutritional parameters. Potassium supplements are often required for patients who vomit or abuse laxatives. However, laboratory values generally return to normal after a very short period of normal eating and cessation of eating disorder symptoms (Rock et al., 1996).

One final cautionary note: the severely underweight anorexic patient, if given a large influx of carbohydrate (particularly via IV glucose), can very suddenly develop re-feeding syndrome, which may require intensive medical care and carries a high risk of death (see Havala and Shronts, 1990, for an excellent overview). It is generally safer to use a normal saline solution if an IV is needed, and to provide calories through foods high in protein and fat, and low in carbohydrate. Once medically stable and rehydrated, there is no need to limit oral carbohydrate intake.

Nutritional interventions

The key to any nutrition therapy in eating disorders is to define and model normal eating through the use of a meal plan. In the inpatient program, three meals and two snacks are provided daily, and patients mark menus on a weekly basis. Numerous guidelines are used to assist them in menu marking in order to promote variety and balance, and to ensure adequate caloric intake. The meal plan itself entails seven food groups: protein, starch, milk, fruits, vegetables, added fats, and satisfying foods. This last category consists of desserts (cake, pie, donuts) and snack foods (potato chips, 'cheezies'). These are foods generally labeled as 'bad' and avoided or only consumed during binges, and it is critical to reintroduce them as part of normal eating.

To help with this, patients create a 'risk list' of their most difficult and phobic foods, and are encouraged to gradually incorporate foods from this list in their menu selections.

This meal plan provides a balance in terms of menu-marking guidelines (i.e. the external controls that provide some measure of relief for the patients, but also contribute to feelings of coercion) and patient initiative (i.e. choices they can make to promote their own personal recovery). While learning this new approach to food choices, it is important to reassure patients and remain sensitive to their fear of uncontrollable eating and weight gain (American Dietetic Association, 1994).

At Toronto General Hospital, calories are set at 1500 upon admission, and are increased by 300 calories/week to promote weight gain of 1–2 kg/week. Often caloric levels of 3600/day or more are needed to facilitate weight gain to a BMI of 20. To reduce the food volume, calorically dense nutritional supplements are included in the meal plan. Upon reaching the low end healthy weight, calories are gradually reduced to a 'normal' level, and provided through food only (no supplements). Research indicates that recovering anorexic patients require a higher caloric intake to maintain a healthy weight when compared to normal controls (reviewed in Rock *et al.*, 1996). Our clinical experience supports our use of the Harris-Benedict equation with an activity factor of 1.6 (see Frankenfield *et al.*, 1998, for a recent review and validation of this equation).

The meal plan must also supply adequate dietary calcium to improve bone mineralization as hormone levels normalize and weight is restored. If this is not achieved through food intake, a calcium supplement is needed. For the chronically ill, a low-dose vitamin-mineral supplement is recommended (Rock *et al.*, 1996).

Patients have a myriad of distorted views about food, eating patterns, normal food portions, nutritional requirements, digestion and metabolism. Providing education about normal nutrition can be enormously helpful. Patients can then use 'scientific facts' to challenge their eating disordered thinking. This can also provide them with 'ammunition' to challenge the overwhelming number of media messages promoting thinness and dieting (Reiff and Reiff, 1992; American Dietetic Association, 1994).

Practical food-related experience is invaluable when teaching normal eating habits. Grocery shopping and meal preparation give patients the opportunity to practice a non-dieting approach to cooking and eating. This also allows for ongoing functional assessments to determine further educational requirements regarding food preparation/planning skills. More practice is gained through weekend passes, when patients are expected to leave hospital and practice eating in a normal, less controlled environment. A critical component for successful weekends is the advanced planning. Knowing what meals and activities are scheduled allows patients to anticipate difficulties and implement coping strategies to deal with urges while staying symptom-free.

By virtue of having an eating disorder, patients are often extremely manipulative regarding any food issues. This is a challenge for the dietician and creates difficulty in establishing a collaborative relationship with the patient. The dietician, as a 'food person', is a threatening concept for the patient, which creates an enormous barrier. It is helpful to be extremely clear with patients regarding any aspect of nutrition care, and to reassure them that there is no hidden agenda (e.g. no one is sneaking extra calories into their meal plan). Allow patients to ask questions over and over, and provide simple, logical explanations about any nutritional interventions. Gradually, as treatment progresses, patients can be challenged to deal with their anxiety around food issues by drawing on their own learning and experiences during therapy (Saloff-Coste *et al.*, 1993; American Dietetic Association, 1994).

Groups focused on addressing eating disordered symptoms

Menu-marking group

The purpose of this group is to provide patients with menus for the coming week. The patients mark their menus according to their meal plan, which is based on a food group system and ranges from 1500 to 3600 calories per day. The group occurs once a week for one hour and fifteen minutes, and is facilitated by two staff members (a dietician and a nurse). Each patient discusses any meal plan changes (for example, a calorie increase) with the dietician. Patients also make decisions as a group, such as where to go and what to eat for meal outings, and what recipes to use in meal preparation experiences. As well, patients review their 'risky food choices' in front of the whole group. This is a highly interactive group, where patients support one another and acknowledge their own hard work; however, this group is often overwhelming precisely because it focuses solely on food.

Grocery shopping

This group, in conjunction with the meal preparation group described below, is designed to provide practical experience around food. It occurs once a week, and generally takes one hour. The group members involved in meal preparation (lunch or dinner) make a grocery list and then walk to a nearby grocery store to purchase the required ingredients. Staff review the grocery list and accompany patients to the grocery store. Often patients are overwhelmed by seeing so much food or stop to read every food label. They may also try to purchase smaller amounts of food, extra foods or low-fat/low-calorie items. They frequently have difficulty spending money on food. Staff assist patients to deal with any of these issues during the outing and also encourage patients to further explore the experience in other groups (for example, ward meetings).

Meal preparation

The goal of this group is to help patients learn to both prepare and eat food in a normal, non-dieting way. Lunch preparation, which takes about thirty minutes, occurs once a week after grocery shopping. Dinner preparation also occurs once a week and may take from thirty to ninety minutes, depending on the complexity of the recipes. Generally, two to four patients are in the kitchen at one time, with one member of staff supervising. Recipes are always non-diet and often include 'risky' foods. Patients need assistance to measure items correctly, to follow recipe instructions appropriately, to include added fats, etc. The member of staff (i.e. the occupational therapist) may use this group to complete a functional assessment of a patient's ability to perform in a kitchen, and may make recommendations for future meal preparation experiences.

Nutrition group

This group is designed to increase patients' knowledge regarding general nutrition and healthy, normal eating. It occurs for one hour every second week. The goal is to provide patients with enough basic nutrition information so that they can challenge the many nutrition-related myths appearing in the media (magazines, TV, advertisements). Often patients will use the material provided in this group to challenge their own food-related 'thinking errors'. Topics include normal eating, normal weights, Canada's Food Guide (a government publication, first available in 1997), meal planning, vitamins and minerals, digestion, the facts about fat, protein, carbohydrates and fibre, fluid, facts and fallacies, metabolism and set point theory.

Supervised meals

Meals and snacks are supervised to ensure meal completion and to coach patients to eat 'normally'. For example, if patients are picking at their food or cutting it up into tiny pieces, staff will redirect them to take normal-sized bites. Meals are also timed: thirty minutes are allotted for breakfast, forty for lunch and dinner, and fifteen for snacks. Staff cue patients at half-time and when five minutes remain for the meal, in order to help patients pace themselves. As well, staff direct conversation away from any topics involving food, weight and shape, which may trigger upsetting feelings for patients. Even so, staff frequently need to assist patients who become overwhelmed during the meal.

As mealtimes are generally very triggering and difficult for patients, specific guidelines for meal supervision have been developed.

Weekend planning

This group is designed to assist our patients in preparing for the weekend, as most of them are outside of the hospital during this time. It occurs once weekly, and is two hours in length. Patients are provided with planning sheets early in the week, and expected to work both on their plan for their eating and also their other activities, bringing their nearly completed plan to the group. Each patient reviews her plan in front of the whole group, who provide feedback and suggestions about difficulties the patient might be anticipating for the weekend to come. More senior group members are often able to be very helpful to more junior members.

After dinner discussion

The purpose of this group is to assist the patients to make appropriate plans for the evening and to strategize around possible difficulties. The group occurs each night after dinner. Supervising staff ask each patient in turn to review her plan for the evening, highlighting areas of difficulty and asking the patient and group to assist in formulating a plan to deal with them. For example, a patient may have strong urges to vomit a difficult dinner: the patient would be challenged to develop a plan to deal with the urges while remaining safe.

Weekend review

The goal of this group is to 'close the loop' from the end of the previous week, and allow for the patient to update the group and staff as to how well they had been able to implement their weekend plan. The group occurs each Monday for ninety minutes. Each patient in turn reviews her weekend, both in terms of eating and other activities.

Feedback group

The purpose of this group is for the team to provide constructive feedback to the patient about her progress in the program. This includes commentary on the patient's eating and other symptoms, and also on the patient's psychological progress. Alterations to the patient's program status, such as changes in calories, switching to day attendance, or upcoming discharge, are also reviewed in this group. The feedback is delivered verbally by a staff member, and the patient is asked to comment on the feedback. A discussion amongst all patients and staff may then ensue.

Groups focused on more general issues

Ward meetings

The purpose of this group is to allow for general, unstructured discussion of issues that are not conveniently addressed at other times in the program. This group occurs Wednesday through Friday, lasting one hour. If there is time left over in either the weekend review or the feedback group on Monday or Tuesday, the remaining time becomes a ward meeting. The group is attended by all patients and as many of the staff as are available. The group is totally unstructured: patients may review any issues they like. Staff will often invite patients to review family meetings or significant individual sessions at this time. More difficult day-to-day feedback, such as addressing problems a patient is having in the program, will often be brought to this group.

Self-image group

This group aims to assist patients to identify and work through self-image issues related to their eating disorder. Occurring once a week, this seventy-five-minute group alternates in format from one week to the next. Psychoeducation and structured experiential exercises are offered on alternate weeks, addressing issues such as body image, self-image, and self-care. A psychodynamic format is utilized on alternate weeks, during which patients are encouraged to bring their own self-image-related agendas. Patients process these concerns within the group context, receiving input from other group members and therapists. Patients report that they find this balance between 'structured' and 'open' groups to be helpful in their efforts to explore self-image issues during the recovery process. Topics include a number of specific exercises to assist patients in normalizing their body image.

Rethinking group

This group is based on a cognitive formulation of eating disorders. It is a structured, goal-oriented and problem-focused group intervention. Collaboration and active participation are emphasized. Psychoeducation is an integral aspect of the group. The primary aim is to teach patients to identify, evaluate and respond to their automatic thoughts and underlying beliefs or assumptions. There is an explicit focus on achieving behavioral, affective and attitudinal change. Patients learn about the cognitive model of eating disorders and complete thought records designed to help them evaluate and change unhelpful thinking. Developing alternative coping strategies to combat eating disorder symptoms is another key focus. Patients devise and carry out behavioral experiments to test their thoughts and beliefs. For example, a patient who believes she will gain 5 kg if she eats a feared food is encouraged to actively test out this prediction. Other topics include structured problem solving, graded exposure to feared foods and situations, assertiveness skills training, building self-esteem, and understanding and coping with anxiety.

Sexuality group

This group serves two distinct functions: to deliver sexual education, and to assist our patients in becoming more comfortable with their own sexuality. We recognize that many of our patients are uncomfortable with sexual issues, or have been traumatized, and thus we provide them with a handout at their first group which outlines some of the reactions they are likely to experience.

The group runs for seventy-five minutes, once a week: topics range from birth control through to intimacy in relationships. Patients are advised at each group that the facilitators are individually available to discuss material that the patient feels uncomfortable raising in a group setting.

Family relations group

This group serves to assist patients in identifying family issues that are relevant to their own situation. The group may be an isolated intervention, if the patient is not having concurrent family meetings, or may work in concert with their family therapy. The group occurs on Monday afternoons, lasts ninety minutes, and is co-led by the two family therapists in the program. The group was initially developed in the day hospital and has been described in detail elsewhere (Woodside and Shekter-Wolfson, 1991).

The group is semi-structured. Each session has a topic, which is introduced by a handout. All of the topics are focused around various aspects of family functioning, presented in a non-pathologizing fashion. Some topics involve simply a discussion, while others may include one or more exercises. The exercises are usually experiential, such as family sculpting.

Relaxation group

The purpose of this group is to guide patients, who often experience chronic states of anxiety and agitation, in the relaxation of mind, body and spirit. The relaxation group occurs once a week, and lasts for fifty minutes. Patients are invited to bring to the group anything that makes them feel comfortable (pillow, blanket, etc.), and to relax on mats in a room with soft lighting and music. The group begins with simple stretches and breathing exercises, and then proceeds to a guided relaxation and visualization experience. Attendance at this group is optional, as some patients with histories of post-traumatic stress may find that relaxed consciousness states trigger traumatic flashbacks. Patients who choose to attend are encouraged to take whatever measures are necessary to maintain their sense of safety and comfort during the relaxation experience.

Reconnection group

Based upon the occupational therapy domains of self-care, productivity, and leisure, the reconnection group was created to assist patients with the process of 'reconnecting' to contexts and situations outside of the intensive inpatient treatment environment. Additionally, this group helps patients re-orient to life skills and activities that may have been lost during a lengthy or acute struggle with illness. The group meets once weekly for fifty minutes and uses a psychoeducation model. Through the didactic presentation of information by leaders, and various group activities and discussions, patients learn about topics such as developing a healthy lifestyle, budgeting, community resources, developing friendships and preparing for the holidays.

Integrative and expressive arts therapies

The integrative and expressive arts therapies are offered in our program to support metaphoric and non-verbal self-expression through art, sound, puppetry, story-telling, movement and music. As health promotion processes, these modalities support the collaborative initiative between the patient and others, to enhance and maintain a positive sense of self-esteem and a healthy experience of self-agency and self-expression.

These therapies are offered in a weekly arts therapies group supplemented by individual art projects. The integrative and expressive arts therapies are also offered on a one-to-one basis from time to time, as patient need dictates.

Other elements of the program

Individual therapy

We currently offer a limited amount of concurrent individual therapy, typically one to three hours per week. While nursing staff provide the bulk of this element of treatment, patients will meet with any of the team members as required.

Foci of individual therapy are patient-specific, and may range from general support to the implementation of a complex protocol for the treatment of an anxiety disorder.

Patients understand that issues discussed with one member of the team are shared with all team members, and patients are encouraged to review important issues in their individual sessions with the group as a whole.

Family/couple therapy

Our model of family and couple therapy has been extensively described elsewhere (Woodside and Shekter-Wolfson, 1991). We provide a specific type of brief therapy, focused on psychoeducation, symptom control, and the establishment of age-appropriate boundaries and autonomy. Our approach is permissive, and our definition of family is broad. Patients are informed that the service is available to those who wish to use it; however, we will normally encourage the patient to allow us to meet with her and her significant others.

Managing medical problems

While many of our patients are admitted with serious medical problems, the majority respond well to brief, focused medical interventions, and the patients usually do not require any absence from the program. Patients who are too ill to participate in the program are temporarily removed until their condition allows a return.

The scope of this chapter does not allow for a comprehensive review of the medical management of inpatients with anorexia nervosa. The majority of the problems that are encountered are dealt with by the medical staff working in the program (psychiatrist, nursing staff) with consultations from other medical specialties as required.

Current experience with the program

Treatment response

Between July 1997 and August 1999, eighty patients were admitted to the program. The diagnostic breakdown of the patients was as follows: 40 (50 per cent) AN (restricting type); 36 (45 per cent) AN (binge/purge type); 3 (3.7 per cent) BN (purging type); and 1 (1.3 per cent) EDNOS (eating disorder not otherwise specified). Nine of the patients had multiple admissions. For the data reviewed below, information from the most recent admission is used.

Descriptive characteristics of the patients meeting DSM-IV criteria for AN (N=76) are as follows. The mean age was 27 years and the mean BMI at admission was 15±2). Seventeen (25 per cent) were classified as drop-outs (defined as length of stay less than four weeks). Of the remaining fifty-two patients, the average length of stay was 13 (±5) weeks. The average weight gain for these patients was 12 (±6) kg and the mean discharge BMI was 18 (±2). Thirty-two (62 per cent) were weight restored (BMI >20); four (8 per cent) had a good outcome (BMI = 18–20); ten (19 per cent) had a moderate outcome (BMI <18 but gained at least 5 kg); and six (11 per cent) had a poor outcome. Follow-up data are not available at the present time.

Special issues

Underweight patients in group therapy

Our current practice is to include new patients in all aspects of the group therapy program from admission, regardless of their weight. While most patients do take some time to recover cognitively from the effects of starvation, there are marked improvements by the end of the second week and cognition is fairly intact by six weeks.

During the first two weeks, when most patients are quite starved, they tend to participate to a more limited extent in the groups, and will have some deficits in their ability to retain information. However, our patients uniformly report that they preferred to be in the group during this phase of their illness. The usual reason cited is a reduction in the sense of isolation that accompanies an admission to hospital.

Self-harm

Our current program policy is that self-harm (such as cutting, bruising, etc.) is not compatible with being in our program. We recognize that individuals require support and time to gain control over self-harm behaviors: thus we implement our policy by focusing on whether the patient is working with us to avoid acting on urges to harm herself, and whether such actions are decreasing in frequency. Thus, we will usually not discharge a patient for a single act of self-harm, but will continue to try to develop a working relationship with the patient focused on safety.

Substance abuse

Along the same lines as self-harm, we expect patients to abstain from drugs or alcohol while admitted to the program. We are not equipped to detoxify patients or to specifically treat substance abuse. We normally ask that a patient who has a substance use problem be dry for three months prior to admission.

Trauma

Many of our patients have been abused sexually and physically, and the period of acute recovery from starvation is often a time when thoughts and feelings related to such experiences become more active. This can occur immediately, or can take a number of weeks to develop.

We provide patients with as much support and treatment for trauma-related issues as possible. This includes the provision of accurate information about the effects of trauma, training in grounding techniques, and individual treatment focused on safety, grounding and the identification of trauma-related symptoms.

While some patients respond very well to this approach, there is a subgroup of patients, usually those with extensive histories of trauma, who become activated very shortly after admission. These individuals present a complex and challenging management problem. Those who do not know the team well often are not prepared to disclose details about their thoughts and feelings, and thus are not accessible to interventions as described above.

Some of these patients gradually become more comfortable with the treatment team over the course of several admissions, and are eventually able to make good recoveries. We are currently experimenting with joint admissions to our program and a local sexual abuse day program.

Patients with chronic illness

As the main provider of intensive treatment for anorexia nervosa in Ontario, we have a large number of patients with chronic illness attached to our program. We have had to make some decisions about how to apply our limited resources to the whole population of individuals suffering from anorexia nervosa, rather than solely to the group who are chronically ill. At the present time we are happy to admit such patients to our program if their goal is to attempt a full recovery from their illness. While we recognize that many such patients might benefit from briefer admissions with more limited goals, at the present time we are hesitant to mix such a group with our patients who are focused on a more complete recovery. This hesitancy relates partly to our concerns that the majority of the psychological aspects of the program might not be relevant to such patients, and to the possibility of undermining of program objectives by such patients. This is a difficult situation, and one that will require some thought and time to resolve. In an ideal world, we would have a separate program for chronically ill individuals focusing on stabilization, maintenance and incremental gains. We lack the resources presently to mount such a program.

Similarly, we do not presently engage in involuntary treatment of tube-feeding. The occasional individual who requires tube-feeding has this performed in either an intensive psychiatric setting, or a medical setting. We are not generally involved in this process. In our jurisdiction, involuntary admission laws permit only relatively brief periods of detention in these types of conditions. Again, in an ideal world, we would have a setting where we would have access to a more tightly controlled physical setting, one where we would arrange for such involuntary treatment as part of our continuum of care. This is not possible at the present time.

Vegetarianism

Societal changes in eating habits over the last thirty years have caused us to re-examine our position on vegetarianism. A vegetarian approach to eating is now an accepted pattern of eating in society at large. As is reviewed in Chapter 12, our day hospital program currently allows for patients to eat in a vegetarian fashion, so long as their food choices fit in with the meal plan and their calories are adequate to those prescribed.

In the inpatient program, we presently attempt to distinguish between those individuals who have a religious reason to be vegetarian, or who have a lifelong pattern of vegetarianism, from those who became vegetarian in the context of their illness. We will accommodate the former group, but not the latter. For example, a Hindu woman who has been a lifelong vegan would continue to eat in a vegan fashion in our program. For the latter group, we currently suggest that the choice to become a vegetarian may have been made as a consequence of having been ill, and that the vegetarianism should be relinquished until the person's eating is normal. At this point the patient can then make a decision about her long-term eating habits unaffected by the presence of anorexia nervosa.

This issue obviously requires more study, both in our own setting and in treatment settings in other centers. It would also be interesting to see some dialogue on this issue at scientific meetings.

Conclusion

This chapter has attempted to review developments in the overall field of inpatient treatment of anorexia nervosa and to describe a single program in considerable detail. Focused academic attention to this element of treatment for eating disorders has been sadly lacking in recent decades. This lack is especially unfortunate given the high costs of inpatient treatment, and the resultant constrictions in funds available for its provision.

Areas that could benefit from ongoing study are many. The role of involuntary inpatient treatment is controversial and the outcome of such treatment is poorly understood. While we favor a more lenient approach, the extent to which patients should be allowed choices of various types when very underweight is a highly controversial topic that demands debate and discussion. The high rate of relapse after inpatient admission suggests that some effort needs to be made to examine the types of interventions that are applied – perhaps several 'streams' of treatment need to be available, some for those wishing to make more significant changes, and others for those wishing stability and palliation.

Study in these areas will be difficult because of the small numbers of patients admitted to most programs, the external constraints applied as to length of stay and other treatment variables, and the long follow-up periods needed to draw appropriate conclusions. It seems most likely that international collaborative studies are the most appropriate technique to try to grapple with some of these issues.

References

Agras, W.S. (1987) *Eating Disorders: Management of Obesity, Bulimia and Anorexia Nervosa.* Oxford: Pergamon Press.

American Dietetic Association (1994) Position of the American Dietetic Association: nutrition intervention in the treatment of anorexia nervosa, bulimia nervosa, and binge eating. *Journal of the American Dietetic Association*, 94, 902–907.

American Psychiatric Association (1993) Practice guidelines for eating disorders. *American Journal of Psychiatry*, 150, 207–228.

Andersen, A.E., Morose, C.L. and Santmyer, K.S. (1985) Inpatient treatment for anorexia nervosa. In D.M. Garner and P.E. Garfinkel (eds), *Handbook of Treatment for Eating Disorders.* New York: Guilford Press.

Andersen, A.E., Bowers, W. and Evans, K. (1997) Inpatient treatment of anorexia nervosa. In D.M Garner and P.E. Garfinkel (eds), *Handbook of Treatment for Eating Disorders.* New York: Guilford Press.

Baran, S.A., Weltzin, T.E. and Kaye, W.H. (1995) Low discharge weight and outcome in anorexia nervosa. *American Journal of Psychiatry*, 152, 1070–1072.

Bowers, W.A. and Andersen A.E. (1994) Inpatient treatment of anorexia nervosa: review and recommendations. *Harvard Review of Psychiatry*, 4, 193–203.

Commerford, M.C., Licinio, J. and Halmi, K.A. (1997) Guidelines for discharging eating disorder inpatients. *Eating Disorders: The Journal of Treatment and Prevention*, 5, 69–74.

Crisp, A.H. and Kalucy, R.S. (1973) The effect of leucotomy in intractable adolescent weight phobia. *Postgraduate Medicine*, 74, 883–893.

Eckert, E. and Mitchell, J.E. (1989) An overview of the treatment of anorexia nervosa. *Psychiatric Medicine*, 7, 293–422.

Eckert, E.D., Halmi, K.A., Marchi, P., Grover, W. and Crosby, R. (1995) Ten-year follow-up of anorexia nervosa: clinical course and outcome. *Psychological Medicine*, 25, 143–156.

Engel, K. and Wilfarth, B. (1988) Therapy results and follow-up of an integrated inpatient treatment for severe cases of anorexia nervosa. *Psychotherapy and Psychosomatics*, 50, 5–14.

Engel, K., Wittern, M., Hentze, M. and Meyer, A.E. (1989) Long-term stability of anorexia nervosa treatments: follow-up study of 218 patients. *Psychiatric Developments*, 4, 395–407.

Ferguson, J.M. (1993) The use of electroconvulsive therapy in patients with intractable anorexia nervosa. *International Journal of Eating Disorders*, 13, 195–201.

Frankenfield, D.C., Muth, E.R. and Rowe, W.A. (1998) The Harris-Benedict studies of human basal metabolism: history and limitations. *Journal of the American Dietetic Association*, 98, 439–445.

Garfinkel, P.E. and Garner, D.M. (1982) *Anorexia Nervosa: A Multidimensional Perspective.* New York: Brunner/Mazel.

Goldbloom, D.S., Kennedy, S.H., Kaplan, A.S. and Woodside, D.B. (1989) Recent advances in pharmacotherapy: anorexia nervosa and bulimia nervosa. *Canadian Medical Association Journal*, 140, 1149–1154.

Havala, T. and Shronts, E. (1990) Managing the complications associated with refeeding. *Nutrition in Clinical Practice*, 5, 23–29.

Herzog, W., Rathner, G. and Vandereycken, W. (1993) Long-term course of anorexia nervosa: a review of the literature. In W. Herzog, H.C. Deter and W. Vandereycken (eds), *The Course of Eating Disorders: Long-Term Follow-up Studies of Anorexia and Bulimia Nervosa* (pp. 15–29). Berlin: Springer-Verlag.

Hsu, L.K. (1986) The treatment of anorexia nervosa. *American Journal of Psychiatry*, 143, 573–581.

Kaplan, A.S. and Garfinkel, P.E. (eds) (1993) *Medical Issues and the Eating Disorders: The Interface*. New York: Brunner/Mazel.

Kreipe, R.E., Churchill, B.H. and Strauss, J. (1989) Long-term outcome in adolescents with anorexia nervosa. *American Journal of Diseases of Children*, 143, 1322–1327.

Kreipe, R.E., Golden, N.H., Katzman, D.K., *et al.* (1995) Eating disorders in adolescents – a position paper of the Society for Adolescent Medicine. *Journal of Adolescent Health*, 16, 476–480.

Maloney, M.J. and Farrell, M.K. (1980) Treatment of severe weight loss in anorexia nervosa with hyperalimentation and psychotherapy. *American Journal of Psychiatry*, 137, 310–314.

Norring, C.A.E. and Sohlberg, S.S. (1993) Outcome, recovery, relapse and mortality across six years in patients with clinical eating disorders. *Acta Psychiatrica Scandinavica*, 87, 437–444.

Ontario Ministry of Health (1991) *Healthy Weights: A New Way of Looking at Your Weight and Health*.

Reiff, D.W. and Reiff, K.K.L. (1992) *Eating Disorders: Nutrition in the Recovery Process*. Gaithersburg, Md:. Aspen Publishers, Inc.

Rock, C.L. and Curran-Celentano, J. (1996) Nutritional management of eating disorders. *The Psychiatric Clinics of North America*, 19, 701–713.

Rock, C.L., Gorenflo, D.W., Drewnowski, A. and Demitrack, M.A. (1996) Nutritional characteristics, eating pathology, and hormonal status in young women. *American Journal of Clinical Nutrition*, 64, 566–571.

Russell, G.F.M. (1977) The present status of anorexia nervosa. *Psychological Medicine*, 7, 353–367.

Saloff-Coste, C.J., Hamburg, P. and Herzog, D. (1993) Nutrition and psychotherapy: collaborative treatment of patients with eating disorders. *Bulletin of the Menninger Clinic*, 57, 504–516.

Sesan, R. (1994) Feminist inpatient treatment for eating disorders: an oxymoron? In P. Fallon, M.A. Katzman and S.C. Wooley (eds), *Feminist Perspectives on Eating Disorders*, pp. 251–271. New York: Guilford Press.

Silverman, J. (1974) Anorexia nervosa: clinical observations in a successful treatment program. *Journal of Pediatrics*, 84, 68–73.

Touyz, S.W., Beumont, P.J., Glaun, D., Phillips, T. and Crowie, I. (1984) A comparison of lenient and strict operant conditioning programs in refeeding patients with anorexia nervosa. *British Journal of Psychiatry*, 144, 517–520.

Vandereycken, W. (1985) Inpatient treatment of anorexia nervosa: some research guided changes. *Journal of Psychiatry Research*, 19, 413–422.

Woodside, D.B. and Shekter-Wolfson, L. (eds) (1991) *Family Approaches in Treatment of Eating Disorders*. Washington, DC: American Psychiatric Press.

Index